Calisthenics & Mobility

The content of this book was carefully researched. However, readers should always consult a qualified medical specialist for individual advice before adopting any new exercise plan. This book should not be used as an alternative to seeking specialist medical advice.
All information is supplied without liability. Neither the authors nor the publisher will be liable for possible disadvantages, injuries, or damages.

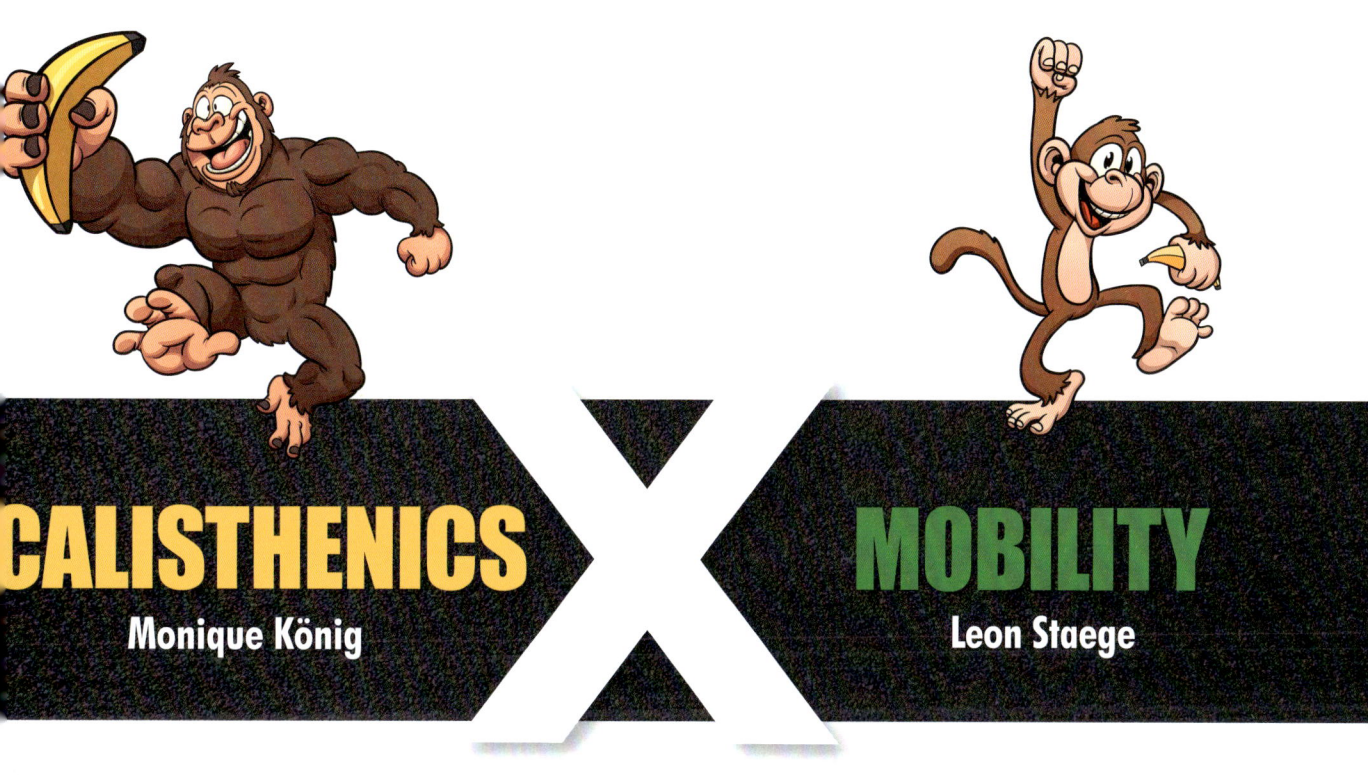

STRONG & SUPPLE

Meyer & Meyer Sport

British Library of Cataloguing in Publication Data
A catalogue record for this book is available from the British Library

Original title: *Calisthenics X Mobility*, © 2019 by Meyer & Meyer Verlag

Calisthenics & Mobility
Maidenhead: Meyer & Meyer Sport (UK) Ltd., 2021
ISBN: 978-1-78255-215-4

All rights reserved, especially the right to copy and distribute, including the translation rights. No part of this work may be reproduced—including by photocopy, microfilm or any other means—processed, stored electronically, copied or distributed in any form whatsoever without the written permission of the publisher.

© 2021 by Meyer & Meyer Sport (UK) Ltd.
Aachen, Auckland, Beirut, Dubai, Hägendorf, Hong Kong, Indianapolis, Cairo, Cape Town, Manila, Maidenhead, New Delhi, Singapore, Sydney, Tehran, Vienna

 Member of the World Sport Publishers' Association (WSPA), www.w-s-p-a.org

Printed by Print Consult GmbH, Munich, Germany
Printed in Slovakia

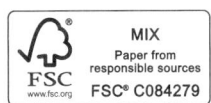

ISBN: 978-1-78255-215-4
Email: info@m-m-sports.com
www.thesportspublisher.com

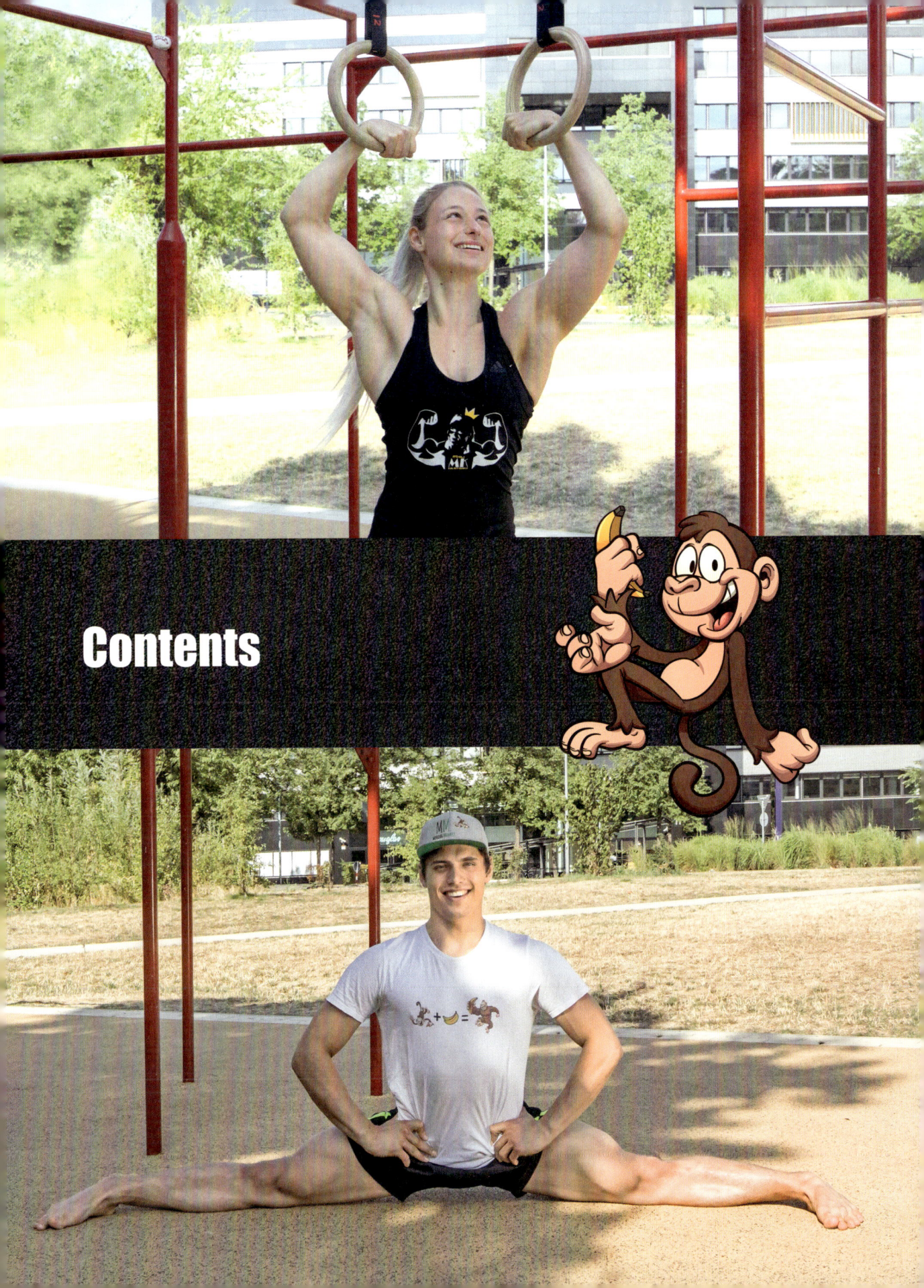

Contents

	Preface	10
	Introduction: Book Layout	12

MOBILITY

		What Motivates Me to Get You Moving	16
1		**Mobility—Modern Flexibility Training**	**20**
2		**Understanding Mobility**	**26**
	2.1	How to Become More Mobile	26
	2.2	The Reason We're So Stiff	29
	2.3	Don't Mobilize Every Joint	31
	2.4	Why Stretching and Yoga Won't Make You More Mobile	34
	2.5	Why Foam Rollers Won't Make You More Mobile	36
		2.5.1 The Foam-Roller Phenomenon	36
		2.5.2 Rolling, Rolling, Rolling	37
		2.5.3 Surface Sensibility versus Proprioceptive Sensibility	38
		2.5.4 Pain While Rolling	39
		2.5.5 Foam Rollers—**Sense or Nonsense?**	40
	2.6	More Exercise Equipment You Don't Need	40
	2.7	How Mobility Makes You Stronger	41
	2.8	Why Stress Makes You Immobile	43
3		**Mobility Fundamentals: What You Need to Know**	**48**
	3.1	Four Easy Steps to Becoming More Mobile	48
		3.1.1 Evaluation	49
		3.1.2 Isolation	51
		3.1.3 Integration	54
		3.1.4 Improvisation	55
	3.2	Pain and Injuries	56
		3.2.1 Pain	56
		3.2.2 Injuries	58
	3.3	Guidelines for Pain-Free Training	62
4		**The Most-Common Questions About Mobility**	**66**
	4.1	How Long Until I'm More Mobile?	66
	4.2	How Can I Become More Mobile More Quickly?	68

		4.3	How Do I Add Mobility to My Strength Training?	69
		4.4	How Do I Integrate Mobility Into My Daily Life?	70

5 Mobility Lifestyle Hacks 74

6 Movement Is Life, and Life Is Movement 82

7 Mobility Exercises 86

7.1	Wrists		87
	7.1.1	Wrist Figure Eights	88
	7.1.2	Wrist Mobilization on the Ground	90
	7.1.3	Backhand Push-ups	92
	7.1.4	Shaolin Push-ups	94
	7.1.5	Wrist Push-ups	96
7.2	Spine		97
	7.2.1	Spinal Rotations (CARs)	98
	7.2.2	Spinal Wave 1	100
	7.2.3	Spinal Wave 2	102
	7.2.4	Neck Mobilization	104
	7.2.5	Three-Point Thoracic-Spine Rotation	106
	7.2.6	All-Fours Rotation	108
	7.2.7	Ball	112
	7.2.8	Prone Thoracic-Spine Rotation	114
	7.2.9	Wrestler Rotation	115
	7.2.10	Table Rotation	116
	7.2.11	Heel-Sitting Rotation	118
	7.2.12	Cross-Legged Rotation	120
	7.2.13	Cobra	121
7.3	Shoulders		122
	7.3.1	Shoulder Rotations (CARs)	123
	7.3.2	Shoulder Rotations Against the Wall	124
	7.3.3	Hanging	125
	7.3.4	Single-Arm Hanging	126
	7.3.5	Wall Slides	127
	7.3.6	Shoulder Crawl	128
	7.3.7	Swimmer	130
	7.3.8	Protraction and Retraction Drill	132
	7.3.9	Shoulder Dislocator With a Band	134
	7.3.10	Shoulder Rotation With a Band	136
	7.3.11	Side Bend	138
	7.3.12	Skin the Cat (Regression)	140
	7.3.13	Skin the Cat	142
	7.3.14	Scapula Push-up Rotation	143
	7.3.15	Arched-Back Pulls	144

CALISTHENICS

8	**My Path to the Pull-up Bar**	150
9	**Calisthenics**	156
9.1	Roots of Calisthenics	156
9.2	The Rain-or-Shine Training Mentality	158
9.3	The Four Types of Calisthenics	158
9.4	From Trend Sport to Business: Calisthenics in Germany	160
9.5	Calisthenics versus CrossFit versus Freeletics	161
9.6	Why Everyone Benefits From Bodyweight Training	162
9.7	Your Prerequisites	163
9.8	Useful Equipment	164
9.9	Calisthenics Parks: The Best Spots for Your Training	166
9.10	Guidelines for Ambitious Calisthenics Beginners	167
9.11	Ditching Familiar Movement Patterns: Embracing the Unusual	168
9.12	Exertion to the Point of Exhaustion: The 80-Percent Rule	168
9.13	Setting Goals the Right Way	169
10	**Calisthenics Fundamentals: What You Need to Know**	174
10.1	Overview of Basic Exercises	174
10.2	Balancing Stability and Mobility	177
10.3	Movement Variations	177
10.4	Movement Specifics	178
10.5	Assistance Exercises	178
10.6	Difficult Exercises Made Easy	179
10.7	Sticking Points	180
10.8	Full Range of Motion	180
10.9	Shoulder-Blade Positions	181
10.10	A Firm Grip	184
10.11	Hollow-Body Position	184
10.12	All About Levers	186
10.13	Repetition: The Mother of Skill	189
10.14	Straight-Arm Strength	189
10.15	Training on Rings	189
10.16	Calisthenics and Leg Training	190
10.17	Shoulder Joint	190
11	**Beginner Basics and Their Possible Progressions**	194
11.1	Healthy Shoulder Balance With a Combination of Pulling and Pushing Loads	195
11.2	Activation Exercises	196
11.3	Pull-ups and Possible Progressions	202

	11.3.1	What Your Pull-up Should Look Like	202
	11.3.2	Typical Mistakes	205
	11.3.3	Frequent Sticking Points	206
	11.3.4	Grip Variations	209
	11.3.5	Overhand Pull-ups versus Underhand Pull-ups	210
	11.3.6	Arched-Back Pull-ups	211
	11.3.7	Pull-up Exercise Regressions	212
11.4	**Push-ups and Possible Progressions**		**216**
	11.4.1	What Your Push-up Should Look Like	216
	11.4.2	Typical Mistakes	218
	11.4.3	Frequent Sticking Points	218
	11.4.4	Grip Variations	219
	11.4.5	Push-up Exercise Regressions	219
11.5	**Dips and Possible Progressions**		**224**
	11.5.1	What Your Dip Should Look Like	225
	11.5.2	Typical Mistakes	226
	11.5.3	Frequent Sticking Points	227
	11.5.4	Dip Exercise Regressions	228
11.6	**Squats and Possible Progressions**		**231**
	11.6.1	What Your Squat Should Look Like	232
11.7	**Regression: The *L*-Sit**		**234**
	11.7.1	Hanging *L*-Sit	235
	11.7.2	*L*-Sit in a Support Position (Arms)	236
	11.7.3	Assisting Exercises	237
11.8	**Rehabilitation and Prehabilitation Exercises**		**239**

12 General Training Structure 244

12.1	**Training Methods**		**246**
	12.1.1	Frequency of Training, Number of Sets, Number of Repetitions, and Breaks	247
	12.1.2	Types of Training	250

13 Goals, Time Investment, and Motivation 254

14 Acknowledgments 258

15 The Authors 260

16 Appendix 262

	1 Glossary	262
	2 Further References	266
	3 Credits	267

Preface

Hey there, bar fans and moving monkeys!

Calisthenics & Mobility is our labor of love. Over the past three years, we've been able to help lots of people acquire a healthier, stronger, and more confident lifestyle by following our workshop series.

In Germany, Austria, and Switzerland we made anyone who trained diligently "as flexible as a monkey and as strong as a gorilla." Due to our participants' exceedingly positive feedback, we thought about how we could inspire even more people to do the same.

This book allows us to bring our movement concept for longevity out into the world to accompany you on your very own Calisthenics & Mobility journey.

Our journeys began in early childhood. To both of us, growing up with competitive sports meant learning early on to work for a physical goal. Character, for each of us, was shaped by discipline, willpower, and performance which could all be accessed anytime. Competitive sports created a positive attitude toward our bodies in motion. Four to five training sessions per week and competitions on weekends taught us that hard physical work can be very rewarding. Our sessions helped us grow physically, mentally, and emotionally.

The joy of movement was so great for us that we both chose a career path that would allow us to share our knowledge and personal experience with you. The essence of our concept is this: reaching your goal healthy and pain-free.

Calisthenics & Mobility refers to the symbiotic relationship between strength and mobility. We'll show you the most-important principles of these two interconnected areas. Both can be viewed as separate elements, but in this book, they should be viewed as an interrelated construct with a correlated and positive effect.

The content of this book focuses on resistance training with one's own body, specifically with calisthenics. This isn't a new type of sport but, rather, a neologism. Calisthenics could be considered the modern gymnastics. It prioritizes progressive strength increase via the basics (e.g., pull-ups, push-ups, dips, and knee squats).

Mobility training as a fitness-related ability is often neglected in favor of strength.

Most underestimate the fact that a greater degree of motion results in more strength.

Mobility training creates the balance between movement without strength and rigid strength.

At the same time, you'll get more long-term enjoyment from your training, due to fewer injuries, and when you are in pain, you'll have the right exercises at hand.

This book is intended to get you to move. For us, it's not about bulging muscles. Rather, we want you to learn to understand your body.

We'll teach you which technical details of the exercises are important so your musculoskeletal system will enjoy long-term good health. We'll provide you with the most-important know-how so you'll be able to use different, helpful tools from your tool kit.

With all the input you'll receive, please keep in mind the following during your journey:

1. *Anyone* can work with mobility and calisthenics, regardless of age and gender.

2. Every person is an *individual* with different abilities.

3. There's *no* single best method.

4. Don't think about the approach—just start.

5. Comparing yourself to others *won't* help you one bit.

This book does away with lots of preconceived notions in order to give you clear guidelines for your training. Calisthenics is only for tough guys? Flexibility is genetically predetermined? Far from it! We'll show you how to find long-term joy in training and get stronger and more flexible, all while staying pain-free.

In this spirit, do the following:

Stay loose, flex your biceps.

Keep moving, stay sexy.

Monique & Leon

Introduction: Book Layout

Before you embark on your *Calisthenics & Mobility* journey, we'd like to give you some tips on how to use this book.

You can choose to read everything in the order it's presented or skip between sections. The many chapter and section cross-references ensure you won't lose the thread and will, by the end, understand the link between mobility and calisthenics.

We've brought the authentic delivery style of our workshops to this book so we can bring the atmosphere of a live workshop to your home. Besides, this is a book about calisthenics and not about traditional German gymnastics from Saxony-Anhalt.

In this book, we talk about front levers and muscle-ups.

The book is divided into a mobility section and calisthenics section, which are further divided into theoretical and practical segments. The practical segments include image-guided explanations of exercises.

In these practical sections of the book, look for the following symbols, which provide simple illustrations of the most-important technical details for the execution of an exercise:

Introduction

 External rotation

 Maintain body tension (hollow-body position)

 Shoulders away from ears (depression)

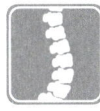 Lengthen your spine

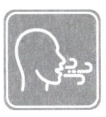 Watch your breath

If you don't yet understand all this terminology, don't panic. We provide detailed descriptions in the following chapters and in the glossary at the end of the book.

Every exercise is also accompanied by a difficulty rating. To be exact, it's a banana scale for Leon's mobility exercises and a biceps scale for Monique's calisthenics exercises.

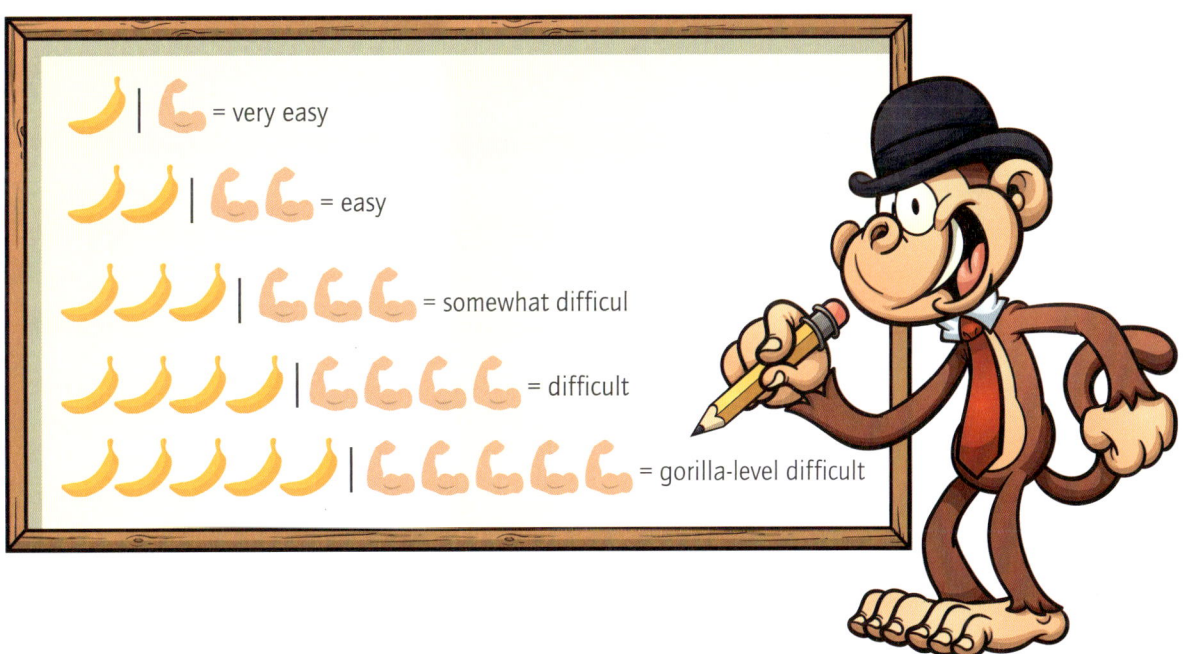

But enough about legends and instructions. By now you're probably impatiently tapping your feet, ready to dive into your adventure.

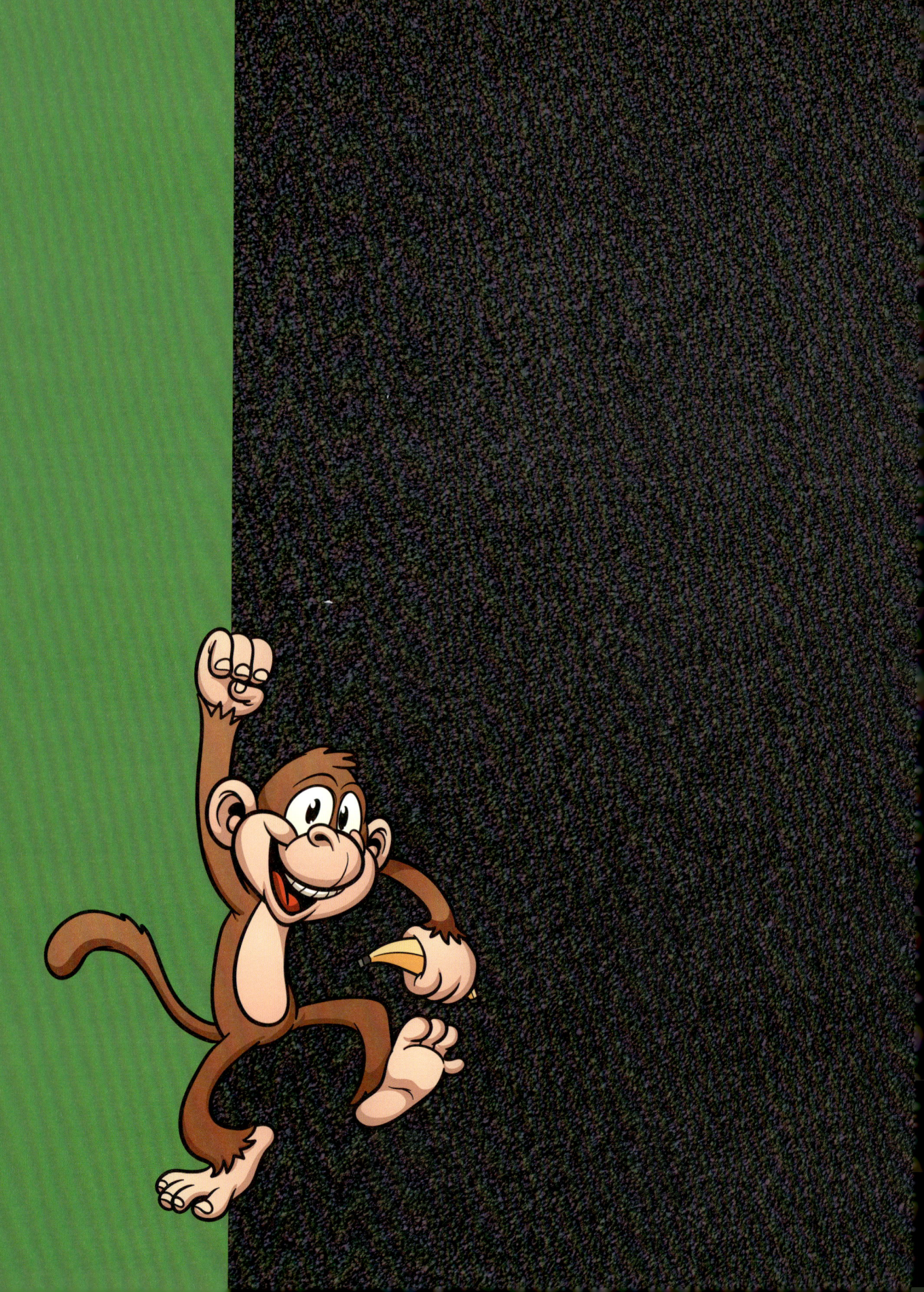

MOBILITY

What Motivates Me to Get You Moving

My exercise path started quite early. At age two, I was on the Wildenrath golf course, which was largely built by and then managed for many years by my father. He often reminded me that I had talent and that the other guests on the driving range spoke of "the next Tiger Woods" in my presence. Surely, they were joking!

Nevertheless, I must thank my parents, who—instead of dressing me in polo shirts and plaid pants—put me in a pair of soccer shoes. I can still hear my father saying, "The boy needs to learn a team sport. It builds character!"

So at age three, I was on the soccer field. Although I spent more time picking daisies (for my mom) during those early years, soccer had a formative influence on me. Then, after playing for fifteen years, I hung up my soccer shoes. By the time I graduated high school, after a move, and several personal changes, I found myself in a deep performance slump, which is why I didn't connect with my new team at Fortuna Köln.

In my first book, *Pragmatisch Gesund*, I talk a little about my health problems, which, among other things, caused my athletic interests to change. In short, my growing interest in strength—or, rather, fitness sports—caused me to adopt a one-sided diet that ended up costing me my performance capacity and, in the end, my soccer career. But as it turned out, this difficult time was the best thing that could have happened to me. When in life does one ever get the opportunity to completely redefine oneself and embark on a new path?

The new path led me to a place where I wanted to learn more about people's health and the human body overall. Where I wanted to help people get out of the hole they'd fallen into, through one-sided diets proclaimed by the fitness industry as panaceas or due to poor exercise habits. During my active soccer career, I tried out lots of different sports, even though I always stayed with soccer.

Thanks to my mom, I was able to try out other sports, such as hockey, tennis, basketball, swimming, judo, and dance. I loved any type of exercise during my free time: table tennis, bowling, cycling, badminton, wrestling with my younger brother, and more. All these experiences with exercise would serve me well on my new path and lead me to where I am today—my small but awesome monkey gym in the space I share with Monique in Cologne.

Nearly every day, clients come from all over the German-speaking world to my 12-square-meter (130-square-foot) gym, where together we search for the cause of their pain and where, in typical Moving-Monkey fashion, I make them strong, flexible, and pain-free. But how did I get from my soccer career to starting my YouTube channel, **Moving Monkey**, and becoming a student of physical therapy?

Next to one of my best friends, Alexander Wahler, who convinced me to upload my first YouTube video, it was primarily one other man's influence that I embarked on the exercise journey, and his name is Ido Portal. Over the years, a number of others have certainly joined the ranks as mentors from whom I've been able to learn, but it all started with him.

After Ido's workshop in Munich in late 2015, my head was practically spinning. I even told him in person that everything was whirling around in my dreams the night after the first day of that workshop. I was effectively able to experience my beliefs, views, and, last but not least, my body get turned upside down, spun around, and newly aligned.

Ido's response, in his typical terse and concise manner was this: **"It's a scary place, the place of change. But it's worth it!"**

In retrospect, I have to admit he was right. My greatest takeaway from my days with Ido was that we should pay more attention to the way we move (quality of movement, variety of movement, and **movement culture**) rather than chasing the next workout.

Even today, this philosophy still guides my actions and way of thinking. Not just with respect to Moving Monkey but also in my everyday life. After all, we humans are made to move, and our greatest gift is that we possess a body that's capable of doing so much.

I want to spark in you the same enthusiasm that burns inside me for movement and the human body. Maybe after reading this book you'll start to add a little morning mobility routine to your day. Or you'll choose to take the stairs instead of the elevator.

Some people start with lots of baby steps, and others prefer to take a few big ones. What's clear is that everyone is on their own journey at their own pace. And every journey begins with movement—namely with the first step.

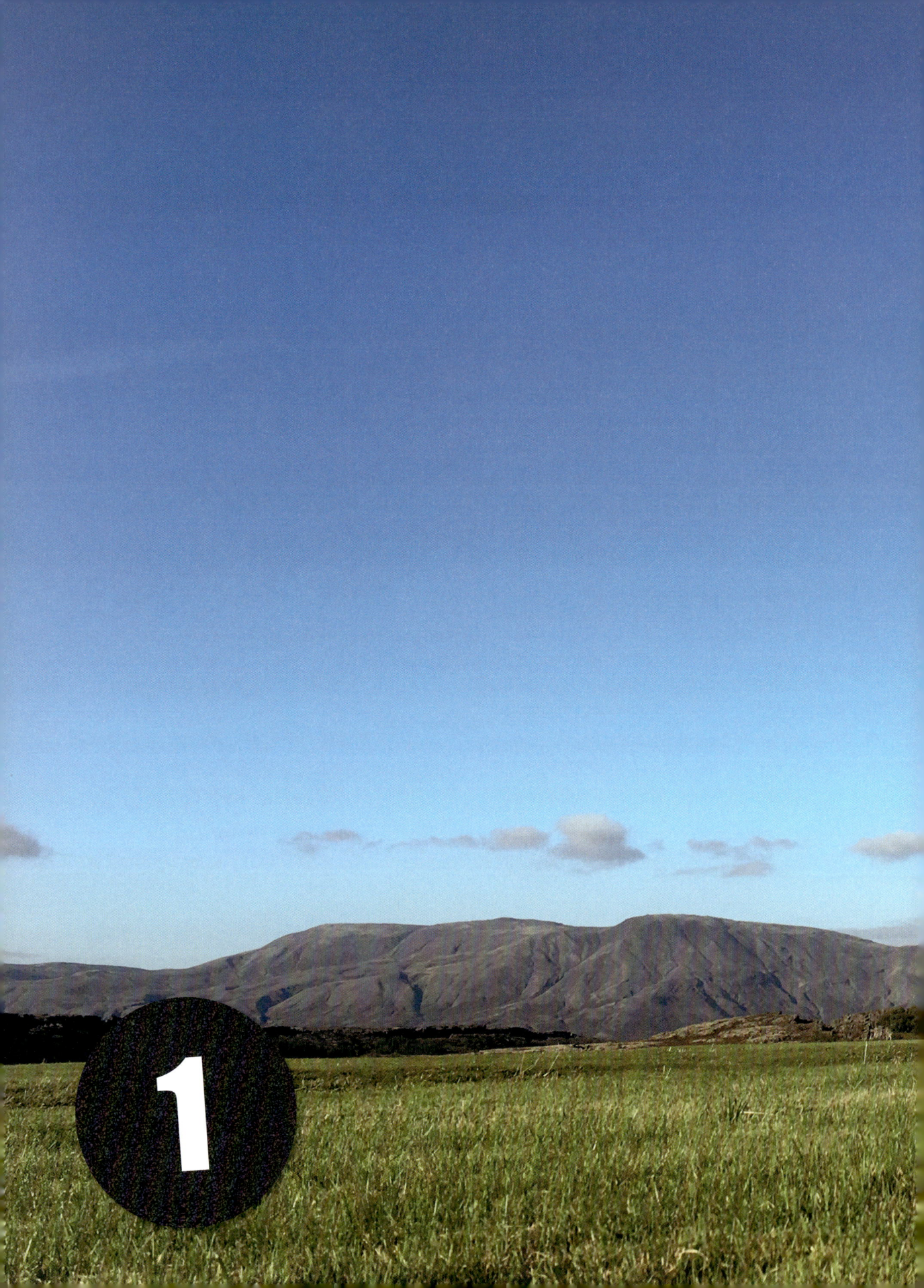

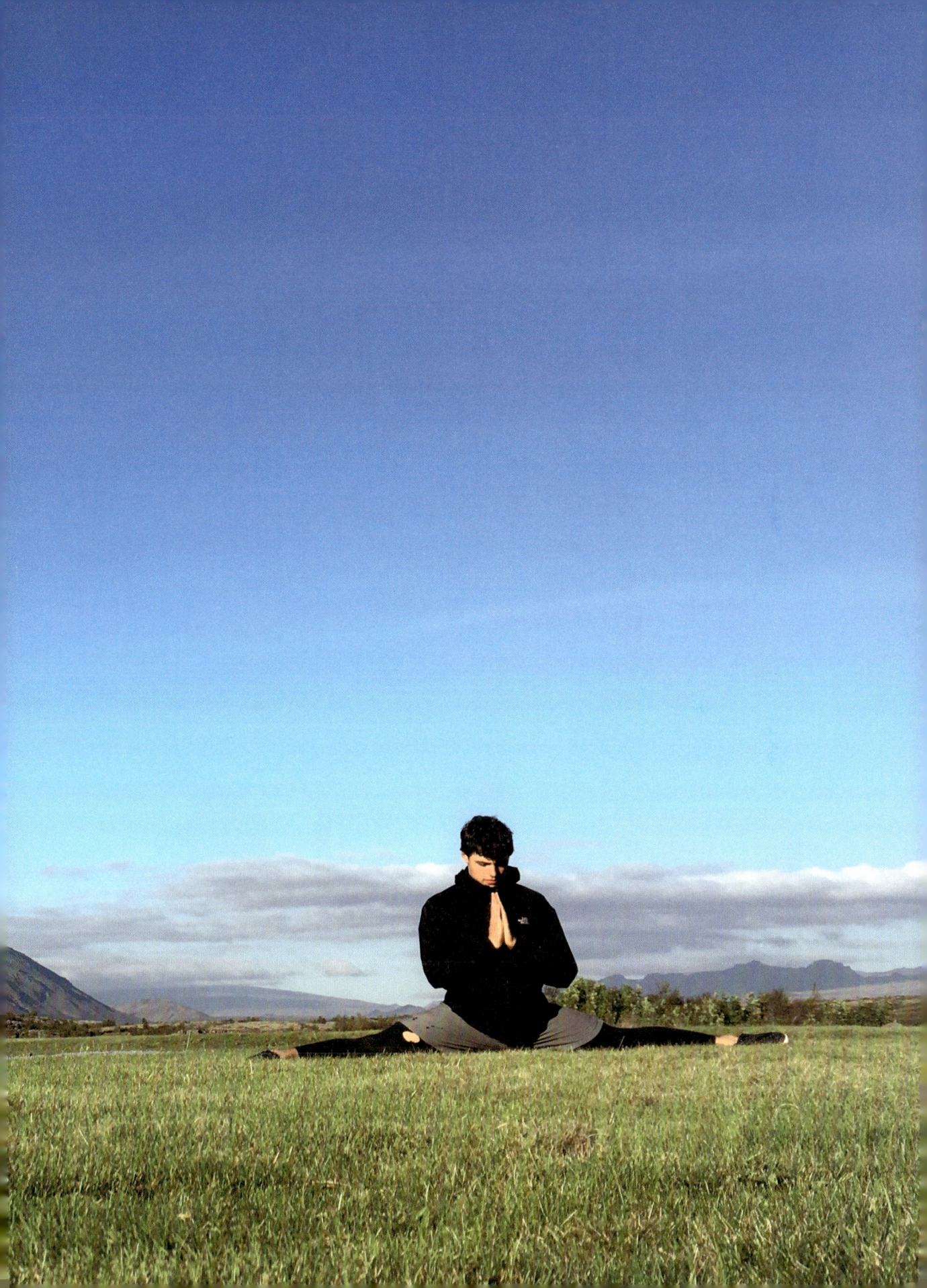

1 Mobility—Modern Flexibility Training

When I start our Calisthenics X Mobility workshop, I always begin with the following question: "Can someone give me the definition of *mobility*?" Almost all our workshop participants have watched one of my videos on YouTube, which is why most of the responses go in the right direction. The following catch phrases are then tossed around:

- "active flexibility training"
- "like stretching, but with strength"
- "range of motion"

Mobility training clearly focuses on movement. Unlike stretching, where a position is held for an extended period, mobility training always requires active control over a certain distance. Here's a simplified formula:

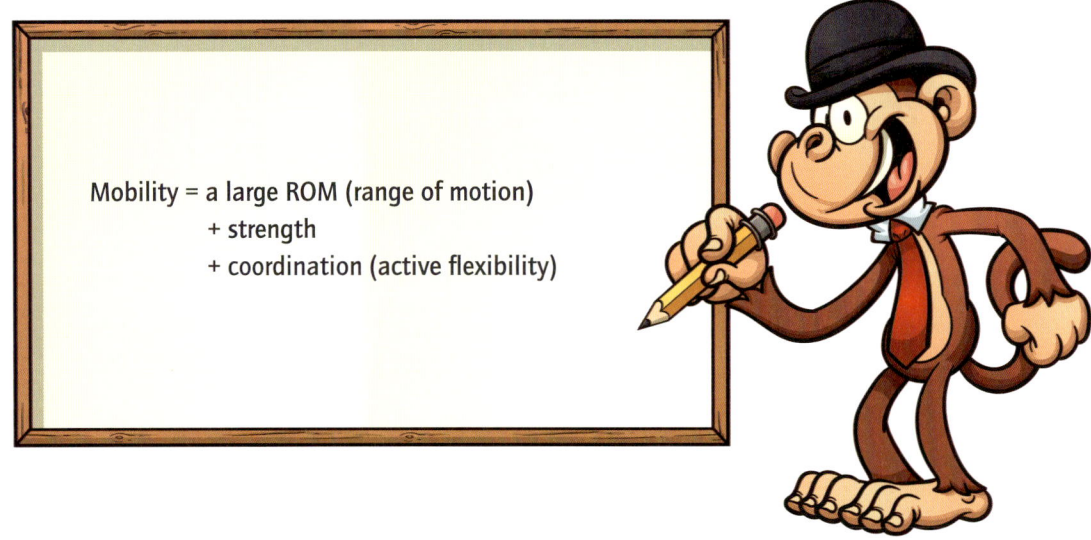

Mobility = a large ROM (range of motion)
+ strength
+ coordination (active flexibility)

Mobility—Modern Flexibility Training

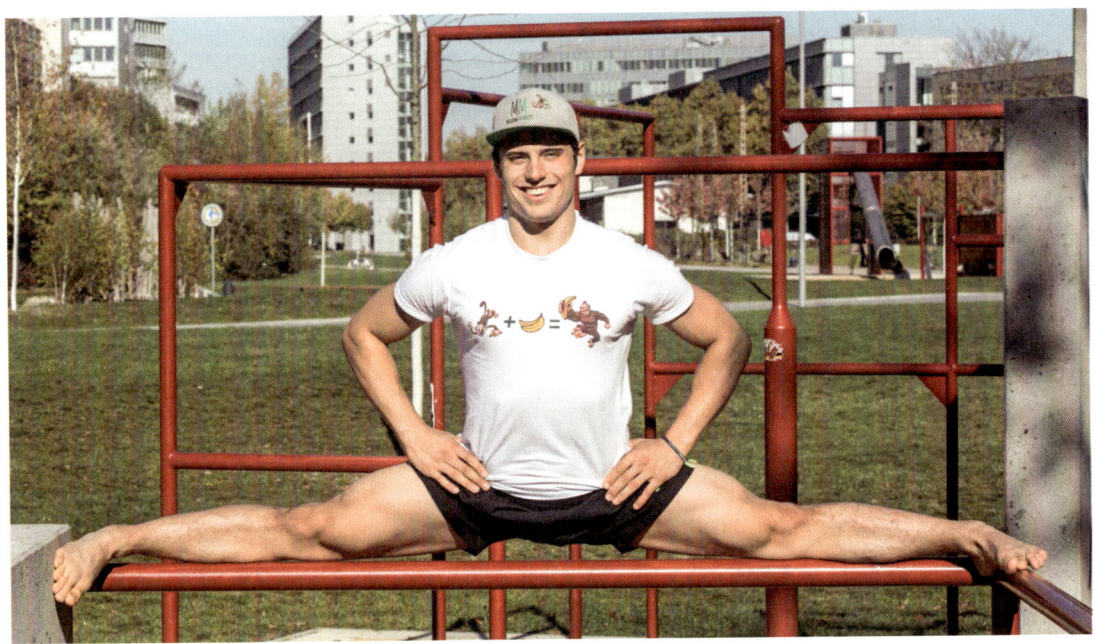

Next, I always demonstrate a practical example. Imagine I let myself slide from a standing position down into the straddle splits and then returned from the splits to a standing position by using only my leg strength.

This type of mobility stands in contrast to passive mobility, which is called *flexibility*. Imagine holding on to one ankle while standing and pulling it toward your backside. You'd be passively holding your leg at this range of motion without tensing the muscles in your legs.

Of course, we don't start the workshop by practicing the splits. To achieve long-term mobility and strength, we must understand how mobile our bodies should really be.

Mobility and strength are always mutually dependent. Imagine a seesaw with flexibility on one side and stability on the other. Since the body is a dynamic system, much like a seesaw, we need a mix of flexibility (passive range of motion) and stability (strength) to keep our balance. The sweet spot is called mobility.

In medicine, we refer to **homeostasis**, meaning a state of equilibrium. By definition, it's subject to dynamic self-regulation.

These are fancy words that ultimately describe the fact that our bodies vacillate between flexibility, mobility, and stability. Thus, our joints also have different functions. Some primarily provide stability, while others primarily provide lots of mobility.

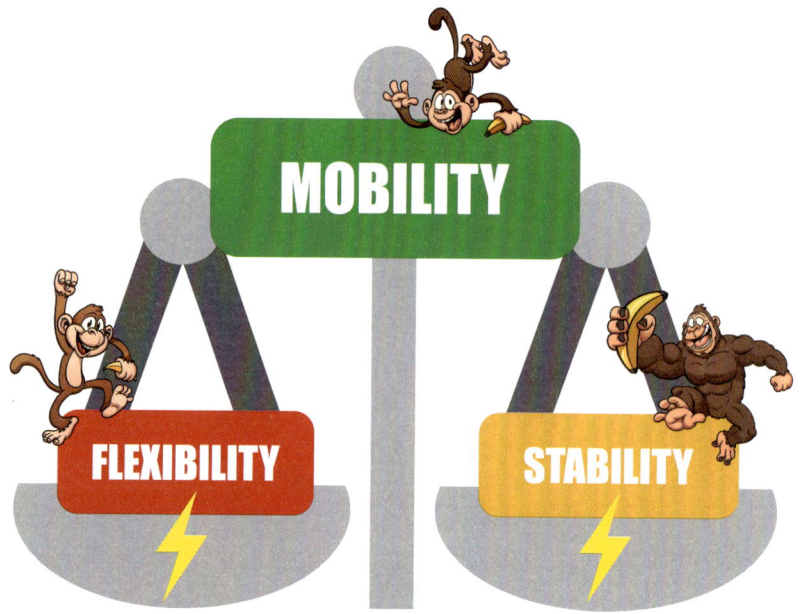

Here's what this teaches us about our mobility training:

1. Not every joint must be pushed to be as mobile as possible. (In fact, in some cases, this can even cause damage and lead to pain.)

2. Feeling less flexible on some days than others is completely normal. We're all subject to natural fluctuations.

In section 2.1, "How to Become More Mobile," I explain how you can create a harmonic balance so you don't have to move through your daily life with tight muscles and pain. But first I want to briefly talk about how mobility training has become so popular.

ORIGINS OF MOBILITY

Mobility training is gaining increasing popularity. With mobility training, the focus is very much on the health-preserving aspect. For an athlete, be it recreational or professional, injuries are always a setback. Injuries lead to a sharp decline in athletic performance and, in some cases, can even trigger depression. An athlete's sport is often a huge part of his or her identity and is directly linked to self-confidence and overall satisfaction.

Someone who loves her sport and is injured will do anything to quickly return to her previous performance level.

For a long time, the problem was that the subject of "prevention" was written off as rather boring. People preferred to push the limits of their performance capacity and to do so at every training session. Until they couldn't.

Once the injury had occurred, the search for the cause and a solution began.

In the past, this was a real problem. In 2009, YouTube didn't yet have the number of high-quality help videos about pain that it has now. The first descriptive videos about sports came from bodybuilding, a sphere that still provides the bulk of sports videos on the internet.

The bodybuilding hype has always motivated more people to go to a fitness center. Due to the influence of social media, the makeup of that population got increasingly younger. And then they started to "pump away," having only a smattering of knowledge.

Here's the problem: just working out all the time doesn't make for a healthy body.

Then, a few years ago, the alleged savior of injured shoulders, backs, and hips came on the market: the foam roller.

Now, apparently, every pain was caused by tight muscles, connective-tissue adherences, and trigger points. No one had an actual plan as to what to do with these rollers and, later, the trigger balls. So people lay down on the rollers and pushed and rolled everything that hurt.

Whether foam rollers make sense or not is discussed in more detail in section 2.5, "Why Foam Rollers Won't Make You More Mobile."

Over time, it became clear that foam rollers weren't the answer, and the search continued. Yet many still used the rollers for warm-ups or for mobility training. Despite their questionable effectiveness, the rollers were part of a very positive development. More and more athletes were thinking about preventative health measures. This also helped introduce the concept of mobility.

And then there was a second major influence on making mobility more popular:

MOVEMENT CULTURE

Created by Ido Portal, movement culture is a philosophy of movement that's characterized by much of what has to do with movement. Because of him, I landed on this topic also, and he's one of my greatest role models with respect to my work as a trainer and athlete. Movement culture made a couple things popular, including **animal moves** and a movement concept that added the strength component to mobility training.

Most athletes now include mobility training in their training regimen, though unfortunately, they often still prefer static stretching to active mobilization, completely missing the effect of mobility training. Nevertheless, it's good that more and more people are opening up to the idea of mobility training, thanks to rolling and more. It doesn't matter whether they're bodybuilders, CrossFit athletes, or calisthenics athletes.

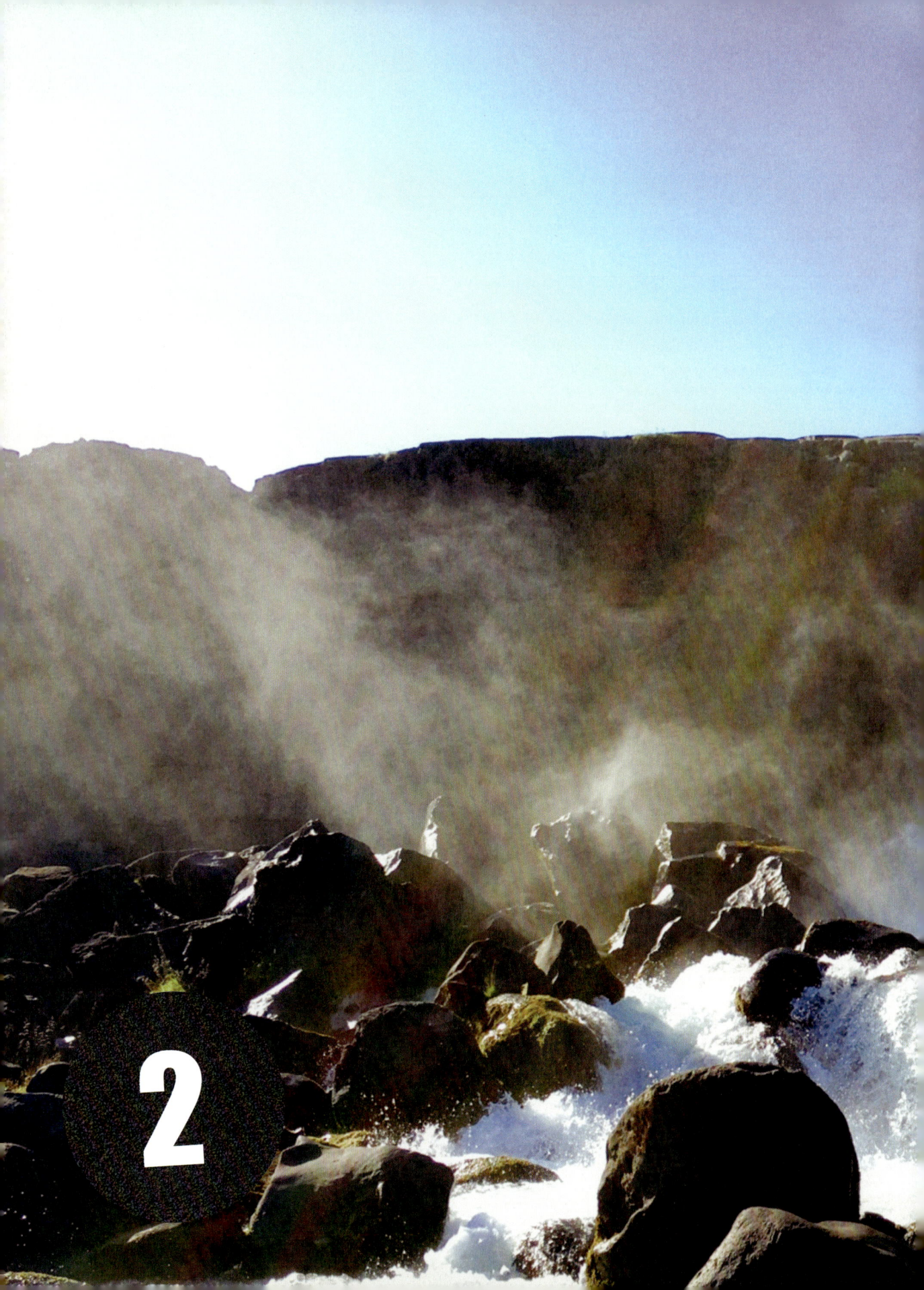

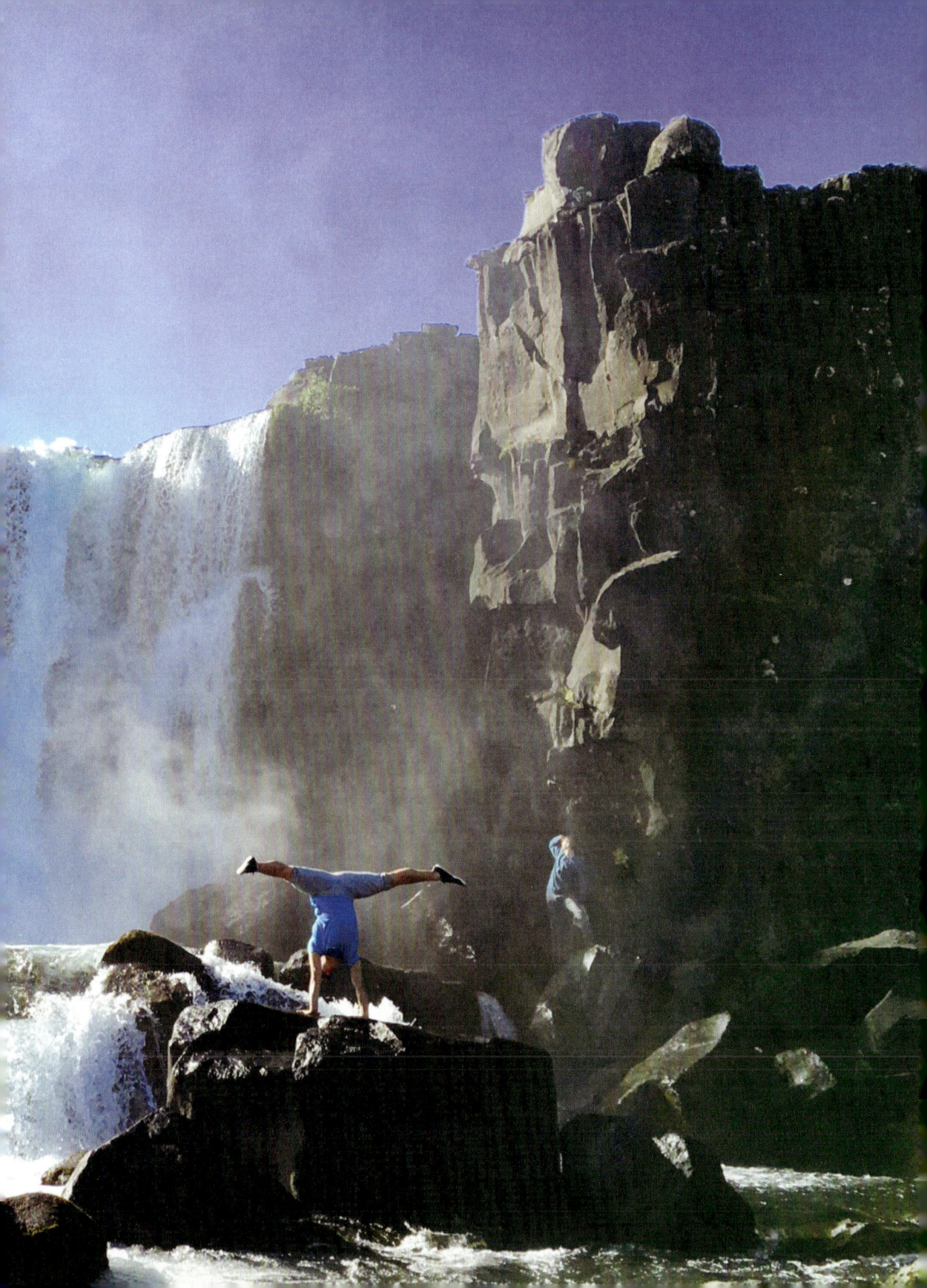

2 Understanding Mobility

2.1 HOW TO BECOME MORE MOBILE

For many, flexibility is a blind spot. Yet there are thousands of books about strength training.

Nearly everyone involved in fitness has held a dumbbell at some point.

But when it comes to mobility, most people think only of stretching. Actually, the ability to achieve a certain amount of mobility isn't just another type of training but also a very good indicator of the body's overall exercise capacity.

To better understand this, let's take a look at which factors affect mobility and why some athletes are very stiff despite doing strength training.

Mobility is grounded in the brain.:

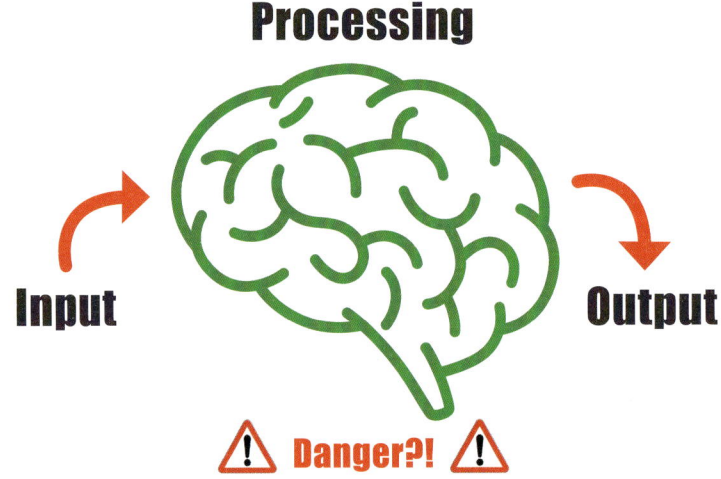

Everything we do in our daily lives or in sports is subject to the brain's processing of information.

Despite our modern society, our "software" still operates based on the very important survival mechanism, the question our brains pose for everything:

Am I safe, or am I in danger?

This also means our brains must be able to correctly assess movements and situations. What do I mean by *input*? Input is all the information that's routed to the brain:

1. Eyes (different ways of seeing and eye movements)
2. (Inner) Ears (hearing and balance)
3. Mouth and throat (taste, tongue position, and jaw movement)
4. Nose (smell)
5. Joints
6. Muscles
7. Skin

This information is handled within fractions of seconds.

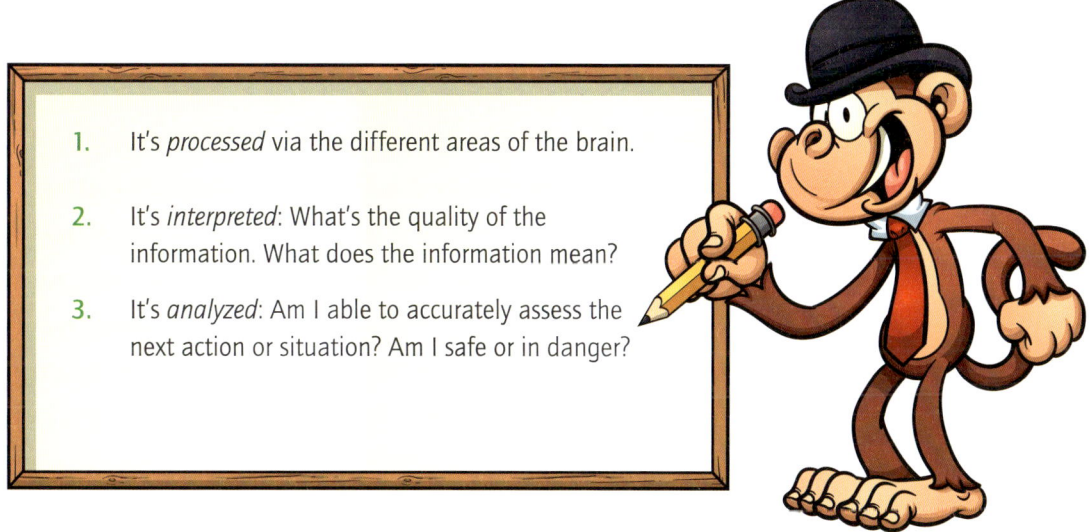

1. It's *processed* via the different areas of the brain.
2. It's *interpreted*: What's the quality of the information. What does the information mean?
3. It's *analyzed*: Am I able to accurately assess the next action or situation? Am I safe or in danger?

When your brain experiences ambiguities during this process and the final analysis determines that your brain is unable to ensure full functionality, your brain protects you by taking the following measures:

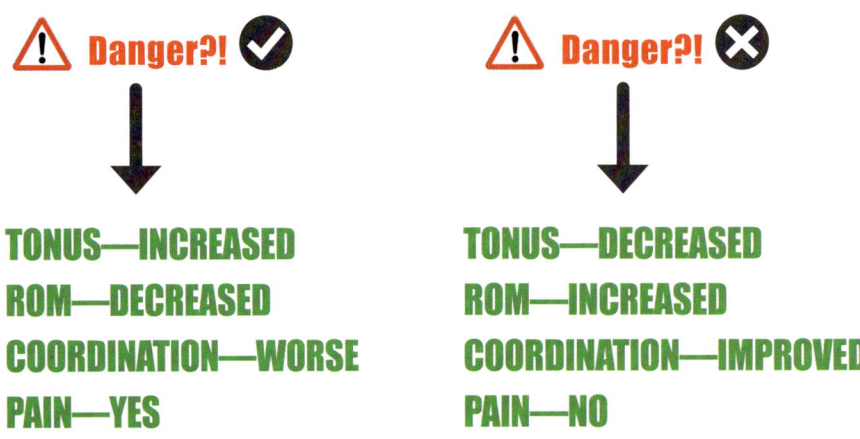

As you can see, when you improve the input, the ROM also improves.

With respect to mobility, here's an example:

When you practice moving your shoulders through their full range of motion (**FROM**) without crossing the pain threshold, such as doing a swimmer (see chapter 7, "Mobility Exercises"), your brain registers that you have control over every portion of the movement. The more you practice the activation of your shoulder joints and the joints involved in the movement (thoracic spine and shoulder blades), the clearer the image of the movement you're practicing becomes to the brain.

This takes us to the concept of a **body map**. Body mapping describes how well your joints and the surrounding muscles' ability to contract (tighten) are anchored in the brain, because moving a joint also includes the ability to adequately contract muscles and relax them again at the right moment.

Here's a word picture to help you better visualize this:

Imagine the path to the bakery nearest you. It doesn't matter if you're in Tokyo, New York, or your hometown. You know exactly which streets you need to travel to get to that bakery. In your head, you have a "map" to the bakery. But if you were a tourist in New York and someone asked you where to find a bakery, you'd have to resort to Google maps, an external map to show you the right way because your personal map (in your head) doesn't have a plan.

That's how it is with movement—or, to be more specific, with your joints' range of motion. If you always train and move your joints—or, rather, your body—in only one way, these paths will be better anchored in the brain than movements you rarely or never perform. For instance, for a strength athlete, this would mean training with in different ranges of motion.

Disrupting homeostasis is a trigger for lots of pains and limitations. This means possible imbalances in strength and flexibility and can even cause an issue with balance. When you learn to activate your joints and muscles, meaning having sensory and motor control, you'll become more flexible.

Of course, it doesn't sound particularly motivating when I tell you that you should practice improving your body's motor control. That's why my goal with this book is for you to learn to enjoy mobility training and then practice moving in different ways.

SUMMARY

Your brain determines your mobility (and strength). When you learn to control your joints and muscles, you also control your movements and make your brain feel more secure. The more secure your brain feels, the more flexible you'll be.

2.2 THE REASON WE'RE SO STIFF

Eyes, ears, mouth? I thought I had to move to become more mobile!

Absolutely correct. Ultimately, moving is always a priority. From an evolutionary standpoint, when someone doesn't move, that person becomes easy prey!

When it comes to mobility, I don't wish to confuse you but, rather, to provide clarity in the jungle of diverse methods and opinions in order to make you mobile and pain-free.

You can greatly change your mobility and performance by affecting your eyes, ears, and your tongue. But this falls into the area of applied neurology training.

Although the transitions are fluid, in this book I want to offer you a simpler and more familiar approach to exercise.

HOW MOBILE ARE YOU?

As I see it, an overwhelming problem today lies in the fact that we don't move enough or that our movements are overly one-sided. Not to mention that we have the ability to use our body to perform movements that should be easy to execute for a normal locomotor system, such as the following:

- Sitting cross-legged
- Squatting
- Hanging from a bar for at least 30 seconds and even up to 60 seconds
- Bending over
- Jumping to a knee-high surface
- Running backward
- Circling each arm in two different directions while standing

These movements aren't a valid test of your biomechanics. Apart from any scientific and evolutionary rationales, they're movements that, in my opinion, are part of normal functionality.

Our modern daily lives require us to use our body less and less. The lack of mobility and loss of body awareness take on a disastrous toll as early as elementary school.

As an elementary-school teacher, Monique can tell you a thing or two about that reality. In elementary school, students certainly sing a lot of songs, and alongside early musical instruction, reading, writing, and math remain, of course, a very important part of our lives.

But with elementary-school PE classes already being cut and only the advancement of the "intellect" being made a priority, we'll soon live in a society overrun by academics, with everyone suffering from joint pain.

Of course, this is a very one-sided picture, and in my opinion, we won't experience such a grievous societal change like the one portrayed in the Disney movie *WALL·E*. Nevertheless, we can't ignore exercise and health. A person can be extremely educated, but if she's unable to move her body, she'll neglect a large portion of her potential.

Physical work greatly supports mental work, as many studies on learning and exercise show. This aspect represents the biggest deficiency—or, rather, the greatest imbalance—in our education system, since the only physical ability we're taught from kindergarten all the way to high-school graduation is sitting.

In a society in which the education system ignores physical development and the healthcare system prioritizes disease control over preserving and promoting health, we have no choice but to become proactive.

Our body constantly alternates between buildup and deterioration. At some point deterioration will win, but we decide the speed at which this process advances and the quality of life with which we age. Do we aspire to wheeled walkers and being in constant fear of being trapped—of falling and not being able to get up again on our own? Not being able to do even half a squat to get up from the toilet without help or not having sufficient arm and core strength to be able to break a fall and prevent a hip fracture?

Or do we aim to age with a resilient body that allows us to play with our grandchildren and be strong enough to master everyday challenges and live autonomously until the final day of our existence?

2.3   DON'T MOBILIZE EVERY JOINT

As I mention in chapter 1, "Mobility—Modern Flexibility Training," we shouldn't mobilize every part of the body.

When someone mobilizes everything and forgets to create tension in certain areas, that person will experience symptoms similar to someone who only strengthens the muscles but never mobilizes. Pain and injuries occur when we ask too much of our body, exercise in too one-sided of a manner, or forget about balance. I cover more on this topic in section 3.2, "Pain and Injuries."

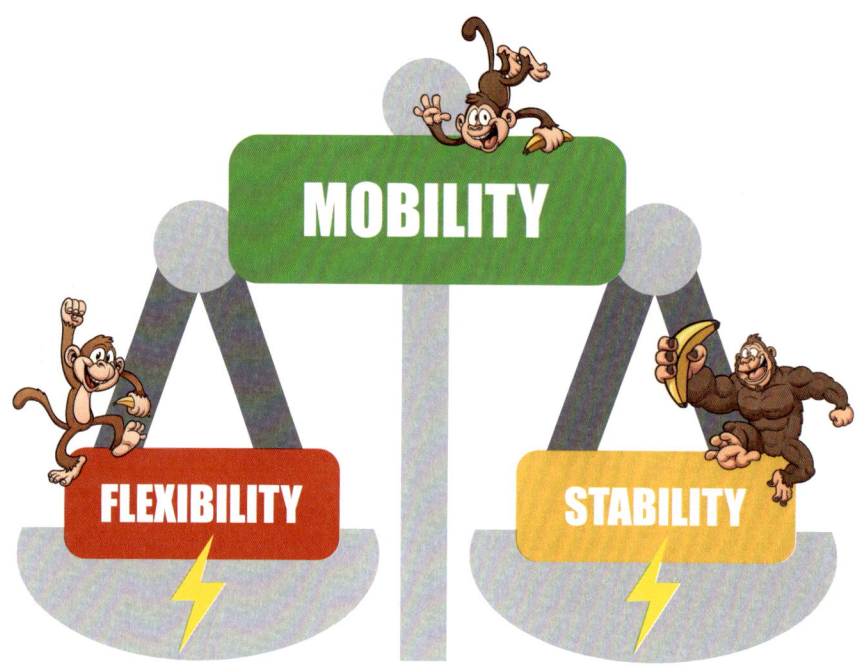

For example, let's think about ball sports, like soccer and tennis. Torn ligaments are common occurrences in these sports. Usually, the problem is that the athlete never practiced the position in which she got injured. Hence her brain and nervous system didn't have the information on how to stabilize her body or the joint in the respective position.

As I mention in section 2.1, "How to Become More Mobile," it's critical that we maintain control over our joints if we want to stay mobile and injury-free in the long term.

The **joint-by-joint approach** helps differentiate between stable and mobile joints. This determines which priorities you should set in your mobility training.:

Understanding Mobility

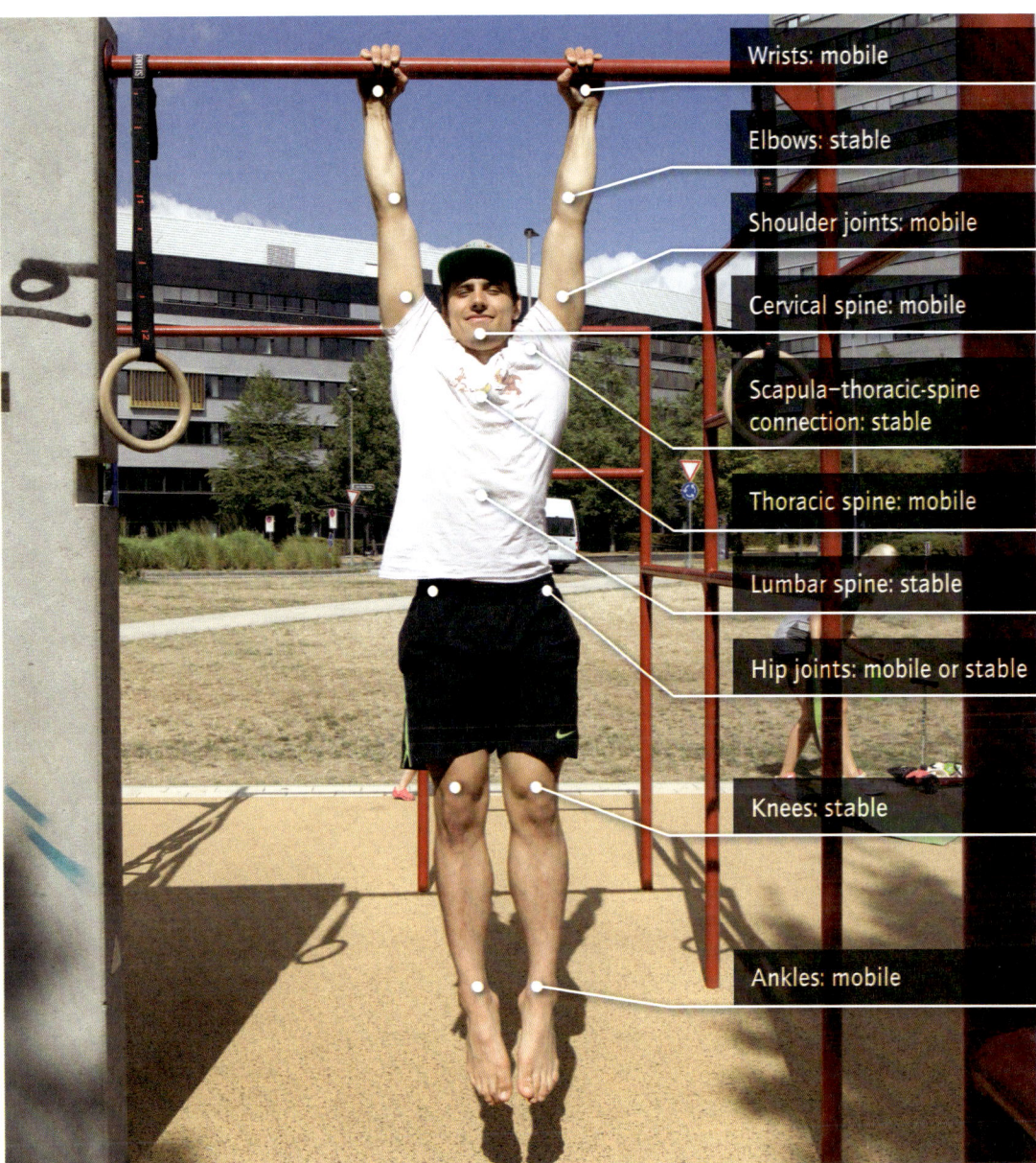

One question I often get on Instagram is this: "How can I make my lower back more mobile? That part of my body feels so rigid when I deadlift or during yoga."

As the joint-by-joint approach shows, your lower back (lumbar spine) should be stabilized. To make your spine more mobile, it'd be better to focus on your thoracic spine and your hips. These two areas are crucial to your upper body's overall mobility, which is why they must be mobilized when there are limitations. By contrast, the lower back links the upper and lower body. When there's too little stability in that area, the other joints must work harder to maintain the body's basic stability.

One reason why some of my coaching clients are stiff is having too little stability in their core, which is why all other joints are producing an excess of tension. I cover more on that in section 3.3, "Guideline for Pain-Free Training."

2.4 WHY STRETCHING AND YOGA WON'T MAKE YOU MORE MOBILE

But, Leon, what about the muscles? Don't they have to be stretched and mobilized to be more flexible?

Ultimately, your muscles are simply the executing organs of your nervous system's signals.

It's the job of your muscles to move your joints and protect them. Flexibility happens in the joints. *OK, but my muscles are tight!*

Right. So let me explain.

The purpose of all mobility exercises is to move your joints into an "unfamiliar" position and to learn to control it via muscle tension. When you learn to control your joint position, your nervous system registers this input and responds (output) by releasing your muscles, with efficient tension, at their current length.

This means your muscles no longer resist this joint position—resolving what we know as *tight muscles*. The more you practice this joint position, the better your body is able to release this muscle length faster and with more strength. You'll become stronger at this range of motion and able to move without restrictions.

Muscles are always given obtuse orders on how to behave. But if you want to achieve long-term changes, you must talk to the messengers (joints) and the commander (brain). If you focus only on your muscles during mobility training, meaning you only try to passively lengthen (stretch) your muscles, the communication between messengers and commander is insufficient. After all, your brain wants specific information about what needs to be done.

In physical therapy, we always talk about how training should be movement specific. This is true for strength training as well as mobility training. Regardless of which sport you're preparing for with mobility training or wanting to improve your performance of through better mobility, one thing is certain: strength is always a factor, even if it's gravity that makes it necessary for you to become strong in your mobility.

Lengthening your muscles will, at best, have a very short-term effect that won't be optimally wired in your nervous system. Always think about the input your brain receives, processes, and subsequently creates as output. When your input (e.g., stretches that were held too long) doesn't match the requested output (e.g., a pull-up) you won't benefit from the briefly acquired range of motion.

Lots of yogis have participated in our past Calisthenics X Mobility workshops. Most of them were a bit surprised when I insisted that passive stretching is a waste of time when you're trying to become more mobile. Most of them reported that their usually statically held positions had resulted in increased range of motion.

The explanation is simple: if you practice something often, you'll get better.

For instance, if I practice doing the splits often and long enough, I'll, at some point, master them. Remember, communication with the brain is the decisive factor for long-term adaptations.

Passive stretching and static yoga poses don't provide nearly as much information for the brain as movement does.

When you're moving, you have to concentrate more, the impact on your vestibular system is significantly higher, and your **mechanoreceptors** (sensory receptors in joints, muscles, tendons, ligaments, and the skin that perceive mechanical loading) receive more input.

These and other factors result in the body adapting more quickly to a certain movement or range of motion. But don't get me wrong, I'm not opposed to yoga. This is purely about the differentiation between passive and active flexibility. There are many other reasons why people do yoga, but, in general, I find that yoga doesn't make us as efficiently mobile as structured mobility training does.

IN SUMMARY

Stretching results in inadequate activation of the nervous system and provides to the brain insufficient information about the safety of the movement.

2.5 WHY FOAM ROLLERS WON'T MAKE YOU MORE MOBILE

Let's move on to another topic that's similar to stretching. Ever since the *Becoming a Supple Leopard* hype, foam rollers and trigger balls have been very popular. They're considered basic equipment in the mobility area of nearly every fitness facility.

I continue to announce on my social-media channels that I'm not at all a supporter of the foam roller.

Following is an explanation of the following:

- Why you don't need to roll around *for hours*
- How you *can* use a foam roller
- Why pain during rolling *isn't* desirable

2.5.1 THE FOAM-ROLLER PHENOMENON

When the subject of "fascia fitness" first emerged, everyone packed a foam roller under his gluteus maximus and rolled like there was no tomorrow to release the "adhesions."

Before I enter into this discussion, I must tell you that while the fascia trend has resulted in more people engaging in mobility training, in the area of fitness, some bad habits have crept in. I'd like to comment on these because they'll keep you from doing a clean pull-up and a perfect handstand.

2.5.2 ROLLING, ROLLING, ROLLING

At the fitness studio, I continue to see one unfortunate phenomenon over and over again.

Most people's warm-up looks like this: roll, roll, and roll some more. I think it's great that because of the foam roller many are even thinking about warming up and not going straight to the pull-up bar. But the resulting problem is obvious. You might manage to increase your range of motion by rolling, but you've likely never before properly trained that range of motion. Your nervous system is unable to control that new range.

Remember, the purpose of training is to improve your quality of movement. But when your training preparation takes place strictly on the roller, you don't practice any movements that would be conducive to your training, like activating the shoulder blades before calisthenics training. Thirty minutes with the foam roller isn't an adequate warmup for training.

2.5.3 SURFACE SENSIBILITY VERSUS PROPRIOCEPTIVE SENSIBILITY

When Monique warms up for calisthenics training, she warms up the areas that are critical to her subsequent training. She focuses on preparing mobility-technical movement patterns.

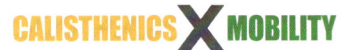

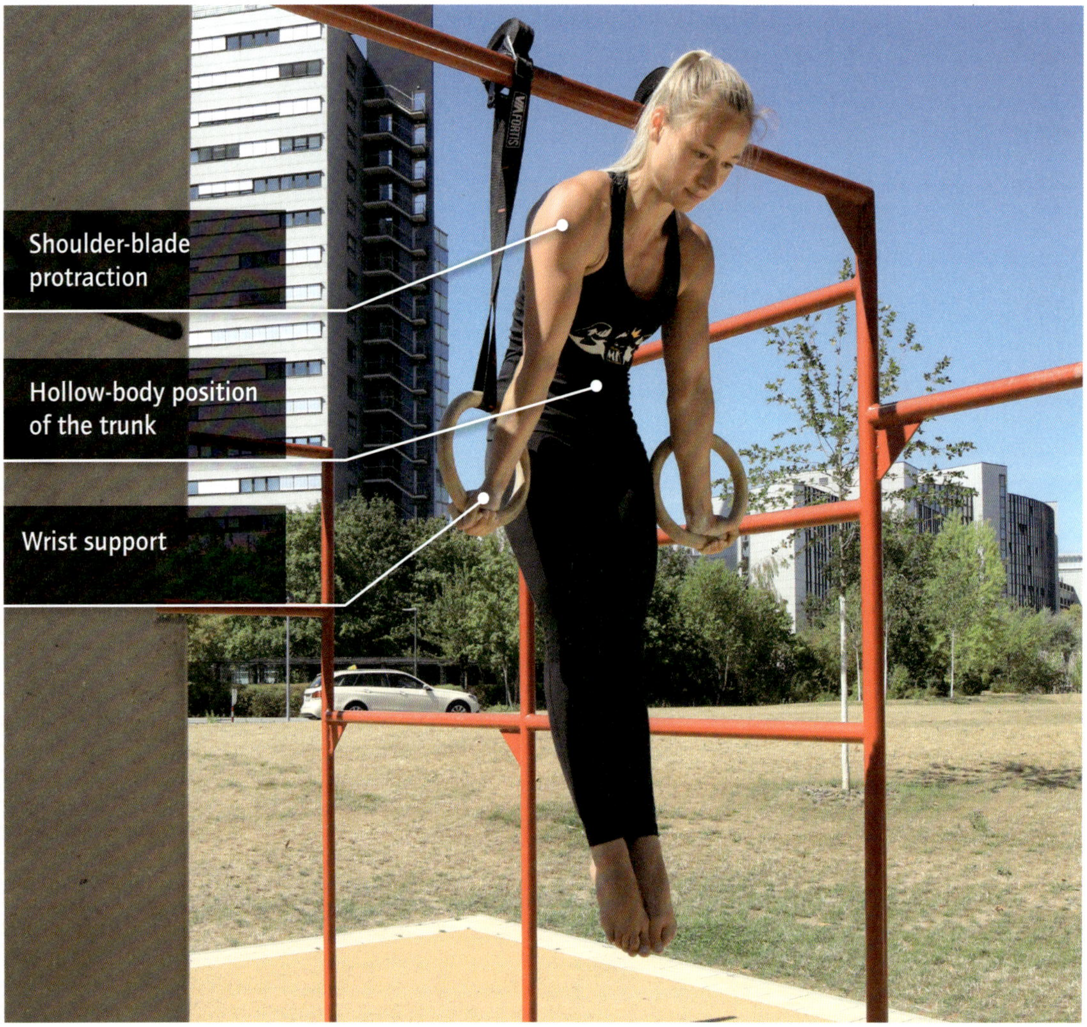

Before her specific warm-up, this allows her to better draw on her movement repertoire during training, because she's practiced her **proprioceptive sensibility** with mobility training.

If she were to spend time only on a foam roller, she'd merely stimulate her **surface sensibility (exteroception)**, which could briefly provide her with an increased range of motion, but she wouldn't practice her movement awareness to the same extent she would by moving.

Each body is unique. The way each one will react to stimulation of its receptors is also unique. The entire debate about needing to work our fascia separately is absolutely moving in the wrong direction. After all, we're always affecting multiple body structures simultaneously by moving, as well as rolling on a foam roller. Affecting only one structure (fascia) is simply not possible.

Thus, I continue to ask myself this question: How can I effectively use my training time to optimize my athletic performance or that of my clients? For instance, when I'm coaching, I try out different methods to help clients move better. Movement is always the central issue when it comes to being pain-free, feeling better in one's body, and being able to perform better during training.

When you focus on practicing your movements, on better activating your joints, and on getting stronger with a big range of motion, you'll achieve 80 percent of the results with only 20 percent of the effort.

You should figure out if the foam roller even works for you. Just because it's generally supposed to be good doesn't mean it's good for you.

Keep in mind the **SAID principle** (specific adaptation on imposed demands). In other words, you always adapt to the stimulus you apply to your body. Passive rolling alone won't make you better.

2.5.4 PAIN WHILE ROLLING

For most people, rolling involves pain—only when you're in a lot of pain and can't move your shoulder for three days does rolling work. This is also true for a lot of athletes and stretching, who think, *I have to lengthen the muscle as much as possible, and it has to hurt!*

While applying this mentality to mobility is a big mistake, many do exactly that: If you want to have bulging biceps, do a lot of curls. If you want strong legs for doing squats, do a lot of squats. If you want to be able to do more pull-ups, do a lot of pull-ups. But do you want to get "better" at pain? Probably not. Our bodies never stop learning. They adapt and remodel themselves as needed. You should therefore provoke pain as little as possible.

Moving pain-free applies to the healthy athlete as well as the injured one. Irritating your body with constant pain impulses isn't beneficial to training or rehabilitation.

When you lie down on the foam roller, it can be unpleasant, but it shouldn't end with a flood of crocodile tears. Pain-free moving is healthy moving. You can find more information in section 3.2, "Pain and Injuries."

2.5.5 FOAM ROLLERS—SENSE OR NONSENSE?

At this point, you're likely asking yourself if the foam roller is a complete waste of time.

Or if you should use it now and then.

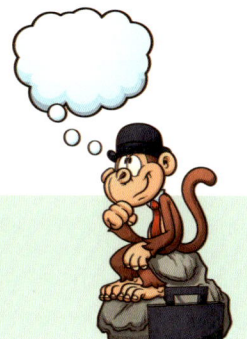

Remember this:

The foam roller is a tool.

No more, no less. It's not a panacea for tight muscles, sore muscles, or achieving a great, powerful range of motion. When you use it, check to see if it was beneficial (did your mobility improve?). And remember that *moving* is the best remedy.

Spend more time with your body (e.g., using mobility or calisthenics) than with any fitness gadgets.

You can learn how to test your movement ability in subsection 3.1.1, "Evaluation."

2.6   MORE EXERCISE EQUIPMENT YOU DON'T NEED

What's true for foam rollers (i.e., they're not equipment you necessarily need) is true for using gloves or a weightlifting belt during training.

At Calisthenics X Mobility workshops, people always ask Monique what she thinks about wearing gloves during calisthenics training. And, similarly, they ask me with respect to weightlifting belts for deadlifts and squats.

The answer is similar to that of the foam roller. All these things are tools. You should know each tool's specific use without depending on any of them. Using gloves during calisthenics training is very popular because gripping the bars causes callouses to form on the hands. In many circles, callouses are considered unaesthetic. Moreover, some look to the example of gymnasts who wear wrist supports so they can swing around the horizontal bar.

If we take a quick look back at human history, it becomes apparent why calloused hands are considered unattractive. In the past, there were working peasants and the nobility. Unlike the working peasants, the nobility didn't have callouses on their hands, because the nobles didn't do hard work. Back then, unblemished skin was considered a beauty ideal.

To reemphasize, if you aren't a world-class athlete, there are no technical, performance reasons for using gloves or a weightlifting belt during legwork, only aesthetics. At best, these tools will lower your performance. After all, humans are creatures of habit. You'll quickly rely on the supposed protection, which can cause the quality of your movements to suffer.

Gloves don't allow you to grip the bar properly, and a belt won't let you maintain proper abdominal tension. This advice applies particularly to beginners and slightly advanced athletes who have maybe one to three years of training experience. All others, if they've completed the proper training, have learned how to control their bodies for a certain movement, which is why these tools can certainly be useful. It's all a matter of performance level and the way you use these things.

2.7   HOW MOBILITY MAKES YOU STRONGER

If you've read up to this point, you already know more about modern mobility training than 90 percent of athletes. But aside from all the useful facts about mobility and movement overall, you're probably asking yourself why this book about mobility is so detailed. Why not, like most strength-training books, describe 10 simple exercises, half of which should ideally be performed with a foam roller, and then sell it as "mobility training"? Mobility is far more than a little warm-up or cool-down. Mobility is the prerequisite for maximum strength development. Here, we can refer to the laws of physics:

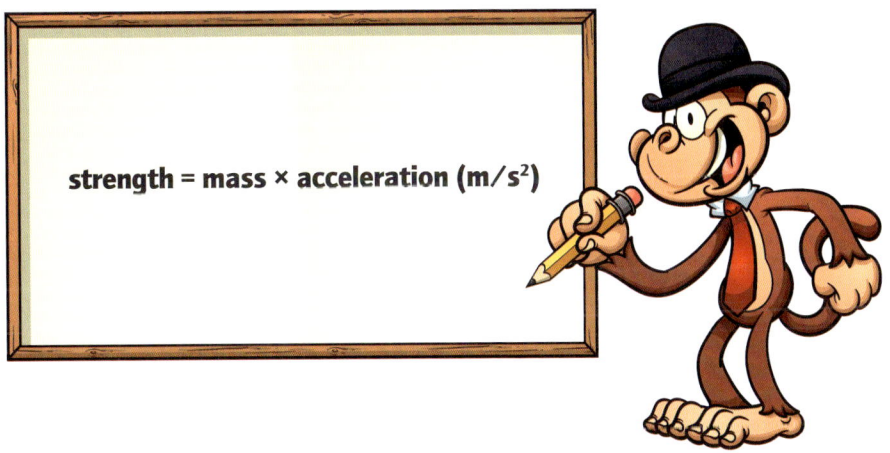

strength = mass × acceleration (m/s²)

With respect to calisthenics, it's quite simple because the mass to be accelerated is your own bodyweight. Now we have two factors that can influence our strength with respect to our bodyweight. For instance, for a pull-up, we can change the distance or the time with which we accelerate upward.

I like to simplify things, so simply put, the more distance (feet or meters) I have at my disposal, the greater the resulting strength potential. Even simpler, mobility has an immediate effect on your strength. But there are additional factors that emphasize the importance of mobility training.

There are frequent debates about the extent to which mobility training tested in this manner has a positive effect on regeneration and injury prevention.

To date, the consensus seems to be that we're not really sure or that occasionally negative results have been ascertained with respect to prevention and regeneration.

I don't wish to engage in an emotionally charged scientific debate on whether the studies are reliable and convincing, but I want to take a more sober approach. In this book, I want to present the arguments in a simpler way than referring to meta-analyses.

Mobility will give you control over your joints. In gaining control, you'll place your joints at all their various angles and give your body what it really needs: variation.

I'll continue to revisit this point throughout this book. After all, variety is what preserves our joints when we keep performing repetitive motions in sports.

So you'll become more resilient against unfamiliar movements and joint positions and will thus reduce the severity of any potential injuries.

2.8 WHY STRESS MAKES YOU IMMOBILE

An often completely ignored aspect of mobility is the opportunity to self-analyze one's performance capacity during training.

Imagine you had a stressful week and worked out only once.

And recently you'd frequently been more stressed. Because you haven't been able to work out regularly, you give 150 percent during your one weekly workout. On the days following, your muscles are correspondingly sore.

You're experiencing multiple factors that are greatly increasing your likelihood of an injury: stress—possibly resulting in a lack of focus during training because you have too much on your mind—and irregular physical exercise). Hence it's extremely important that you're able to assess your performance capacity before a workout. During these pre-workout assessments, you'll definitely feel less mobile. Mobility exercises are even less fun, which can result in a false interpretation of their effectiveness.

Many of my clients have had the problem of doing even fewer mobility exercises during stressful times, when they should have been doing more. They thought mobility just wasn't their thing and were frustrated when they regressed. And yet the cause was merely the fact that their current stress levels were too high. Maybe you've felt the same way and skipped your mobility training.

These words are intended to motivate you so that next time you'll view the whole situation from a different perspective. In doing so, remember this idea of the **stress bucket**: The more stress that flows into the bucket, the fuller the bucket will be. When it overflows, it means your central nervous system is overloaded and performance and mobility will suffer. Next to other effects, these two are the most important when it comes to athletic effort. After all, your body isn't meant to function well for only a few years; it's supposed to stay resilient and healthy for a lifetime.

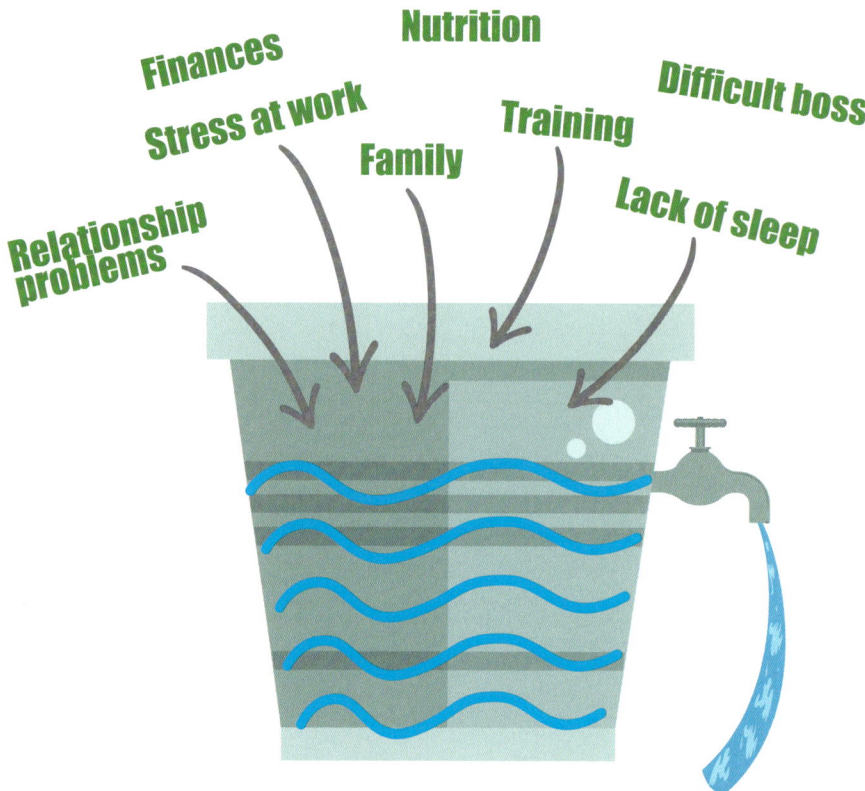

If you take away only one thing from this chapter, let it be that your mobility largely depends on how stressed you are and that, before a workout, mobility can help you determine if you're able to put the pedal to the metal that day or if you should limit your workout to mobility training and an easy endurance session.

Mobility can greatly increase your capacity and strength.

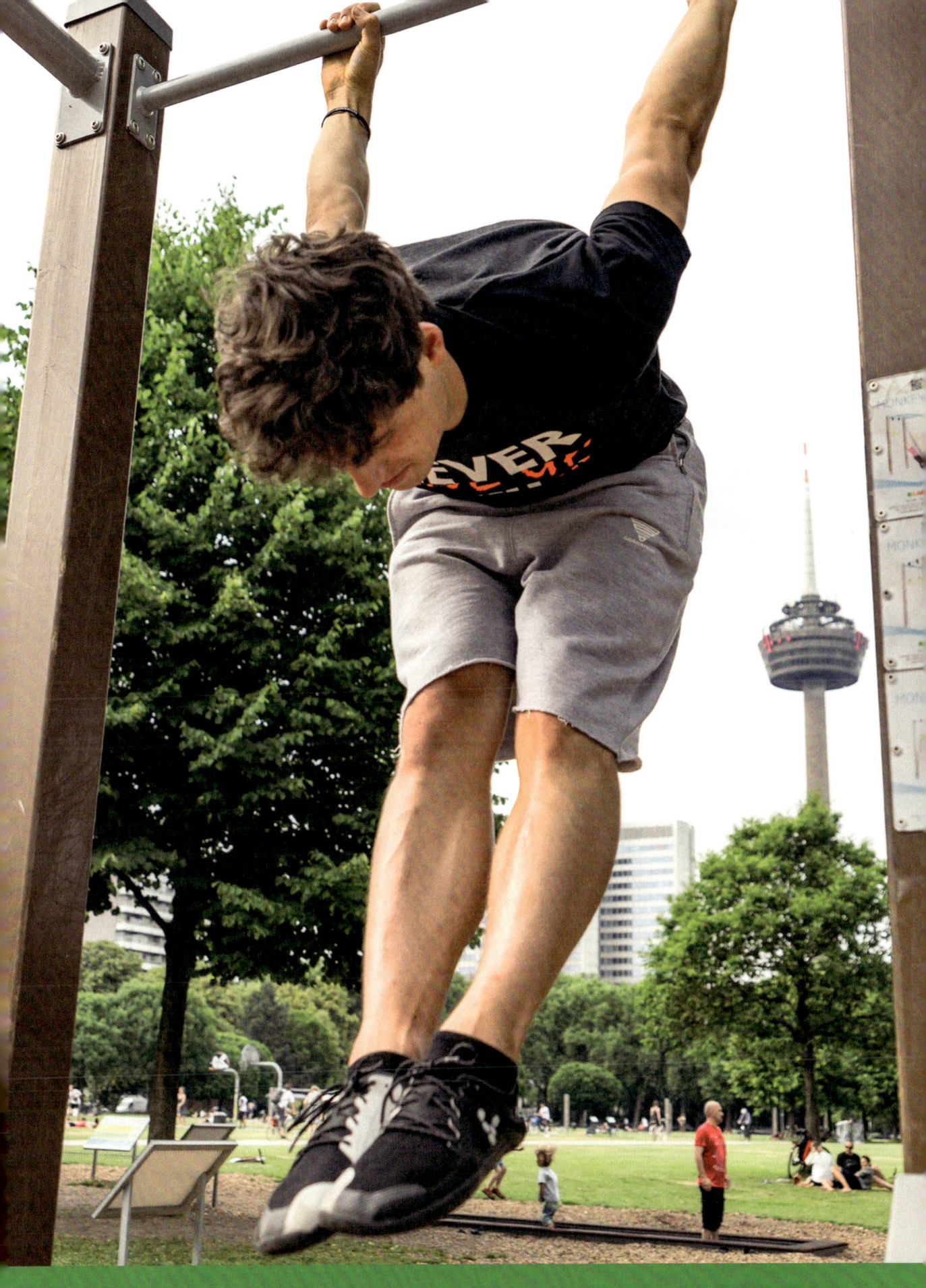

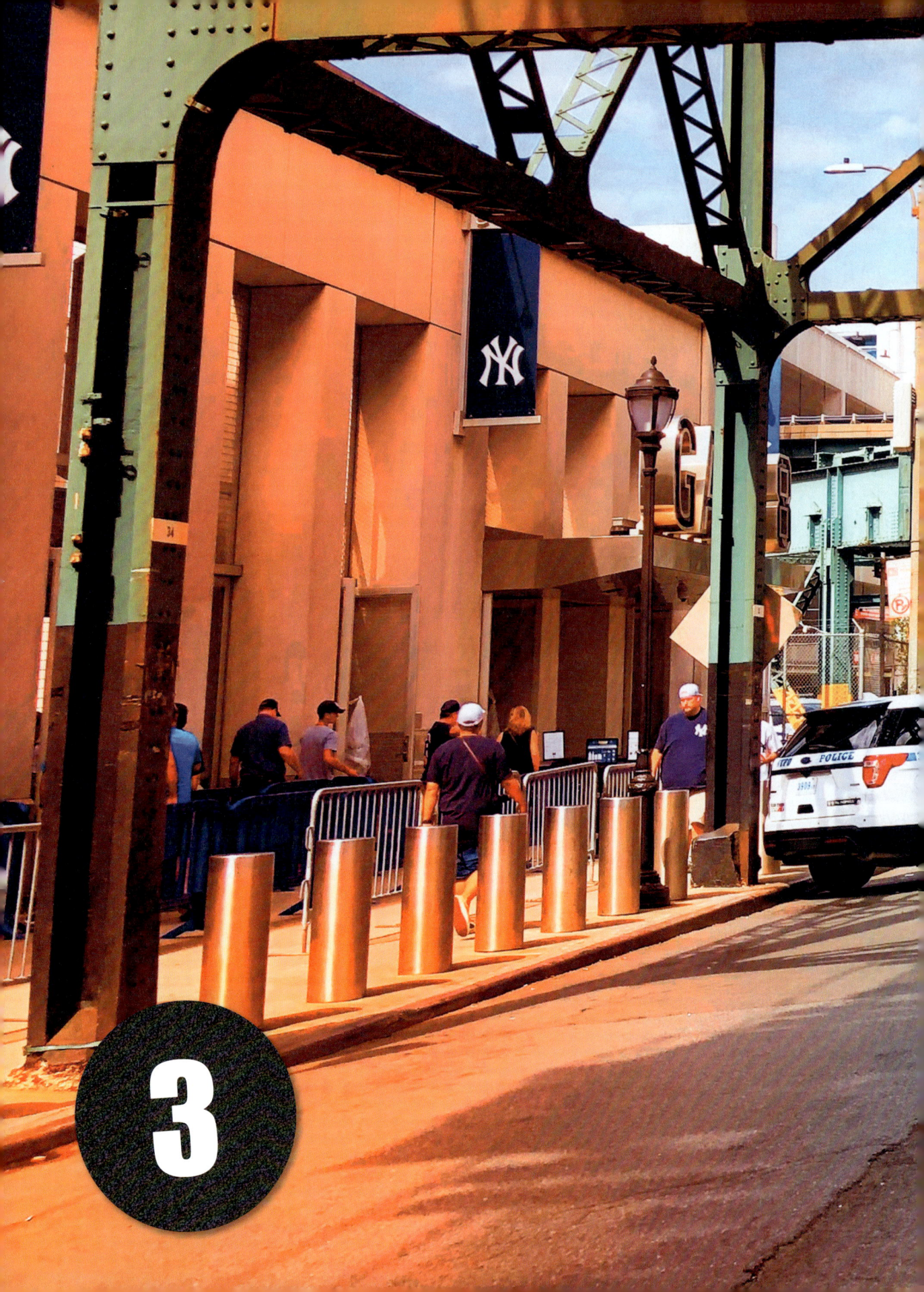

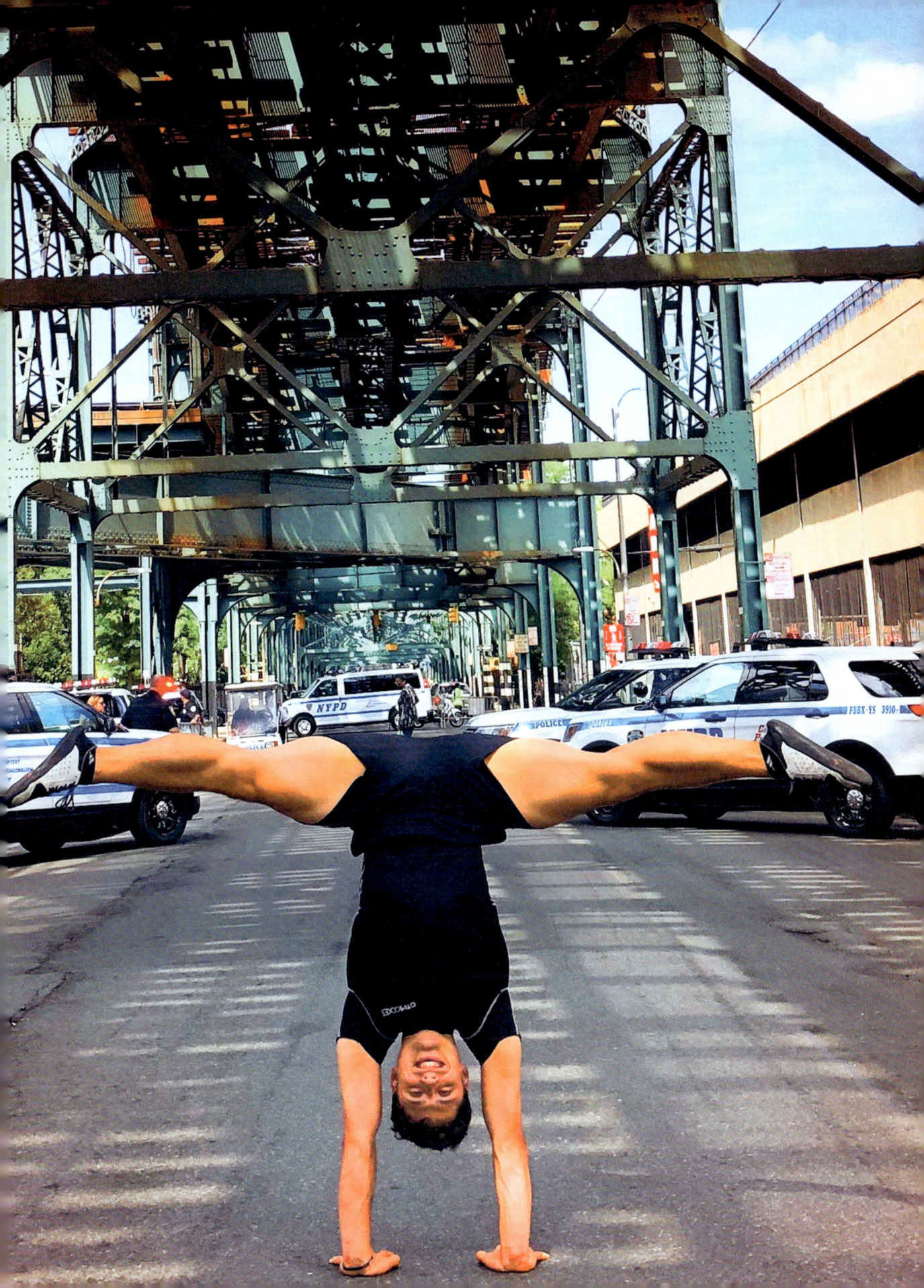

3 Mobility Fundamentals: What You Need to Know

3.1 FOUR EASY STEPS TO BECOMING MORE MOBILE

In workshops, coaching, and my everyday life, I follow certain principles that allow me to work efficiently and effectively and achieve my goals. Regardless of whether they're my own goals or goals I've set together with my clients, one basic idea is always there: How can I simplify the complex?

You now have a good idea of what mobility really means. Next, we concentrate on the arguably best concept for optimally working on your mobility..

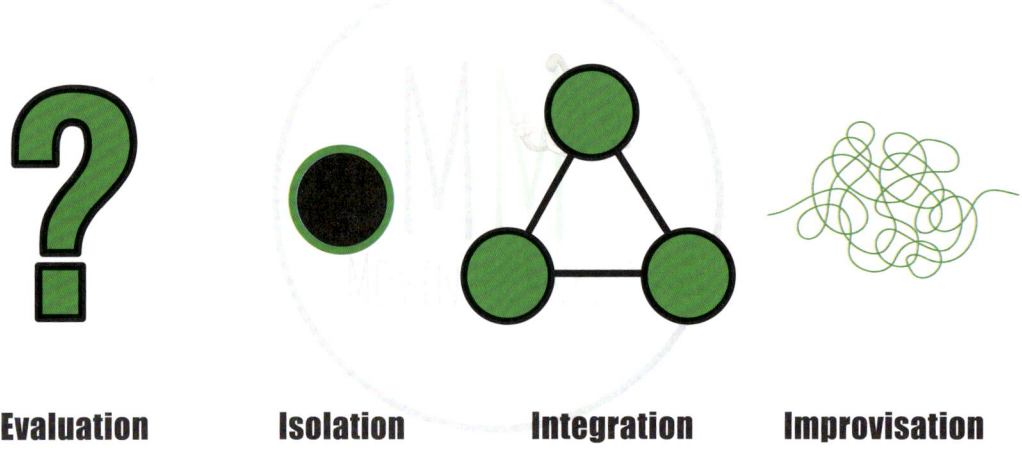

Evaluation   **Isolation**   **Integration**   **Improvisation**

3.1.1 EVALUATION

Evaluation is the absolute foundation of every coaching session with me—and with any good coach. Without evaluation, you don't know what your baseline is, and that means you're unable to set goals. Even worse, a poor analysis and lack of monitoring causes you to, at some point, lose motivation because you're unable to achieve success. Even if you improved, you'd be unable to confirm it, let alone measure it.

The analysis done in this book is certainly not exhaustive but is intended to provide a broad overview so you're better able to evaluate yourself than you were before.

Moreover, I want to encourage you to take photos. Once you've read the chapters on mobility, work out for at least four to six weeks using the exercises in this book.

After that time period, take more photos for comparison. With respect to calisthenics, primarily the following joint functions should be tested:

OVERHEAD MOBILITY

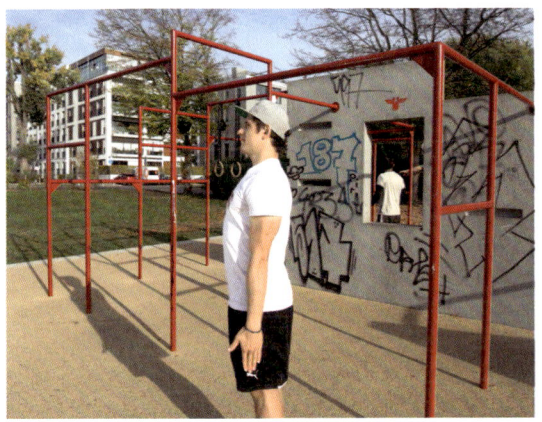 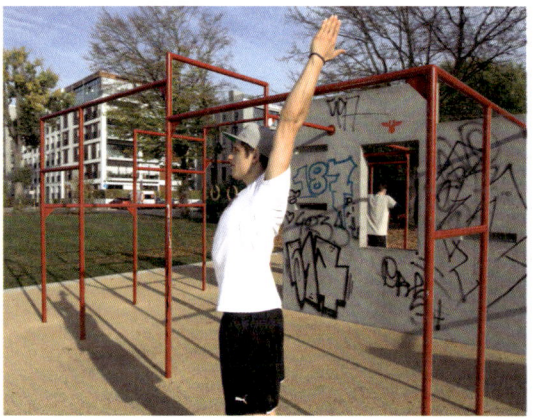

Ensure there are no compensating movements of the spine—keep your arms extended the entire time.

INTERNAL AND EXTERNAL SHOULDER ROTATION

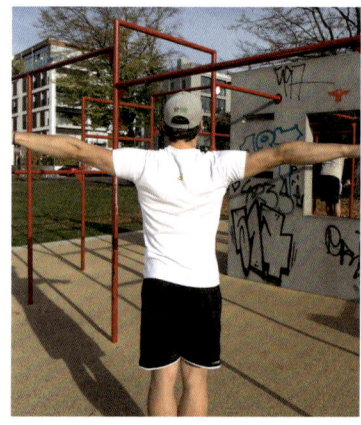 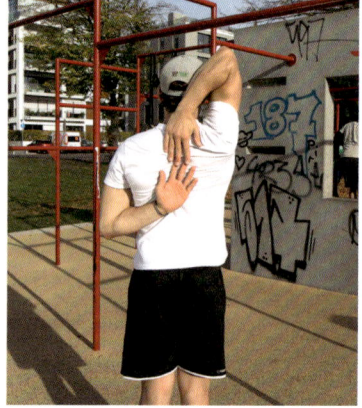 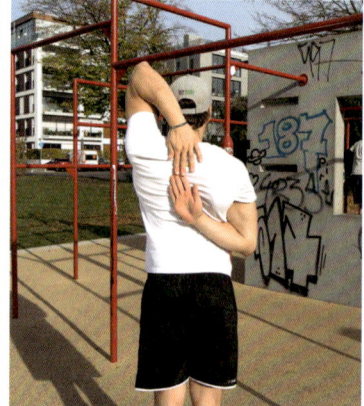

Move easily into the position without trying to force your hands together.

THORACIC SPINE ROTATION

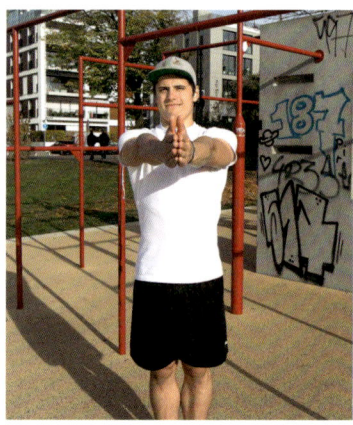 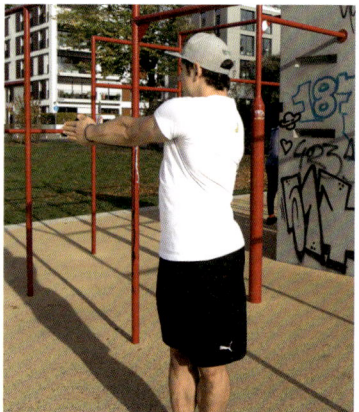 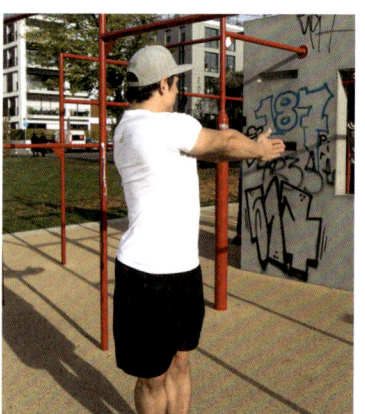

Stand with your feet together and rotate around your body's axis.

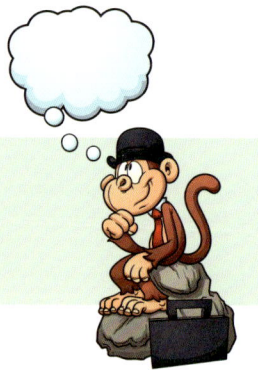

Always remember this:

What gets measured gets accomplished.

3.1.2 ISOLATION

Isolation is the base. Within the context of mobility, isolation means the ability to activate joints separately (without compensating movements by adjacent joints).

ankle – knee – hip – lumbar spine – thoracic spine – cervical spine – wrist – shoulder – scapula

If you're unable to activate a joint, your muscles will always limit your joint's range of motion. Monique also describes this in subsection 11.3.1, "What Your Pull-Up Should Look Like," affirming that the pull-up consists of multiple components. It begins with the simplest step, and the complexity increases with each additional step. Mastering the final result, the pull-up, requires control over each individual step. You'll notice that mobility isn't nearly as easy as you might think it is.

Because activating individual joints is so unfamiliar to your body, this first step is the longest. To really gain control over your joint, you need focus. Don't let other things distract you, and more importantly, perform the exercises calmly. Moving through the isolations quickly won't yield much in the long term. If you can concentrate and put in the effort, you'll get more out of all the mobility exercises. Your ROI (return on investment) will be much higher.

WHAT DOES SUCH AN ISOLATED JOINT ACTIVATION LOOK LIKE?
WHAT ARE SOME PECULIARITIES?

At this point, I like to draw on another concept: controlled articular rotations (**CARs**).

The complete movement a joint can perform is a 360-degree circle. At this point, I regularly get this question from workshop participants: "What about the neck? Should I roll that 360 degrees too? Isn't that dangerous?"

Here, we must understand why this question comes up so frequently. From a strictly anatomical perspective, the neck (cervical spine) consists of the intervertebral joints of your cervical vertebrae, the facet joints.

They're also referred to as the *gliding joints*. In terms of function, a gliding joint can perform only a rotation (looking left and right) and a lateral inclination (moving the ear toward the shoulder). A circular movement is strictly reserved for the shoulder (articulatio humeri), as a ball joint.

Cervical Spine with Atlanto-occipital Joint

- Cranial base
- Dens
- Atlanto-occipital joint
- Atlas (C1 cervical vertebra)
- Atlanto-axial joint
- C2 cervical vertebra
- Intervertebral disk II/III
- C3 cervical vertebra
- Intervertebral disk III/IV
- C4 cervical vertebra
- Intervertebral disk IV/V
- C5 cervical vertebra
- Intervertebral disk V/VI
- C6 cervical vertebra
- Intervertebral disk VI/VII
- C7 cervical vertebra
- Zygapophysial joints
- Artery
- Nerves

This anatomical point of view plays a role in lots of movements—for example, it's damaging when the knee crosses the toe line during a squat, because the sheer forces are unnaturally high and unsuitable for the joint.

Apart from squats and neck circles, we must assume that in sports and in our daily lives our joints can end up in a less-than-optimal position at any time. If we're not prepared, we'll get injured.

Every joint position can be practiced. With regular mobility training and isolated joint activation, you'll internalize the movements and thereby reassure your nervous system that you're able to control the range of motion. As has been frequently emphasized, control is the key here. Another reason why neck circles can be harmful is that they can damage the aorta.

The aorta loops through an arch of the first cervical vertebra (atlas), where the artery could get caught. This happens very rarely. Fast accelerations with terminal rotations can increase the risk significantly. You won't enter this risk area remotely with joint circles. But I'd think long and hard about letting a chiropractor manipulate your cervical spine, regardless of how experienced that chiropractor is.

ADDITIONAL PECULIARITIES

Two joints—or, rather, areas—represent yet another peculiarity: your back and shoulder.

The back consists of three areas:

CS – TS – LS

We should be able to move them independently of each other. Next to having the anatomical background knowledge needed to understand that our back is segmented, one must give particular attention and patience to isolated activation in this area.

Most people simply know they have a back.

The reason for the lack of your spine's sensitivity is primarily the extreme pressure on your back, especially from extended periods of sitting with little variation. Constant pressure and the lack of activation of structures leads to a loss of control, which in turn decreases your mobility.

Mobility Fundamentals: What You Need to Know

But your strength can also be limited considerably. The to-date barely researched **arthrokinetic reflex** means, among other things, a loss of strength, due to severely compromised joints. Next to activation, the solution for a compromised spine is relatively simple:

HANGING, HANGING, HANGING

Ideally two to five times a day.

Hanging from a bar is free chiropractic practice (and much healthier too). Hanging lets gravity bring you back on track. In addition to the positive effects on your spine, hanging is also good for your shoulders. From an evolutionary standpoint, our shoulders are made for hanging. Doing so can have miraculous results.

The shoulder takes us to the second peculiarity you need to keep in mind during the isolation step.

Your shoulder joint consists of three true and two false joints.

True Joints

- ACJ (acromioclavicular joint)
- SCJ (sternoclavicular joint)
- Glenohumeral joint (upper-arm–scapula joint)

False Joints

- Subacromial space (space between the acromion and humeral head)
- Scapulothoracic-bicipital groove (scapula-thorax interface)

You can find more detailed information about the shoulder in section 10.17, "Shoulder Joint."

So we've covered anatomy, but how can we now put that to use? We just need to know that shoulder movements primarily result from a combination of upper-arm and shoulder-blade movements. So, in terms of isolation training, we need to do two different exercises for the shoulder. One exercise in which we focus primarily on the arm and one in which we primarily move the shoulder blade through its range of motion (as described in section 10.9, "Shoulder-Blade Positions").

In section 4.3, "How Do I Add Mobility to My Strength Training?," I talk in more detail about how you can optimally integrate isolation training into your daily life. In addition to the advantages I just told you about, I want to mention one final factor that emphasizes the importance of isolation: body awareness.

In section 2.5, "Why Foam Rollers Won't Make You More Mobile" I talk about the fact that mobility will give you better body awareness. Nowadays, we're so far removed from being even remotely aware of our bodies that we have to practice our awareness before working on complex movements.

3.1.3 INTEGRATION

Once the foundation has been put in place, we transition to integration. Here, I include all mobility exercises that use more than two joints at the same time. For instance, during the all-fours rotation (subsection 7.2.6), we twist primarily from the thoracic spine. But we must also push out from the shoulder along with twisting the cervical spine.

The goal is to develop resilience in doing these diverse movements that we repeatedly perform in our daily lives and while exercising. With the mobility exercises, you specifically target your weak spots or use them as your warm-up.

In order for the exercises to have the desired effect, it's important to be able to feel the areas of the body you're working on. That's why isolation is a requirement. When coaching or in my workshops, I always notice that people do the exercises too fast, based on this thinking: *I'm gonna quickly finish my mobility training so I can start my actual training*.

The best tip for achieving the best results during integration is to link your movements to your breath. I provide more specific details on how to breathe for each exercise in subsection 7.2.6, "All-Fours Rotation."

Why is breathing so important?

By breathing, you create two positive effects at once:

1. You're more focused and calmer.

    Your breathing calms your movements because it's directly linked to your parasympathetic nervous system.

2. You're automatically a little more mobile.

    Controlled breathing stimulates, among other things, an area of the brain called the **cerebellum**. It controls movements and coordination. It also controls your core's **reflexive stability**. As I mention in section 2.3, "Not Every Joint Should Be Mobilized," to achieve more **ROM**, it's important for your core to be stable. One way to influence that is by breathing. This principle is called *proximal stability for distal mobility*. I explain this principle in more detail in section 3.3, "Guideline for Pain-Free Training."

3.1.4 IMPROVISATION

Improvisation is the supreme discipline. Regardless of the type of sport, we all admire top athletes who make the difficult look easy.

Whether it's a gymnast performing an iron cross on the rings or a ski jumper jumping record distances, the art behind top performances is nothing less than years of training. There's no secret or shortcut to long-term excellence. It's the same with your mobility. No one wants to accept this truth, because it implies discipline and patience. The quick way is usually the more attractive one but definitely not the sustainable one.

When someone is passionate about a subject, at some point, she no longer has to think about how certain procedures work. The subconscious takes over.

Our goal isn't to become world champions in mobility training.

But I still like to compare mobility training to competitive sports.

After all, many people imagine they'll become mobile as quickly as they build muscles or strength (more on that in section 4.1, "How Long until I'm More Mobile?").

The comparison is merely intended to help you set realistic goals. Wanting to be able to do the splits within six months won't do you any good. It's similar with being pain-free. Rarely will there be a secret exercise that will make your pain simply go away.

Of course, lots of companies want to sell you this concept of twenty minutes a week being enough. But neither mobility nor foam rollers nor TPST nor TENS will be able to immediately relieve your pain. After all, pain is often a symptom triggered by a long chain of processes (more on that in the next section).

To sum up, you can think of improvisation, as it relates to mobility, in the following ways:

- Mobility flows
- Adopting habits in your daily life that will automatically let you work on your mobility
- Having developed body awareness and reacting accordingly when your body sends itself a message

3.2 PAIN AND INJURIES

3.2.1 PAIN

Many people suffer from pain. Who hasn't had a sore back, shoulder pain, or a headache. It's often difficult to identify the cause. Even with shooting or stabbing pain and subsequent medical examinations, we're often unable to find the cause on an MRI.

Maybe you're one of those people who picked up this book because you're coming off a long injury layoff and are now ready to "really" dive back in. Or you want to get rid of your current pain and are hoping that this book will offer one-to-one tips for getting rid of that annoying pain at the front of your shoulder.

To all of you who've already suffered a few injuries or are currently in pain, I say the following: your MRI won't help you.

Before I lay out my arguments in detail, I want to briefly address why we have pain and what pain actually is.

POTENTIAL CAUSES

- damaged tissue
- limited predictability of a situation*
- unfamiliar movement patterns
- too much stress (mental or mechanical)

* Look back at the diagram in section 2.1, "How to Become More Mobile."

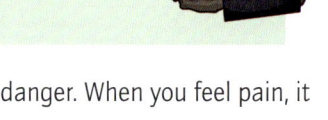

Pain is merely a warning signal from your brain to protect you from greater danger. When you feel pain, it means your brain thinks the body is in acute danger.

Pain is also a call to action by your brain. Thus, this sensor serves only to protect us, whereas most people think of pain as only a nuisance. This should be good news to you.

Another piece of good news is that the most famous pain researcher of our time, Dr. G. Lorimer Moseley, figured out that the level of pain we feel isn't proportionate to the degree of injury, as he and David S. Butler talk about in *Explain Pain*.

But what does that have to do with an MRI? Multiple studies done on pain-free people between the age of twenty and eighty show that imaging revealed one or more signs of degeneration or wear in a large percentage of test subjects.

In physical therapy, I've all too often seen colleagues providing treatment based only on a doctor's diagnosis. But as Butler and Moseley's study shows and as they describe in their book, we aren't able to say precisely why pain occurs where it does.

There's not always a direct link between pain and the injury. Although an MRI is certainly not completely obsolete, treating the pathology on the scan shouldn't be the entire focus.

What we're able to see on an MRI is the status quo and potentially only the cause of the pain. And the pathology, as in the case of the often-diagnosed **impingement syndrome** (structures of the shoulder caught under the acromion), is also not always the cause of all evil.

You don't simply catch impingement syndrome like you do a cold. A pathogen enters the body from outside and thereby triggers a cold. Many doctors and physical therapists apply this logic to said syndrome: you did the [movement name] movement too much (which really isn't healthy), which is why the structures are now overloaded and caught.

But the cause isn't the external load or even the movement but, rather, the lack of control over your joints, the lack of mobility and strength, or imbalances in muscle-tension patterns triggered by your brain.

When you look at your injuries that way, you quickly figure out that the cause of your pain is often very different than what your structures allow you to perceive in any given moment or what an MRI might suggest.

> ### IN SUMMARY
>
> Pain originates in the brain, and the cause of your pain doesn't always lie in the structures that are currently hurting.

3.2.2 INJURIES

As I mention in section 2.7, "How Mobility Makes You Stronger," we can't prevent pain. We also have no absolute guarantees in other areas of life, so why should it be any different for moving our bodies?

Why?

An injury involves more than damage to a structure. The cause can be so multifactorial that no one can pay attention to everything in order to avoid injuries. To some extent, the reason for an injury lies outside our scope of influence. Such as when an opposing player goes for the ball but, unfortunately, your foot is between his cleats and the ball. Or when you're doing push-ups and a careless tourist looking through her camera lens trips over you and you end up with a pulled muscle in your shoulder.

Of course, some things are more likely than others, but again, there are many more factors involved in getting injured than you can prepare for.

But what you can achieve with mobility is that you can limit the extent of the injury simply because you've trained your body for more-complex movement patterns, especially controlling complex joint positions. Because without control—doing merely passive movements—you'll possibly even worsen the extent of the injury.

CHECKLIST

HOW TO PROCEED DURING AN ACUTE INJURY

If you're currently injured or suffer an injury in the future, heed the following advice:

1. DON'T PUSH THROUGH THE PAIN

If some pain gurus on YouTube are telling you that you should do you exercises "at pain level eight but not level nine or ten," stop watching their videos immediately. Stay in a pain-free range to communicate safety to your brain.

2. DON'T TAKE A BREAK, BUT ADJUST YOUR TRAINING AND YOUR MOVEMENTS

Many of my clients have come to me in the hopes that I'll give them two or three exercises to do during their physician-directed exercise hiatus so they don't get too rusty while they wait for the pain or injury to go away. This phrasing alone should make you realize that no pain will be healed this way.

Taking a break means it'll be harder for your body to regenerate. It causes your metabolism and thereby the regeneration processes to proceed more slowly. After a certain amount of time, your activation, mobility, and strength will also decrease. Of course, you won't be able to maintain 100 percent of your performance level, but it's still important that you keep moving and work around your injury.

After all, you're probably not limited in all directions of movement. So, keep moving within the pain-free range and adjust your exercises and training. This definitely requires a certain amount of exercise experience. The reason so many doctors prescribe exercise breaks isn't just that, during their studies, they didn't learn different approaches to moving with pain but also that many patients aren't responsible enough when it comes to their bodies. They're unable to assess what would or wouldn't be too much exercise.

3. GO FROM MICRO TO MACRO

Even though the cause usually isn't in the area of the painful structure, start your rehabilitation measures there.

First, try locally with hot and cold applications, gentle massages, and vibration therapy devices on the muscles surrounding the joint or around the painful area.

You'll thereby stimulate the receptors on the skin and, to some extent, below the skin. Hilton's law tells us that the nerve that innervates a muscle also supplies the associated joint and overlying skin area. Thus, by stimulating your skin, you can also generate an effect all the way to the joint.

Next is *joint mapping* in the painful area (i.e., CARs—see subsection 3.1.2, "Isolation"). Move from the affected area over to adjacent joints.

Mobilization is one side of the coin; strengthening is the other side. Where one muscle is too tight, there's often an **antagonist** that's too weak. Having muscles that are too tight or too weak is very individual, and I can't make a blanket statement on the subject. But you should at least know that there are multiple approaches to solving your problem.

If you don't make any progress with your pain, either the cause lies with a different body system or you didn't choose the right exercises for your circumstances. An analysis like the one I do as a coach can give you more information.

> By the way, Hilton's law is one of the few human-science laws that still endure today and haven't been disproven. It's astonishing, since John Hilton declared this law around 1860.

4. PRETEST, EXERCISE, RETEST

Your brain is very smart. You probably already knew that. As soon as it feels safe or perceives a stimulus as positive input, it signals your body (see section 2.1, "How to Become More Mobile").

Here, pain is a good comparative parameter for you. Do the following to find out if an exercise works for you:

- Test your pain with a provoking movement (it should be controlled and not maximal) and your mobility in the painful area (see subsection 3.1.1, "Evaluation").
- Do one set of an exercise.
- Retest your mobility and pain intensity.

If mobility has improved and pain has lessened, the exercise is a positive stimulus for your nervous system. If you have a negative or neutral result, it'd be worth continuing to search for new exercises or a different system that needs input (maybe your vestibular system instead of muscles or joints).

5. AVOID "PARALYSIS THROUGH ANAYLYSIS"

As a coach, I frequently encounter people who despair after searching the internet or YouTube.

There are thousands of exercises, and each one of them is the best and most amazing for [insert specific pain]. Experimenting with one's body and trying different exercises in itself is a great opportunity to develop better body awareness. But your frustration limit shouldn't get too low. When it comes to mobility, we want to maintain a positive attitude. It's therefore important to have someone—for instance, a coach—who'll turn you upside down and purposefully look for your weak spots and the root of your problem.

You should always maintain a positive basic attitude so you can stick to your mobility goals for the long term.

3.3 GUIDELINES FOR PAIN-FREE TRAINING

PROXIMAL STABILITY FOR DISTAL MOBILITY

Proximal means close to the body; *distal* means away from the body.

In physical therapy, we like to apply the principle "The trunk trumps" to describe that in order to be strong, mobile, and fit you need a strong core.

Here, it's less about tightening your abs all the time or working on your six-pack by doing lots of crunches. Stability is reflexive, which means that it's a quick and spontaneous reaction to an external stimulus (e.g., shifting the center of gravity during a movement).

It also has nothing to do with wobble-board training (see subsection 2.5.3, "Surface Sensibility versus Proprioceptive Sensibility," regarding the SAID principle).

In subsection 3.1.3, "Integration," I offer the tip that you can improve your stability with breathing.

From a neuroathletics point of view, there's more one can do to improve reflexive stability, but that is outside the scope of this book. But if you're interested in this topic, there are some interesting YouTube videos and podcasts out there on the subject.

WE WANT FLEXIBLE STRENGTH, NOT RIGID POWER

Here, we must further differentiate the definition of *tension*.

Tension is always movement specific. We need as much as necessary but as little as possible. Maximum tension makes us immobile and rigid. Adapted tension allows us to efficiently perform the necessary movements in our daily lives or during training.

Our bodies always search for the path of least resistance. That's why we must be able to perform the movement tasks in our workouts as efficiently as possible.

It's similar with calisthenics, as Monique explains in her half of the book.

Otherwise, we overload ourselves too quickly and use some joints in not the best physiological way, which, in turn, can lead to injuries.

YOU SHOULD END YOUR WORKOUT BETTER THAN YOU STARTED IT

Pushing yourself to the limit during workouts is often a glorified goal. "You have to feel the pain. Only then was your workout effective." This No Pain, No Gain mentality has had its day.

If you want to stay pain-free long-term while training, you need to apply the 80-percent rule. While you can increase the degree of difficulty during 80 percent of your training time, you never push past your max.

When we exercise, we strive for a real workout (maximum workload, after which you spend ten minutes just lying on the floor) only 10–20 percent of the time. Maximum loading isn't desirable in strength training nor mobility training. Since most athletes still practice classic stretching, mobility training is also associated with pain. This is, unfortunately, completely counterproductive. One basic rule is this: **don't push through the pain**. Of course, here, too, we must differentiate. You can generally differentiate between pathological pain and stress-induced pain.

But being able to differentiate between these two types of pain requires good body awareness and a certain amount of exercise experience. If you're already experiencing some pain, initially stick with the tip of not pushing through the pain during mobility training. Our brains are programmed to improve with recurring signals. We learn to do the things we perform repeatedly more efficiently.

Unfortunately, there's also negative conditioning. We get "better" at pain, meaning our pain perception becomes more sensitive, and the area of the brain responsible for pain becomes more highly developed.

In short, we want to avoid pain while working out.

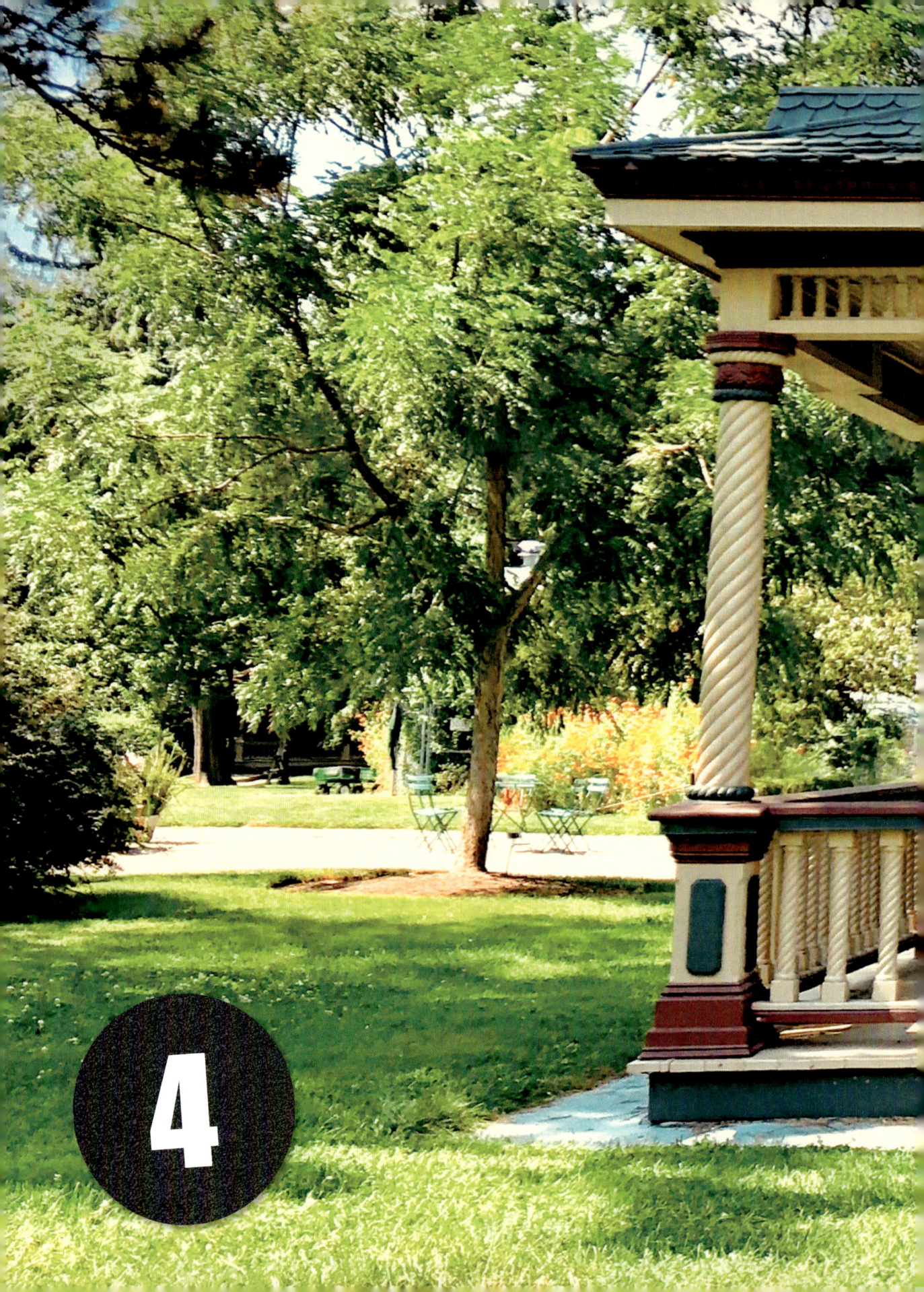

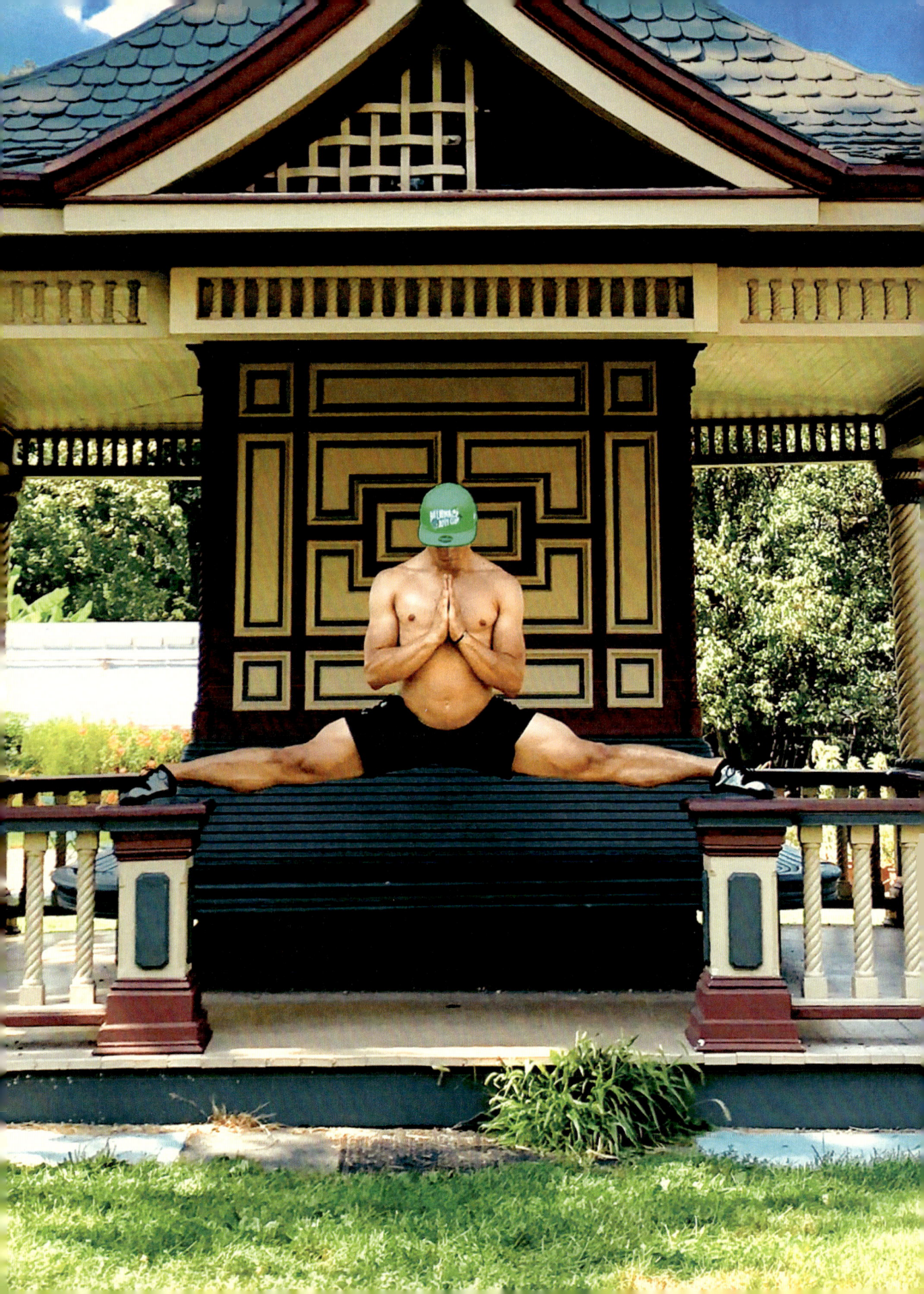

4 The Most-Common Questions About Mobility

4.1 HOW LONG UNTIL I'M MORE MOBILE?

Every good trainer knows this answer all too well: "It depends."

Of course, this statement is rarely satisfactory. So let me briefly outline it with the following two illustrations:

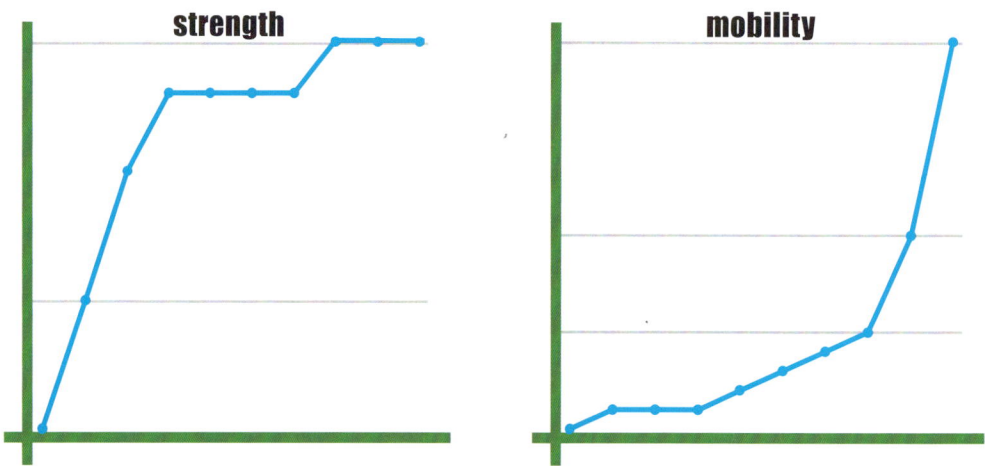

As you can see, the two illustrations look very different. That's because when you first start to do strength training you have to only look at the weights or the bar to get stronger and achieve what are called *noob gains*. Of course, there are major individual differences, but a strength adjustment to a regularly applied stimulus generally happens relatively quickly

The feeling many people have during mobility training can be described as follows:

At first, nothing happens for a lonnng time . . .

then . . .

you make small advances, and you think you're on the right path. But . . .

then there's another long drought phase . . .

but you keep noticing a few subtle but noticeable changes . . .

and then a week of nothing and you feel like you're all the way back at the . . .

beginning.

Well, I had a similar experience. I practiced mobility for a long time without getting a whole lot more mobile. I knew mobility was essential to maintaining a healthy body long-term with a high training load. Here, the adjustment in mobility training relates to the amount of time it takes for fibrous structures (tendons and ligaments) to adjust to the load.

For the average person (without previous experience in gymnastics or calisthenics), one of the well-known US gymnastics coaches, Christopher Sommer, sets a goal of 250–260 days until an adequate foundation has been created. Based on that, I anticipate that it'll take most people a year to become more mobile and reach the initial bigger mobility goals in the book.

Of course, this timespan depends on your objective. If you want to be able to do the splits, you need to adjust your patience accordingly.

As I mentioned at the beginning of the chapter, all adjustments are subject to individual differences.

One factor that shouldn't be ignored is your everyday life. If you sit all day and get hardly any exercise, you'll need considerably more time than someone with a physically active job.

At this point, I absolutely need to dispel the myth that ten minutes three times a week before training is enough to reach your mobility goals.

Let's assume you work in an office and go to calisthenics training three times a week for one hour each time. That's 1.8 percent of your week. If you spend thirty minutes a week working on your mobility, that's 0.3 percent on top of the 1.8 percent..

TRAINING

MOBILITY

3 hours per week = 1.8%

30 minutes per week = 0.3%
(10 minutes before each workout)

Imagine eating only fast-food all week. But once a week, for Sunday brunch, you eat a small side salad instead of french fries.

This approach won't help you get healthier nor lose weight.

It's the same with mobility. Working on mobility 0.3 percent of your time will maintain your status quo but won't significantly improve it.

4.2 HOW CAN I BECOME MORE MOBILE MORE QUICKLY?

I could write books by the dozen about mindset, because proper mobility training starts in your head. As the successful US entrepreneur, trainer, and bestselling author Tony Robbins likes to say: it's 80 percent psychology, 20 percent mechanics.

Everything starts in the head and not only in your neural pathways, which are an integral part of your strength—and mobility potential, as you already know. Before you improve your mobility, you need to be able to accept that it may take a while before you'll see results.

Next to the question of whether or not you'll have enough patience, you should also ask yourself what attributes you associate with mobility training, such as the following:

- boring
- painful
- strenuous
- necessary evil

None of these attitudes will get you very far. You might stick with your mobility routine for a week or two and then return to your old habits. Instead, try to focus on your goals. You want to be able to go through your day without pain, be able to return to working out without worrying about your aches and pains, and be able to achieve new levels.

Mobility will get you there!

Remember this:

"Where focus goes, energy flows."

4.3 HOW DO I ADD MOBILITY TO MY STRENGTH TRAINING?

To help you integrate a mobility routine into your daily life, let me briefly say that not all mobility is the same. If you practice mobility every day, you'll most likely quickly hit your limit because you're doing the wrong exercises.

The difference is simply the intensity of the exercises you choose. If you've already tried doing swimmer (see subsection 7.3.7, "Swimmer"), you know how strenuous a mobility exercise can be. And I stress this again and again: Mobility is like strength training—only, in the other direction. Instead of actively shortening (like strength training), we're actively lengthening.

Take that statement figuratively, because movement happens only when we trigger shortening or lengthening the muscles—or, rather, the prerequisite for movement is the interplay between the shortening and lengthening of the musculature.

So if your routine consists only of exercises with a similar degree of difficulty as swimmer, you'll quickly overload yourself. I therefore differentiate between two types of exercises to work on mobility. (You won't find this concept in other literature. While coaching a new client, I got this idea to help him visualize the training plan after he came to me extremely frustrated because he wasn't making progress.)

MOBILIZING AND MOBILITY TRAINING

The latter should be viewed the same as strength training is.

As a beginner, you should have mobility on your schedule at least twice a week, with exercises that challenge you and possibly even make you sweat.

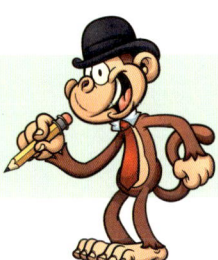

> **TIP**
>
> Choose exercises with a banana rating of three or four from the practical section.

4.4 HOW DO I INTEGRATE MOBILITY INTO MY DAILY LIFE?

It's very important that you don't think of mobility as additional training that you must also build in extra time for. We all already have too little time, and adding something else causes more stress, and stress leads to . . . exactly: immobility and pain (see section 2.8, "Why Stress Makes You Immobile").

To optimally integrate mobility into your daily life, focus on *mobilizing*.

To me, *mobilizing* means nearly all types of joint circles (see CARs in subsection 3.1.2, "Isolation") or swinging.

By *swinging*, I mean the movements we often see gymnasts or dancers do during their warmup (swinging the extremities forward, backward, or sideways). When swinging, the intensity is relatively low, but you're still causing increased joint metabolism, which is essential to arthritis prevention and overall joint health. Ultimately, mobilizing is "toothbrushing for your joints." You can maintain your status quo with a short routine of ten to fifteen minutes a day.

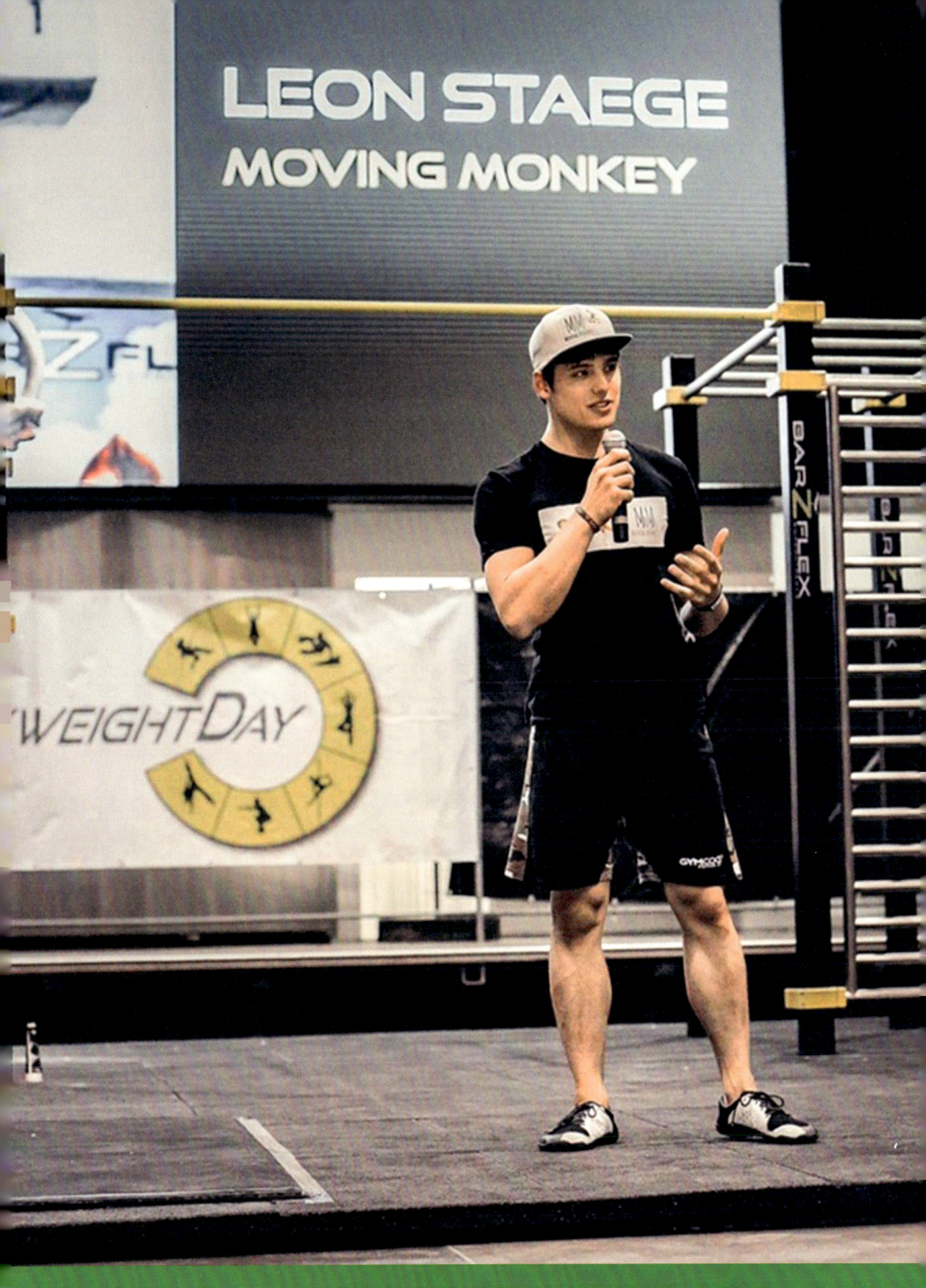

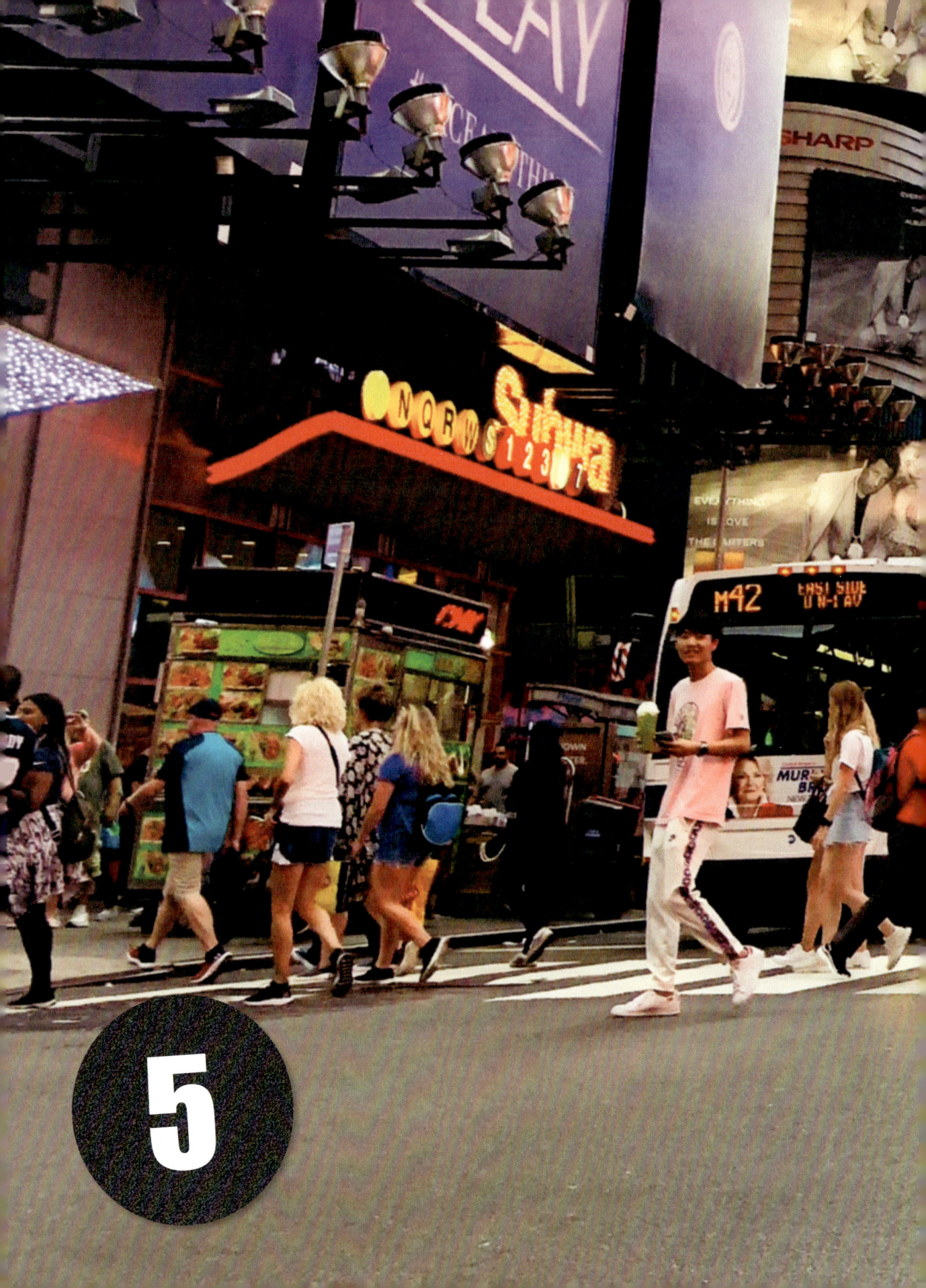

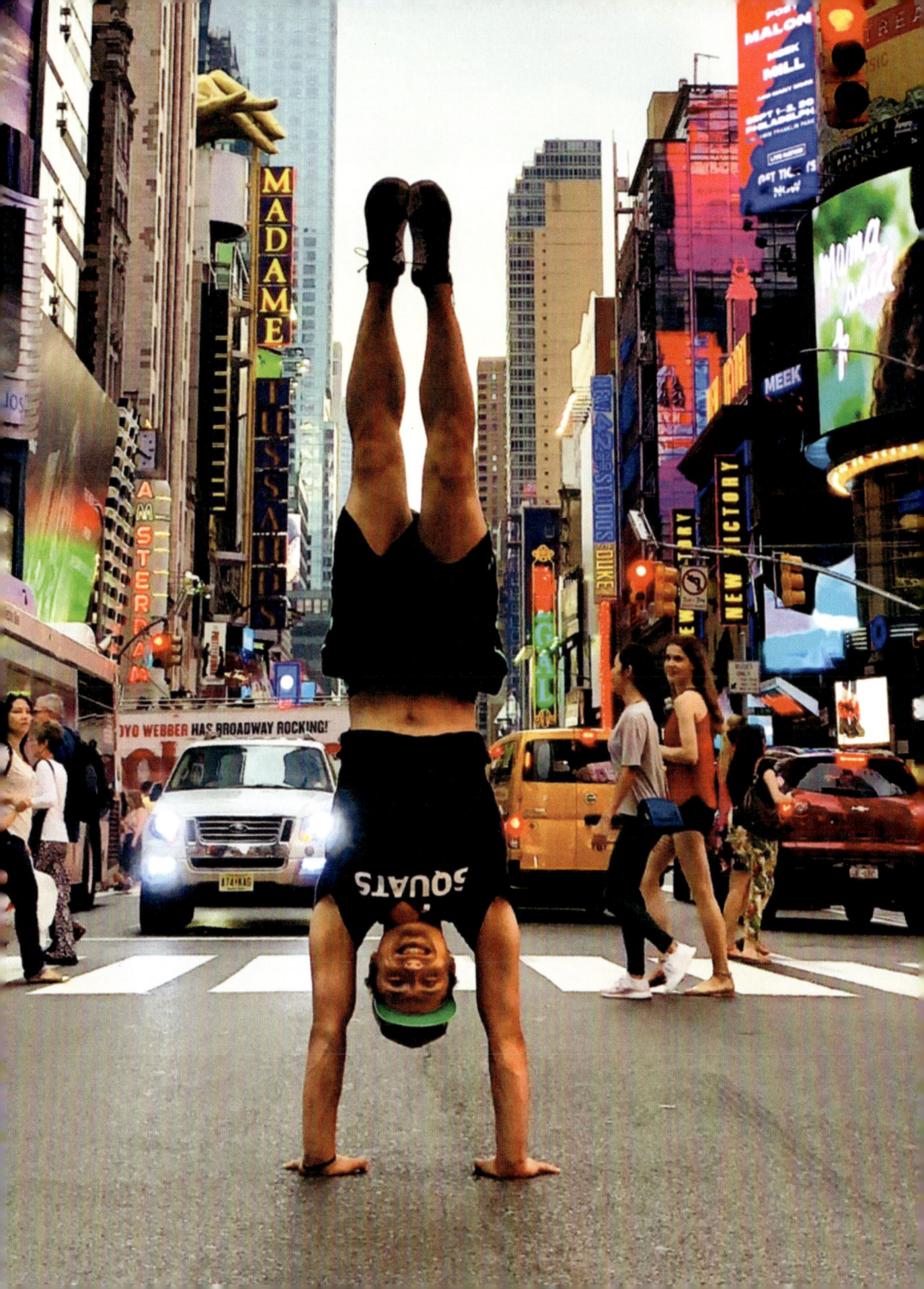

5   Mobility Lifestyle Hacks

As I establish in chapter 4, setting aside only 0.3 percent of your time each week is too little. Now, if you were to do your CARs (see subsection 3.1.2, "Isolation") every day, you'd already be at 1 percent (ten minutes of mobility in the morning, daily, and ten minutes three times a week, as part of your training, equals 100 minutes). So now we're gradually approaching an adequate amount to really make progress. Still, most people's days look like this:

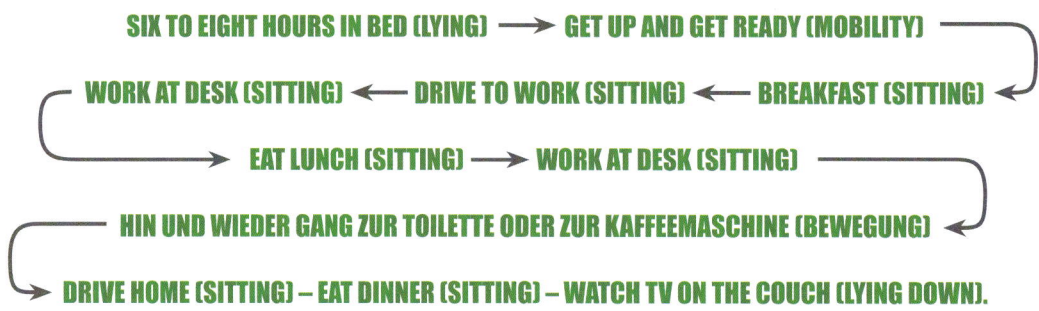

EASY CHOICES, HARD LIFE—HARD CHOICES, EASY LIFE

I can't imagine what causes your back pain when you exercise all day sitting down.

How's that for sarcasm? Hopefully most of you will get it. But it might help some of you realize for the first time how little we move nowadays. Or, more precisely, how little we're required to perform physically. Our ancestors did strenuous work in the fields and had to walk for miles to get to school, shop, or visit friends and relatives. Our modern world has made many things easier. But one thing we can't give up is exercise. You have to continue to take your own steps, regardless of which smart watch, fitness bracelet with pedometer, or calorie tracker you wear on your wrist.

Take the stairs instead of the elevator.

Ride your bike instead of driving your car.

Most of the time, it's the simplest decisions that are most effective. You just have to follow through.

SITTING VERSUS STANDING (BUT NOT JUST STANDING)

When I first launched my YouTube channel, the book *Deskbound: Sitting Is the New Smoking*, by Kelly Starrett, had just been published in the US, and the trend of working while standing was becoming increasingly popular.

Today, still, I make videos about working while standing as one of the most effective methods for avoiding sitting diseases (i.e., weakness of posterior chain—the hamstrings and gluteal muscles—and the hip flexors and the resulting bad posture).

Regardless of where you are, there's almost always a way you can build a standing desk. I've even used upside-down waste baskets, a large stack of magazines, my backpack, chairs, or coasters, among other things, to raise my table.

STOP

Before you decide to send me exasperated letters or leave a bad review of this book on Amazon because none of these tips help you at your workplace, allow me to make one more point.

Standing isn't the cure-all. I emphasize standing only because we're a sedentary society. We redefine the term *settled*. Nonetheless, standing for too long isn't brilliant either.

Here, we must understand how this "sitting trend" began.

After all, a few decades ago, it was just the opposite. Tons of people had problems because they stood at the assembly line all day. Most jobs were performed while standing. Offices came, along with advances in industrialization and the extensive automation of assembly-line work. This somewhat explains the transition from standing to sitting.

The human race is simply very good at overturning a plan and changing direction without learning from mistakes.

THE SOLUTION

You're probably wondering what the best and healthiest solution might be.

VARIATION

Our body wants variation. Sitting isn't inherently unhealthy—nor is standing inherently healthy. The enemy is imbalance. When your input is too one-sided, your output can't be good. Our environment is characterized by constant change. Nothing is certain except for change.

SOME POSSIBLE VARIATIONS TO INSPIRE YOU

Sitting

- Upright
- Bent over
- Cross-legged
- Cross-legged with one leg
- Squatting on a chair (yes, it's possible and one of my favorite positions)
- With ankles crossed
- Straddle-legged
- On one leg
- On the ground (in different positions)

Standing

- With one foot propped on a raised area
- In a straddle
- With a closed stance
- With one leg extended back and resting on a chair

I know, not all variations are office-appropriate. Nevertheless, I encourage you to get a laptop or a standing desk. Based on my conversations with frustrated Moving Monkey followers, I know that many companies allow the use of a standing desk only after the employee has suffered a ruptured disk or the like.

Regardless of the red tape and which decisions are involved, there's no logical argument that aftercare is better than prevention. Do I visit the dentist to prevent getting cavities, or do I wait until I already have cavities?

If you're an employer, please take these words to heart. The best investment you can make in your employees isn't yet another weekend training course during which your staff are away from their families but an investment in their health..

SQUAT – SQUAT – SQUAT (IT'S SQUATTING TIME WHILE YOU BRUSH YOUR TEETH)

Squatting is humanity's most natural, basic position. Just take a look at Eastern Europe and Asia. There, people often sit in a deep squat—while waiting for the bus, taking a quick break, or eating. When I squat at the train station, I always get strange sideways looks. I then return the look, puzzled that the looker choose to sit on an uncomfortable metal bench.

But all joking aside, I want to briefly explain why the squat is so healthy. I often hear the following argument: "That can't be healthy in the long term—it's worse than sitting."

No one said you have to squat for hours. It's all in the dosage. Besides, it's a way to prepare your joints for more varied movements. I just want to stress again that having healthy joints and a functional body requires two things: homeostasis and variation.

And there's the suitability and efficiency for everyday activities that you can achieve only in a squat. Like how when you're cleaning your home and have to vacuum under the furniture you inevitably have to get into a tilted squat. When you come home from grocery shopping and put the food away, you can bend over awkwardly with your back or simply squat. You can even squat while you fold laundry, change a tire, and pull weeds in your yard—and especially while you brush your teeth.

At our Calisthenics X Mobility workshops, I always tell participants that brushing your teeth is "squatting time." We want squatting to become a habit. Habits are best implemented when we associate them with something we do anyway. Hence we associate the new habit (squatting) with an old habit (brushing our teeth) to effect long-term changes.

Surely, we all brush our teeth at least one to two times a day. Continue to look for actions or places you visit multiple times a day—like whenever you go to the coffee machine during a break, when you get home, and when you read, text, and talk on the phone. These are all great moments to implement more movement, like squatting.

And of course, there's the psychological component. Whenever I squat in public places, people stare. I don't even notice those looks anymore. The looks don't matter, because I don't make my health conditional on the opinions of others. If it's just too difficult for you to squat in public despite all the good reasons, that's perfectly fine. Similar to my principle on everyday life and mobility, we don't want to create a negative association with mobility (see section 4.4, "How Do I Integrate Mobility into My Daily Life?").

Since you have a number of different options at home for squatting, now you just have to be able to do a full squat. Here are some very easy tips for you for if, to date, you haven't been able to do a complete squat (heels on the ground and back straight)

Use a book to raise your heels.

Why books?

Books are the perfect **progression** parameter. After a while, you can use a thinner book and objectively see your progress. Imagine how motivating it would be if you started with a huge tome and arrived at a small paperback. At some point, that elevation will be nothing more than a softcover children's book, and from that day forward, you can completely eliminate a heel lift.

HANGING – HANGING – HANGING

Hanging can be seen as similar to the squat. From an evolutionary point of view, our shoulders aren't designed for pull-ups, push-ups, and muscle-ups but are primarily designed for hanging and moving hand over hand. For this reason, the shoulder is also the most mobile joint in the body. You can learn more on this subject in section 10.17, "Shoulder Joint."

One of my mentors once said to me, "The subject people have researched best and most thoroughly to date is evolution. Something that doesn't make sense from an evolutionary point of view doesn't make sense from today's point of view."

After all, our structures are still built the same way as those of our ancestors. What's changed is our environment and how we move through that environment. Our environment is sedentary and one-sided. But our bodies desire complexity (i.e., variation).

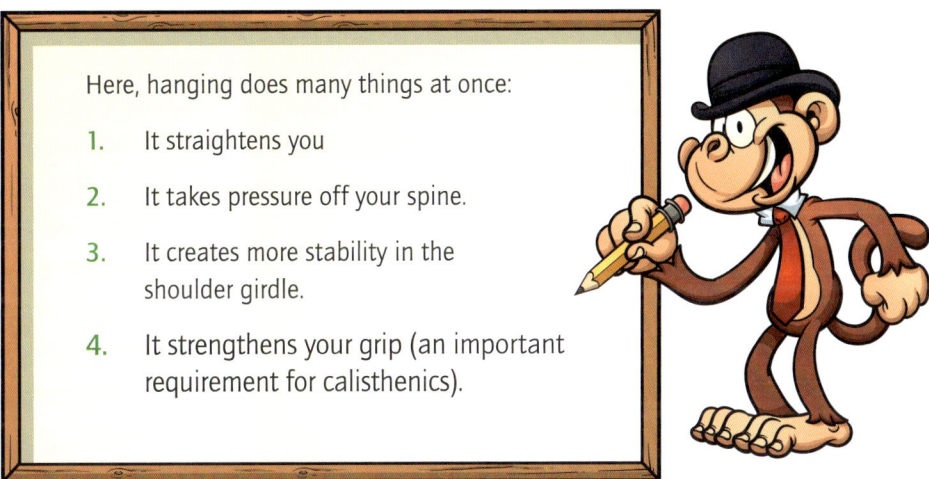

Here, hanging does many things at once:

1. It straightens you
2. It takes pressure off your spine.
3. It creates more stability in the shoulder girdle.
4. It strengthens your grip (an important requirement for calisthenics).

If you build these factors into your daily life, you'll quickly notice that your mobility is improving without you feeling like you have to do a whole lot for it. The requirements are merely good habits.

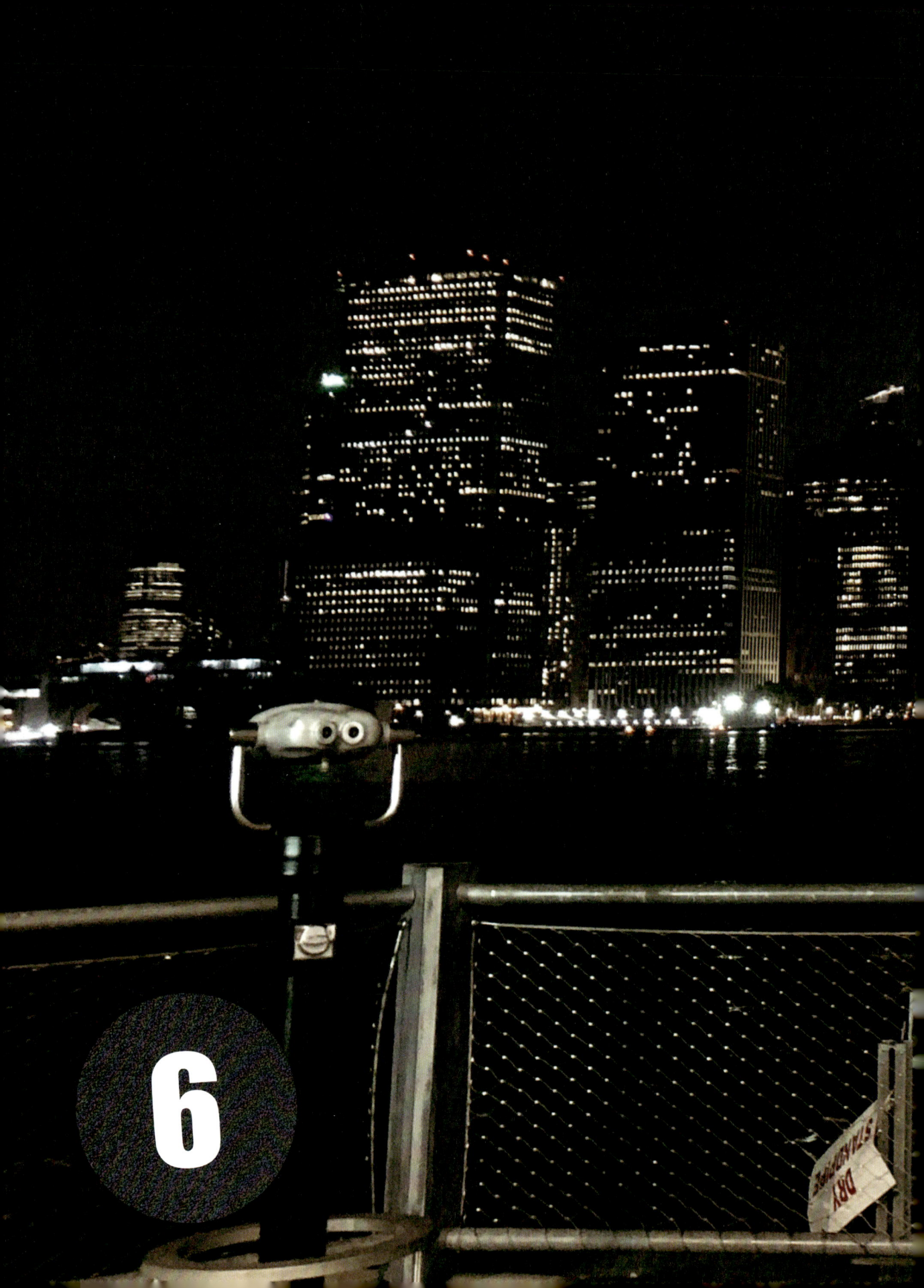

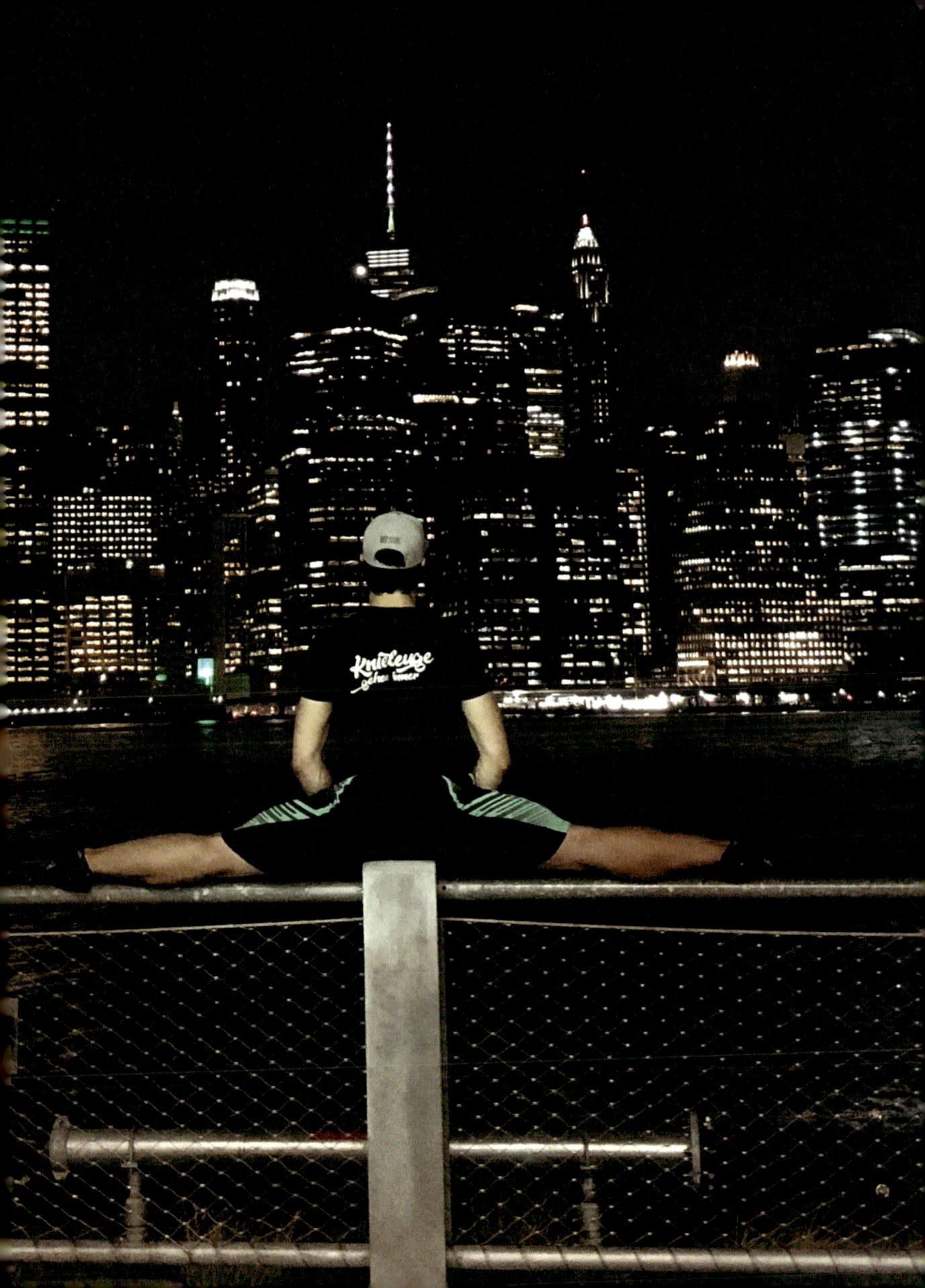

6 Movement Is Life, and Life Is Movement

To me, mobility training isn't just a way to become strong, mobile, and pain-free. Mobility teaches me a new sense of body awareness.

During a conversation I had with Monique about exercise and training, she said (in passing), "He's in the process of discovering his body." This beautiful sentence describes better than any other what mobility can do for you. Next to all the science surrounding this subject and all the discussions about different methods and the multimodular interpretations, mobility does primarily one thing:

IT TEACHES YOU A NEW BODY LANGUAGE.

This is not body language, not in the sense of gestures and facial expressions, but as a metaphor for the engagement with one's own body. We very often only make demands on our body. We wear it to work, to exercise, to the movies, and in the shower. We constantly demand that it function.

But with everything we have to do, we unfortunately forget to give it something in return. Always performing and not giving also leads to pain, like working out full throttle without warming up.

Keep the stress bucket (see section 2.8, "Why Stress Makes You Immobile") in mind.

When you learn to speak your body's language, you'll learn to better evaluate yourself. You'll learn to read signs that, at first, look like hieroglyphics. The body is more intelligent than the mind.

Our mind wants . . .	But our body wants . . . :
SAFETY and COMFORT	**GROWTH and ADVENTURE**

When you learn to listen to your body and control the voice of your mind, you'll stay healthy and pain-free long-term.

When we're healthy and pain-free, we feel good. By implication, good feelings result only from moving. **Motion creates emotion.** The reason we pace while having an important phone conversation or when we're happily anticipating something is that our bodies and our brains function better in motion. For this reason, all my clients tell me this after I've been coaching them for a while:

"I suddenly have the urge to move more."

This is because, with mobility, you're giving your body what it needs. Most people have simply forgotten what it's like to have a body that functions—one that doesn't annoy us all day but is agreeable.

This book is meant to help you shift your focus to qualitative exercise so you'll once again enjoy moving. Nothing is more valuable than your body.

Keep moving, stay sexy!

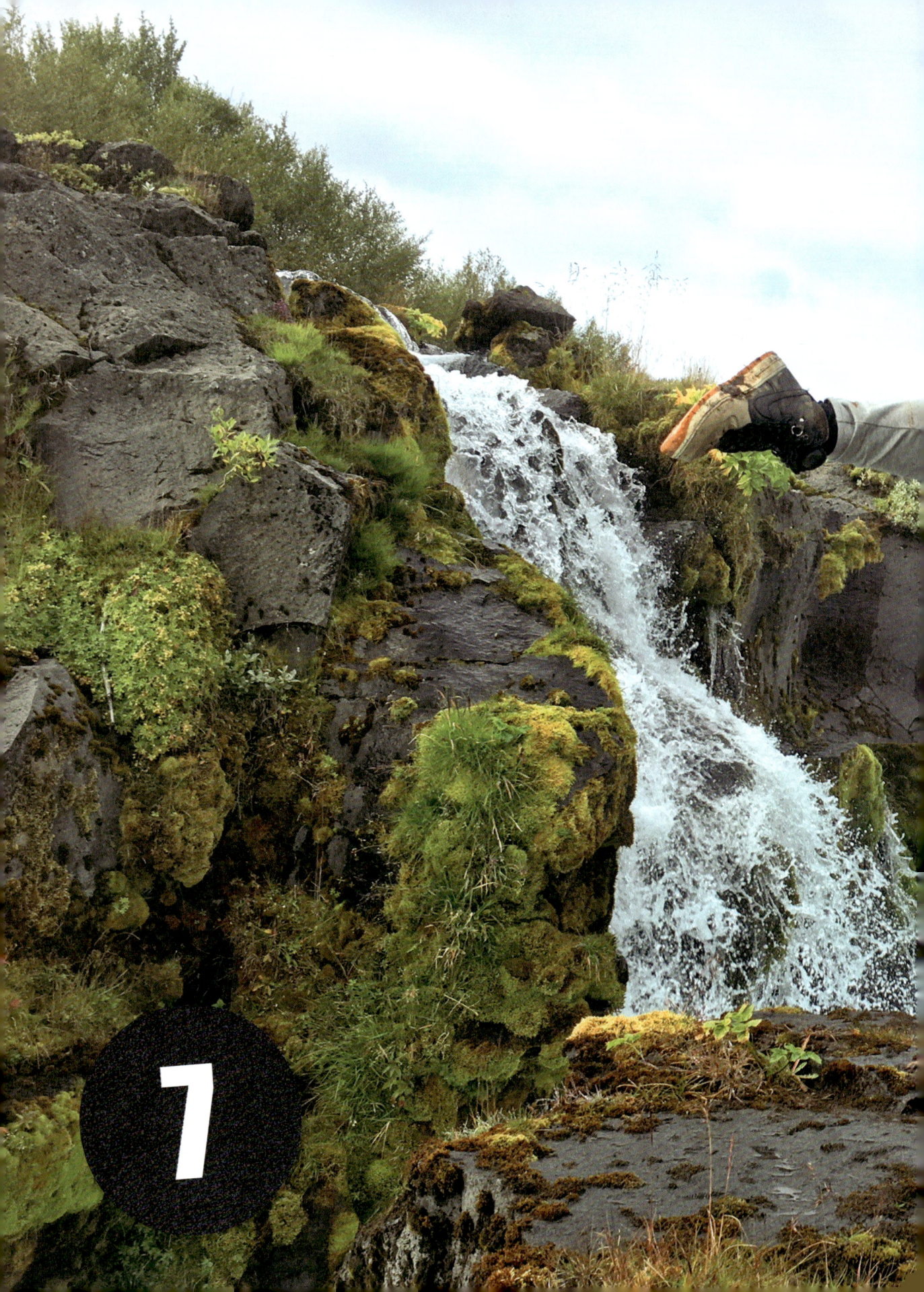

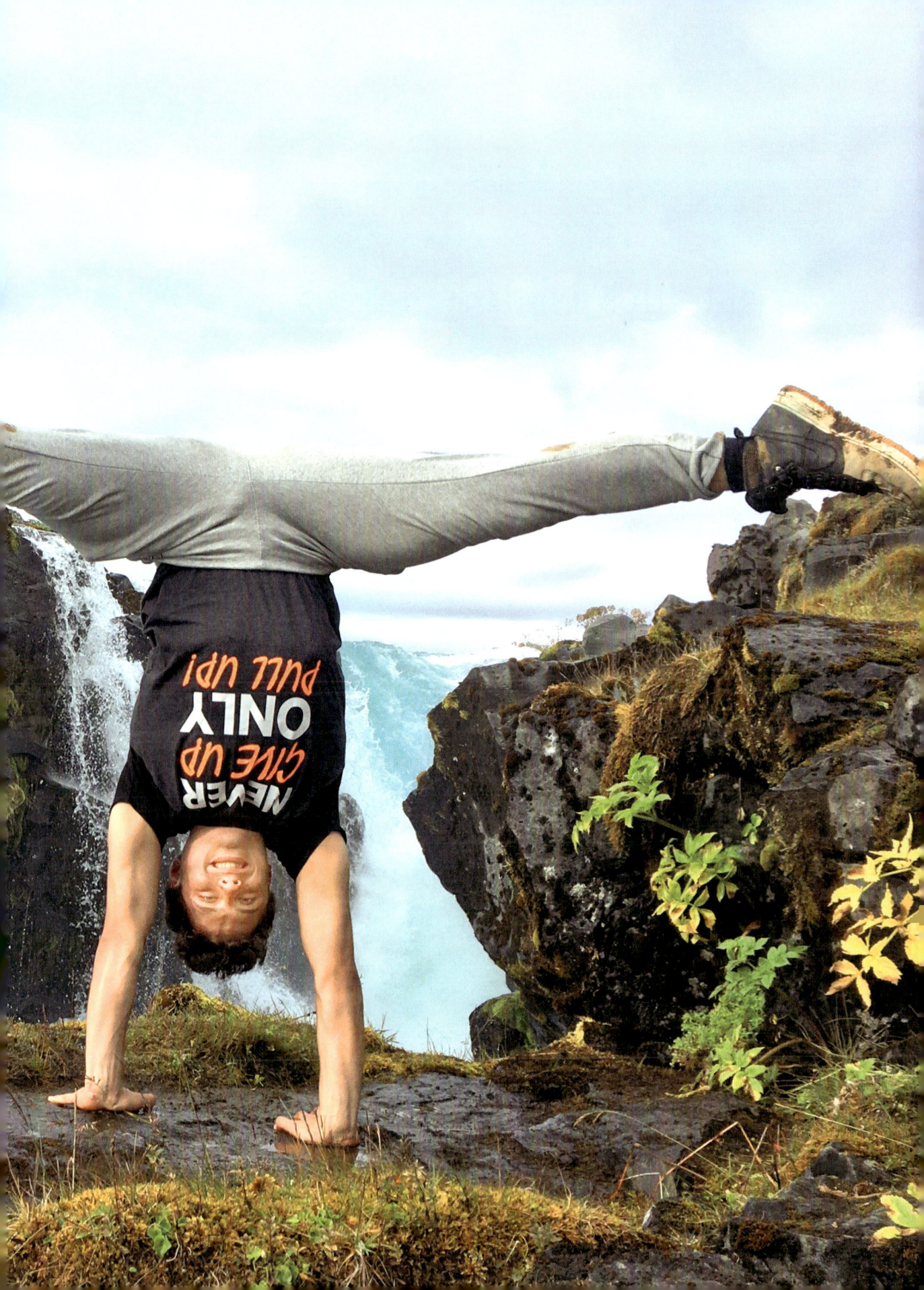

7 Mobility Exercises

Before we get into the exercises, please take note of the following:

Pain, particularly **closing-angle joint pain**, should be avoided during any exercise. That means that during the exercises you'll always want to feel traction on the open side and not where your joint's angle closes. If you do feel pain, avoid the pain and slowly work your way toward the pain threshold with the mobility exercise, but never cross it.

On page 13, we show you some symbols that briefly summarize the most-important technical details with respect to exercise execution. The symbols for *external rotation, maintain body tension* (**hollow-body position**), and *shoulders away from ears* (**depression**) are explained in greater detail in the calisthenics half of the book.

The symbol for *watch your breath first* appears with the spinal rotations (7.2.1). The first exercise will include directions regarding this symbol.

The final symbol is for *lengthen your spine*. Imagine someone pulling you out of the water by your hair. Your spine, including the cervical spine, automatically extends, and you straighten up. This doesn't mean that your posture should be exaggerated or that you have to strain to keep your chest puffed out like a gorilla.

It's just a slight straightening against gravity and against the habitually hunched posture we so often assume nowadays.

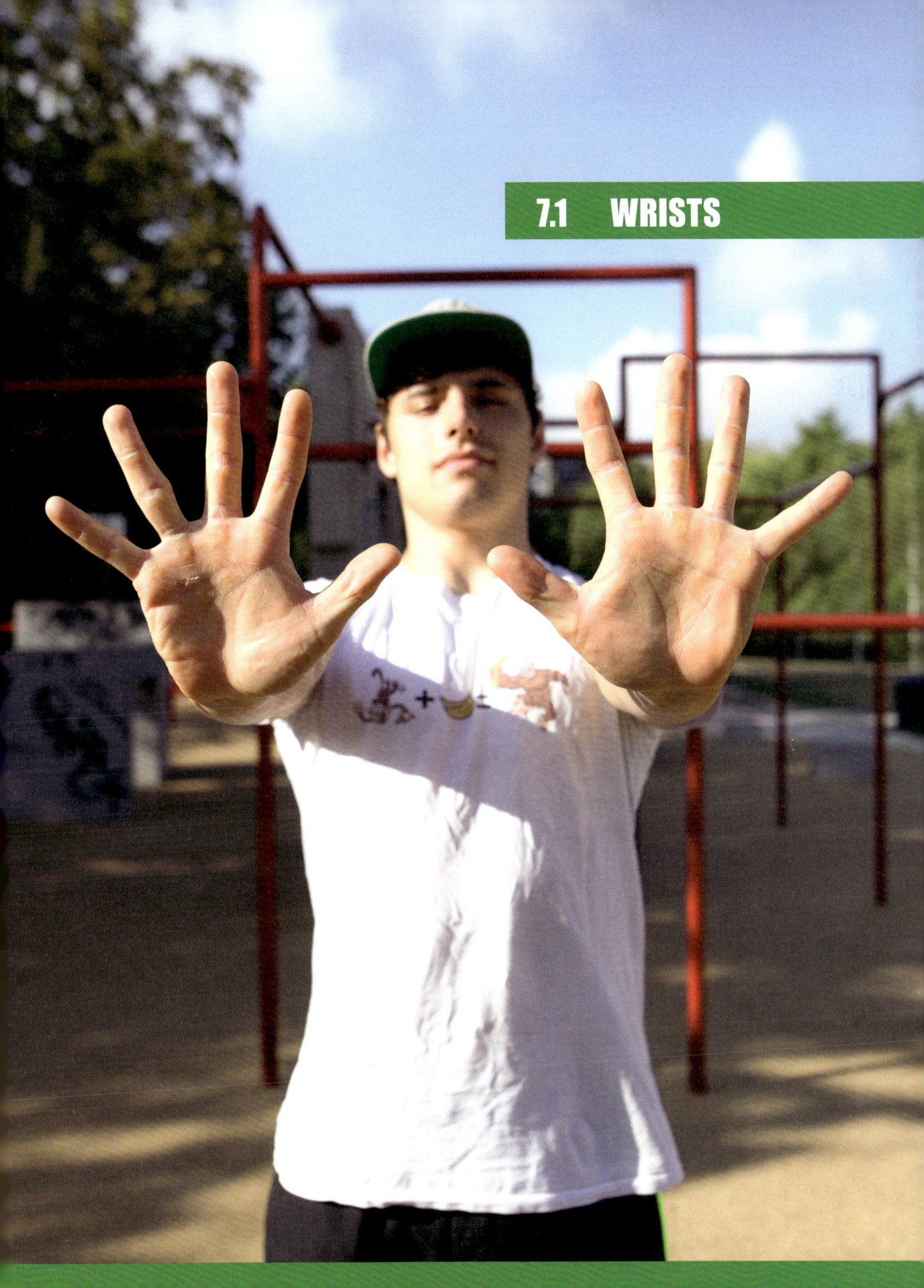

7.1 WRISTS

7.1.1 WRIST FIGURE EIGHTS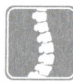

1. Start by extending your arms in front of your body, parallel to the ground, with your fingers spread.

2. Stretch your hands as extensions of your arms.

3. Make yourself long—shoulders in depression (pulled down)—with your arms remaining extended throughout the exercise.

4. Flex your wrists by pulling your fingertips back toward yourself as far as you can; you should feel a significant stretch.

5. Rotate your fingertips outward until your pinkies are pointed down, keeping your wrists flexed.

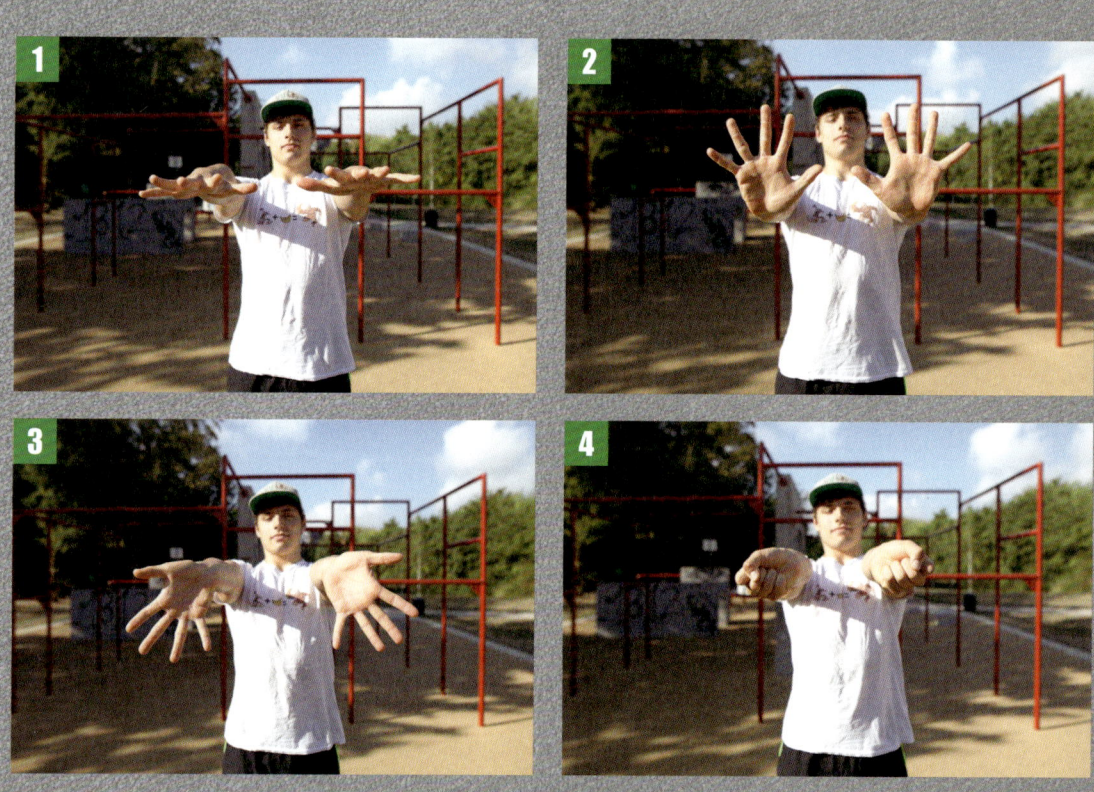

Mobility Exercises 89

6. Keep your wrists in maximum flexion.

7. Close your hands into fists and, without rotating your arms, pull your fists toward you.

8. When you can't pull your wrists any farther, turn your fists inward until your knuckles point down.

9. Open your hands and spread your fingers. (Make it difficult for yourself. Imagine that gravity's effect on your hands has increased tenfold.)

10. You've now finished one repetition. Repeat the movement or change direction.

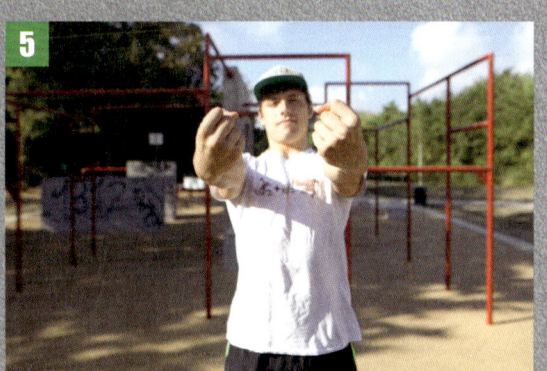
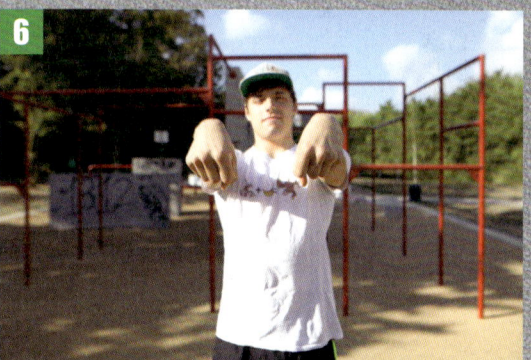
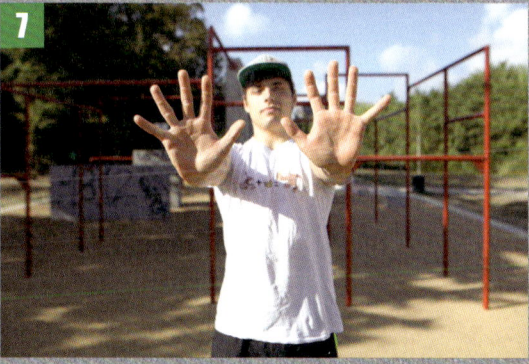

7.1.2 WRIST MOBILIZATION ON THE GROUND

1. Start in an all-fours position (wrists under shoulders and knees under hips).

2. Spread your fingers and grip the ground. (Maintain your grip on the ground throughout the exercise). **Variation:** Try to lift your fingers.

3. Keep your arms extended throughout and keep the inside of each arm rotated inward (imagine screwing your arms into the ground to achieve an external rotation of your shoulders).

4. Move your shoulders in a large circle over your wrists, while the heels of your hands remain on the ground. When you're in the back position, imagine that you're trying to push the ground away from you.

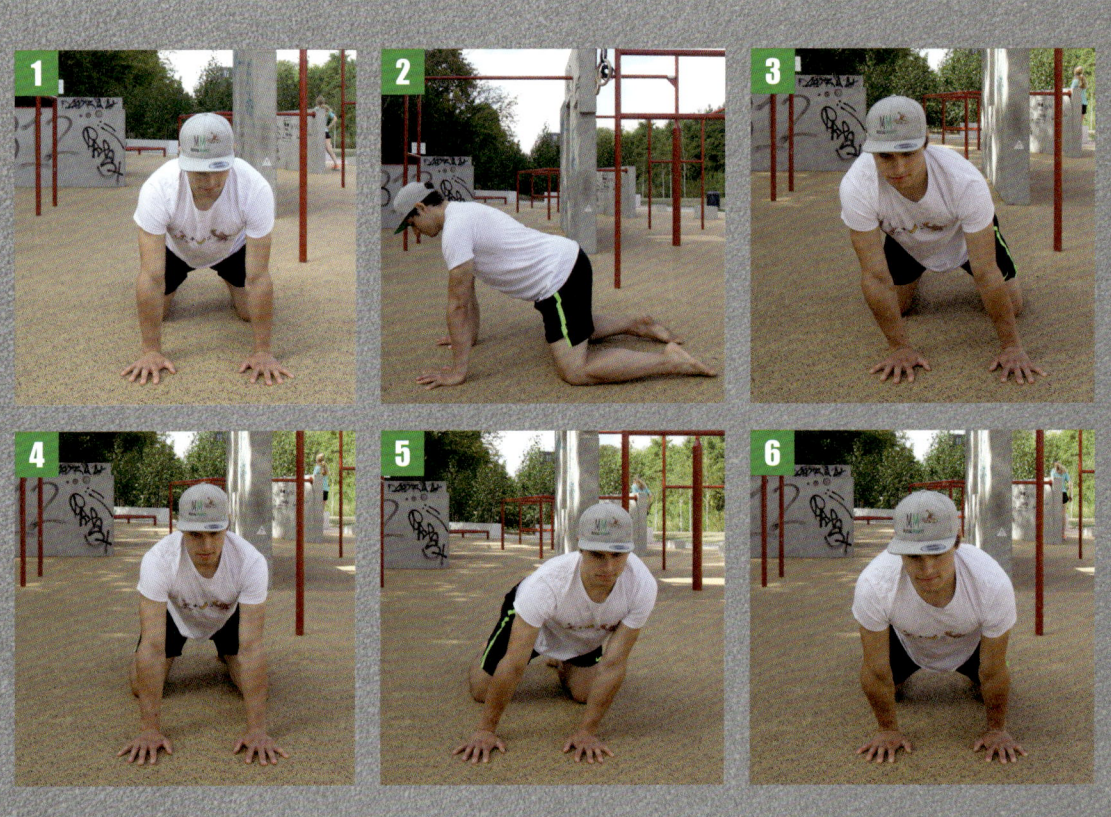

Mobility Exercises

5. After a few repetitions, change your hand position by turning your fingers outward. Start again at step 1.

A THIRD POSITION

- Point your fingers inward.
- Move your hands closer together.
- Instead of circling motions over your wrists, move your body forward and backward.
- In the back position, push the ground forward and away from you.
- When you lean forward over your thumbs, continue to press your thumbs into the ground.

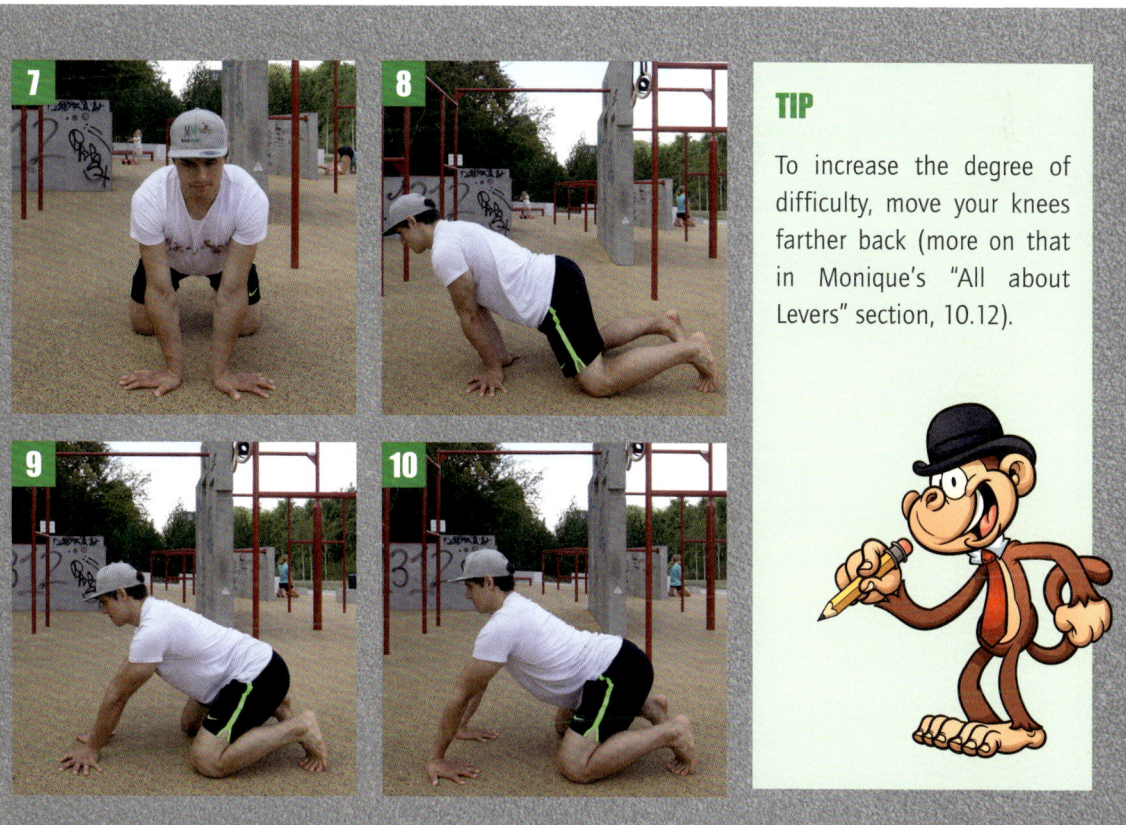

TIP

To increase the degree of difficulty, move your knees farther back (more on that in Monique's "All about Levers" section, 10.12).

7.1.3 BACKHAND PUSH-UPS

1. In an all-fours position, rest on the backs of your hands.

2. You should ideally be able to lock your elbows and turn the inside of your arms forward. Most people won't be able do so at first, and it's more likely that it'll hurt than that you'll be able to use your FROM. If it does hurt, take another look at the beginning of this chapter on how to handle closing-angle joint pain.

3. Bend your elbows so they point back rather than to the sides and do a push-up.

4. In the lowest position, close your hands into fists, and keep your fists firmly closed.

5. Slowly straighten your arms so, ideally, you end up in the starting position, with your arms completely straight.

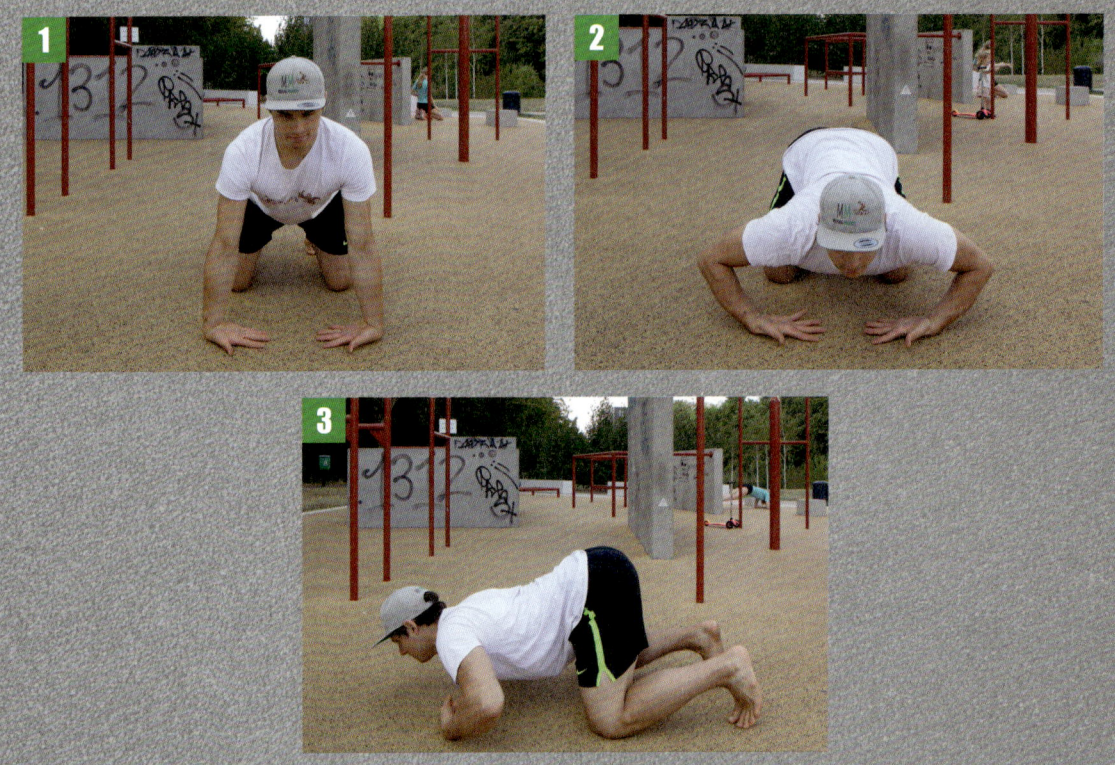

Mobility Exercises

TIP

Most people have a lot of trouble with straightening their arms, because they're in an unfamiliar position. Don't try to force it but practice it, do it regularly, and be patient. You can also increase the difficulty level by performing this exercise in the full plank position.

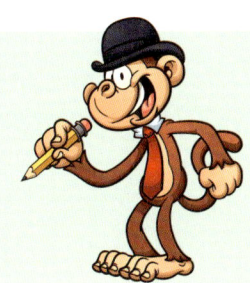

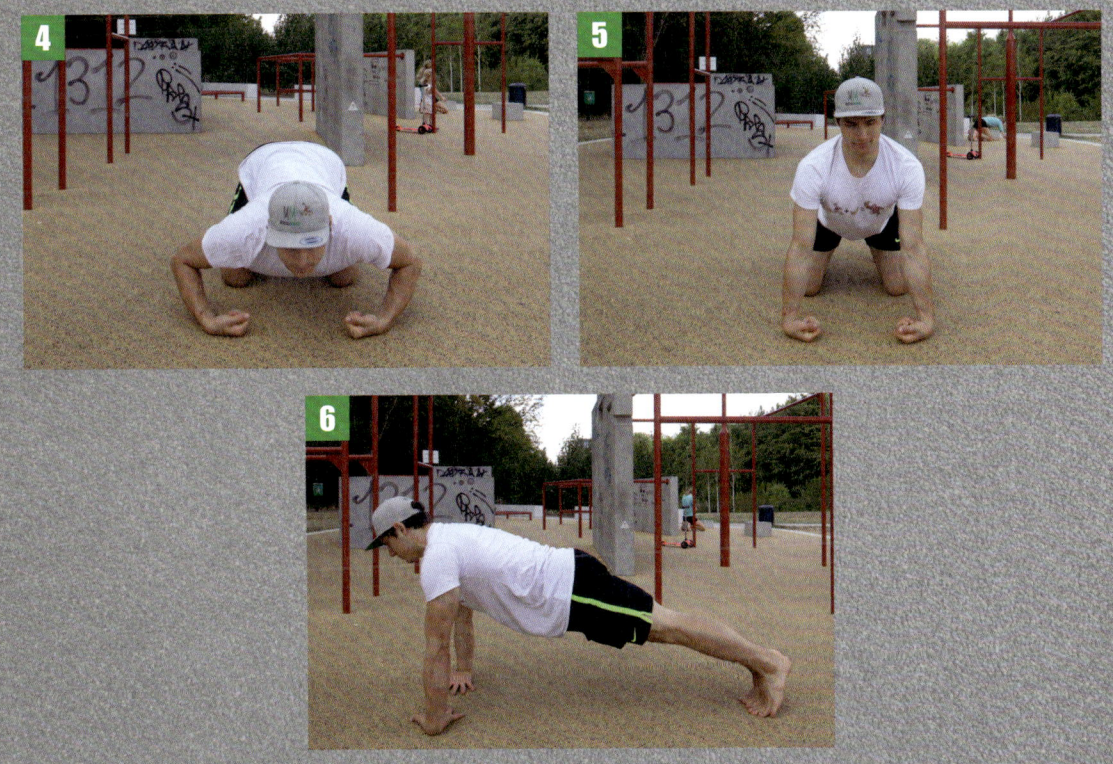

7.1.4 SHAOLIN PUSH-UPS 🍌🍌🍌

1. Start in an all-fours position.

2. Rest on closed fists on the ground.

3. Slowly shift your center of gravity over your fists and then tilt so the backs of your fists lift off the ground.

4. Hold the final position for a moment and then shift your center of gravity back to the middle, lowering your fists back to the ground.

5. Bend your elbows so you're parallel to the ground.

6. Continue to press your fists into the ground and return to the starting position.

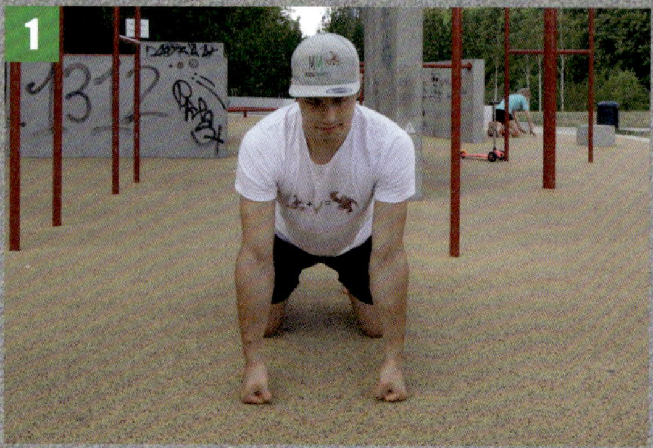

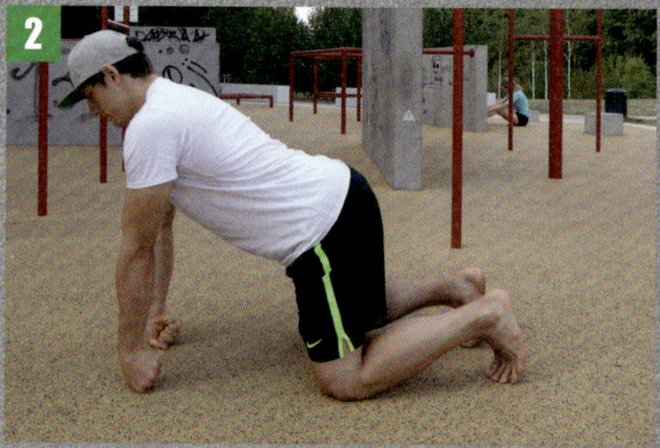

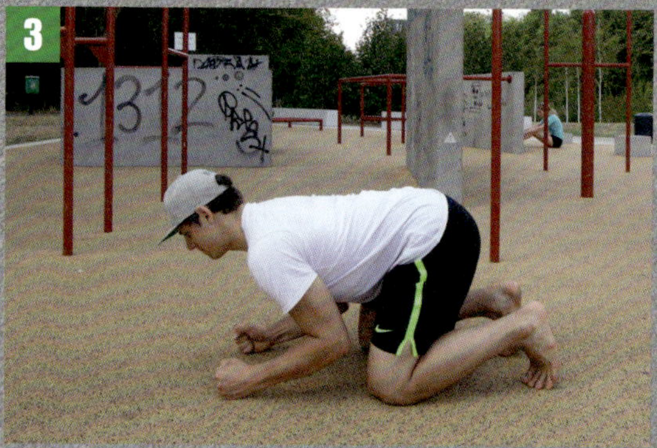

Mobility Exercises 95

TIP

To increase the degree of difficulty, you can also lengthen your lever by straightening your knees until you're in a full plank position.

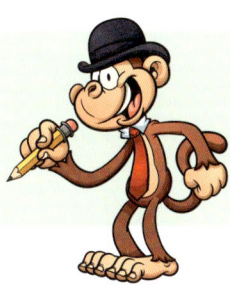

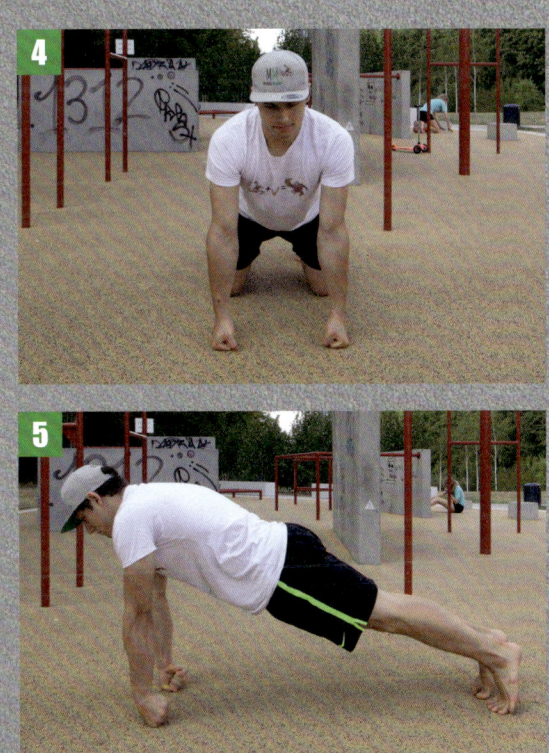

7.1.5 WRIST PUSH-UPS 🍌🍌🍌

  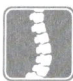

1. Start in an all-fours position.

2. Spread your fingers and press them into the ground.

3. Press your hands into the ground even harder and lift your wrists off the ground (ideally the pressure from your hands against the ground will cause your wrists to lift).

TIP

Shorten your angle by moving your knees closer to your hands. Increase difficulty by performing the exercise in the full plank position.

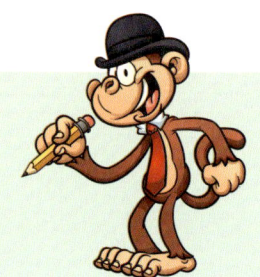

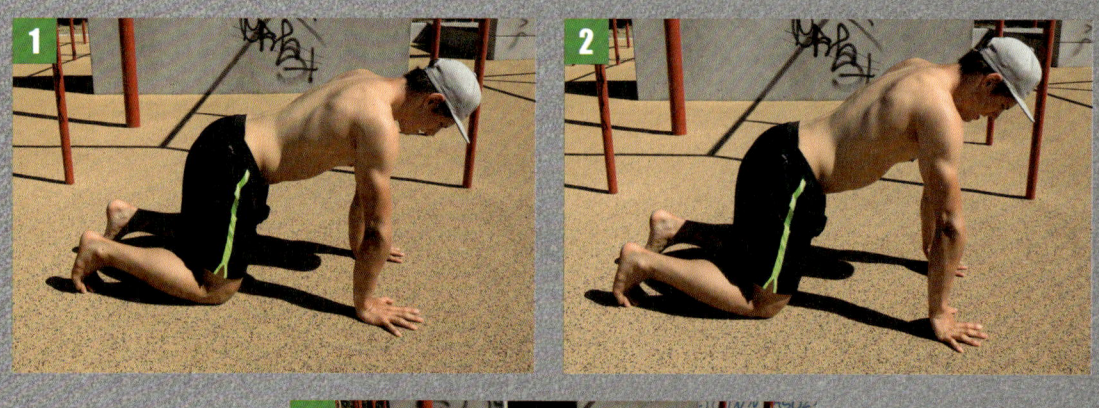

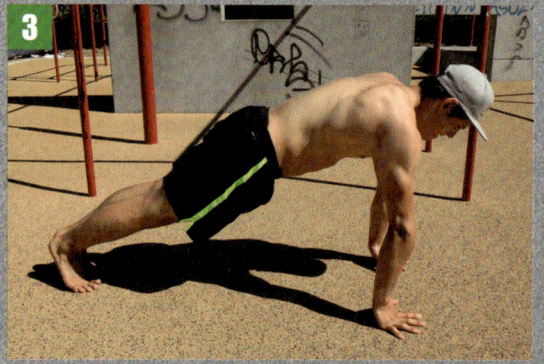

7.2 SPINE

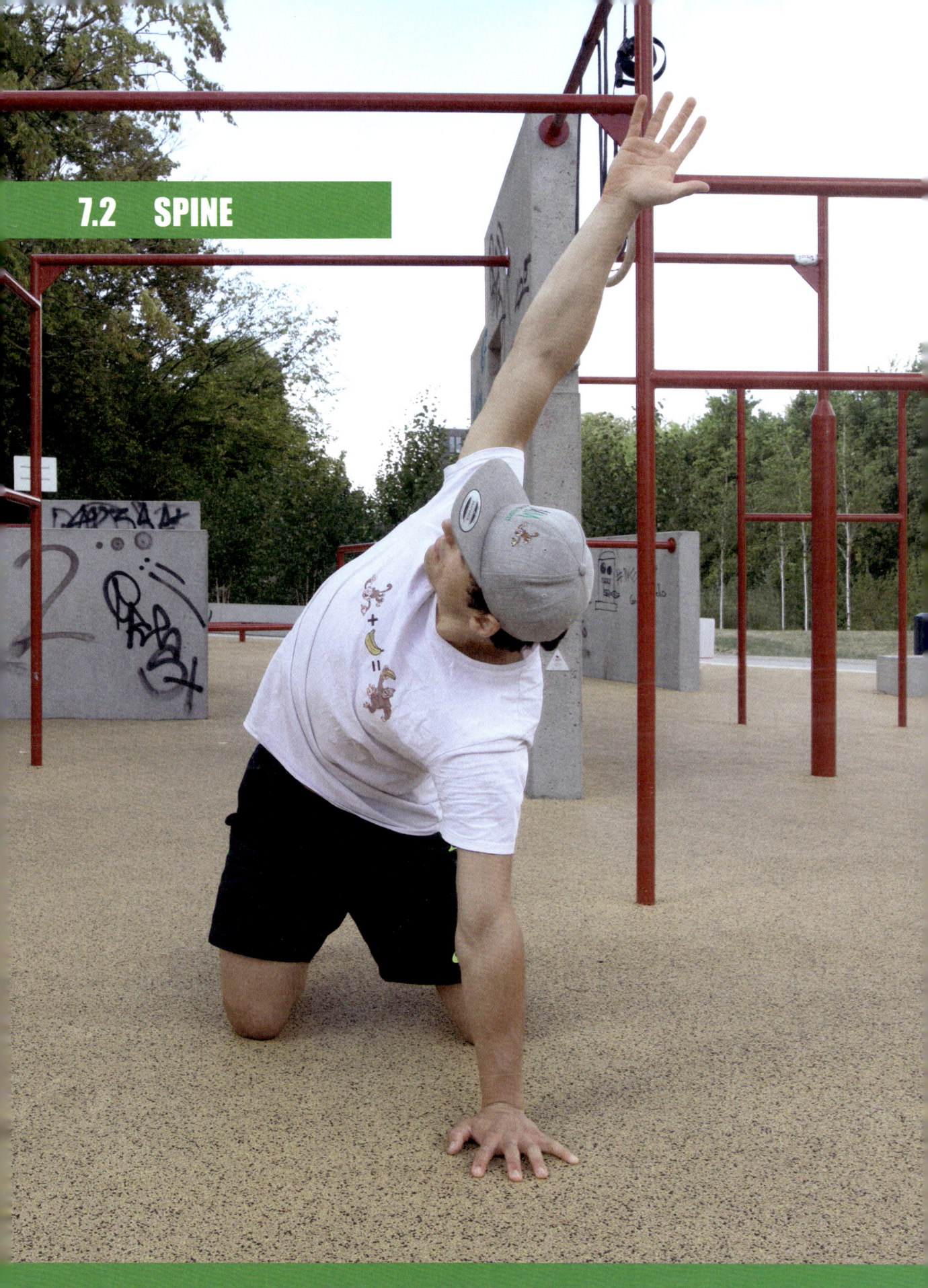

7.2.1 SPINAL ROTATIONS (CARS) 🍌

1. Begin by kneeling and sitting back on your heels.

2. Move your arms into a praying-hands position in front of your sternum (middle of the chest). Your fingertips should touch your chin.

3. Maintain contact with your chin throughout the exercise to make sure you don't bring your head into the movement.

4. Imagine you're drawing a large circle on the ceiling with your head.

5. Make sure you don't move too much with your lower back. Avoid leaning forward or backward. Only bend and straighten your spine.

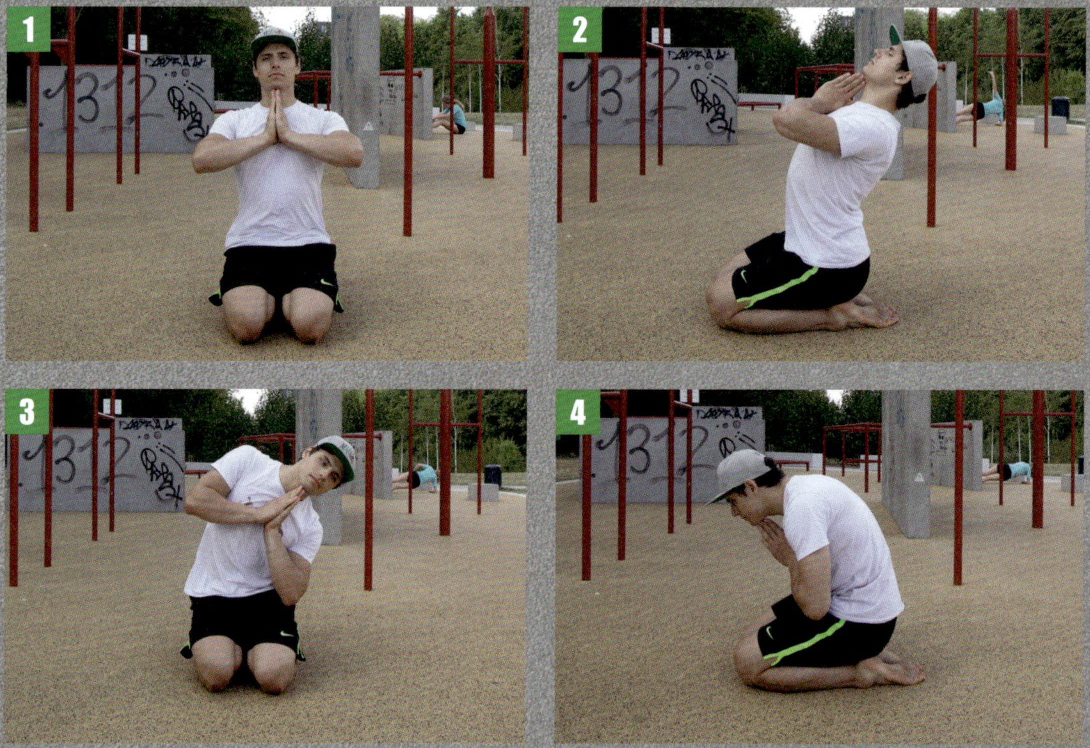

Mobility Exercises

6. Begin by rounding your spine. Think of the uppermost position of a sit-up.

7. Bring your ribs and pelvis together (lateral spinal tilt).

8. Push your chest out and move into the rearmost position. You want to be able to see the ceiling or sky without moving your neck.

9. Do the second lateral tilt (hold a ball between your pelvis and your ribs).

10. End the movement with another forward bend (like you're trying to pull your ribcage over a ball).

TIP

If you're unable to sit back on your heels, you can place a foam roller or a thick pillow between your heels and your posterior.

If that doesn't work for you, do the exercise from a standing position. But in terms of control, that's more difficult.

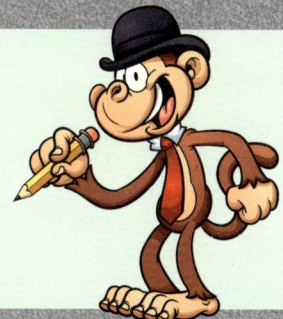

7.2.2 SPINAL WAVE 1 🍌🍌

Most likely, you're familiar with the cat-cow yoga pose, in which you bend and straighten your spine. Spinal wave 1 is similar to cat-cow but more effective.

1. In an all-fours position, bend and straighten your spine vertebra by vertebra, or one vertebra at a time

2. Begin in the neutral position. Imagine a caterpillar crawling along your spine from your neck to your lower back, and round your back in the places the caterpillar has been.

3. Once your spine is completely rounded, press a little more into the curve. Often, you end up losing tension in the area that's already bent. But the idea is to build up tension along the entire curve.

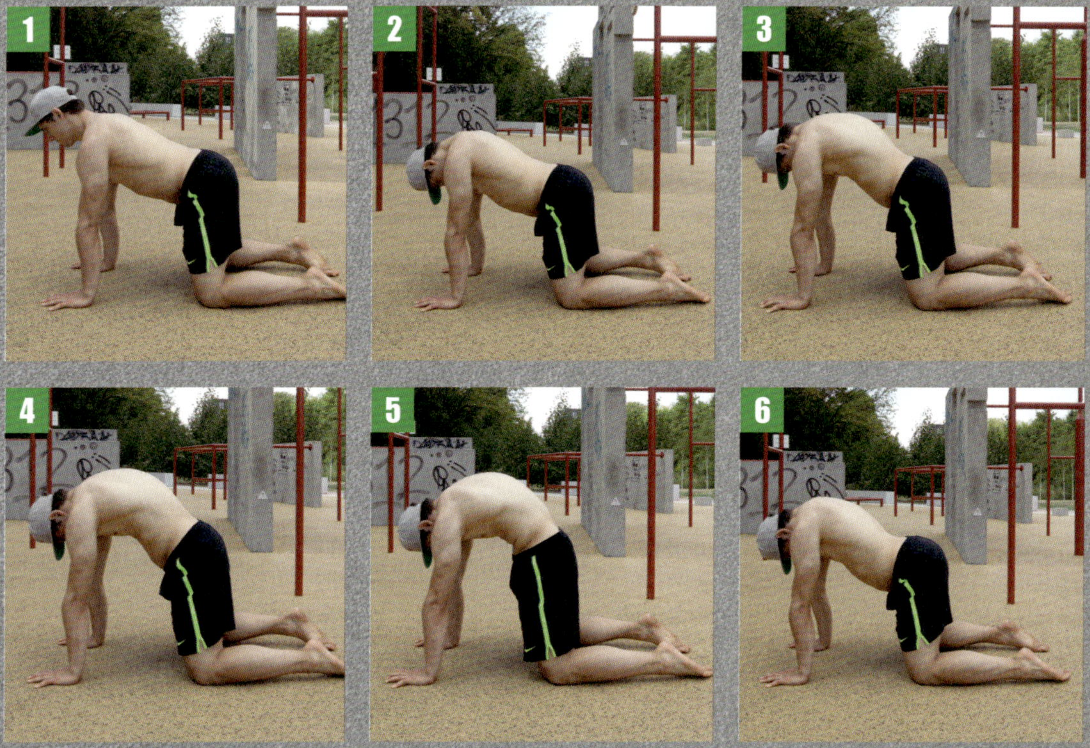

Mobility Exercises

4. Once your spine is completely rounded, begin to straighten the spine, starting at the lower back.

5. First, arch your back, then slowly straighten your thoracic spine and pull your shoulders back.

6. Once everything else is straight, pull your head back. Most people lift their heads too soon. Make sure you straighten your neck last.

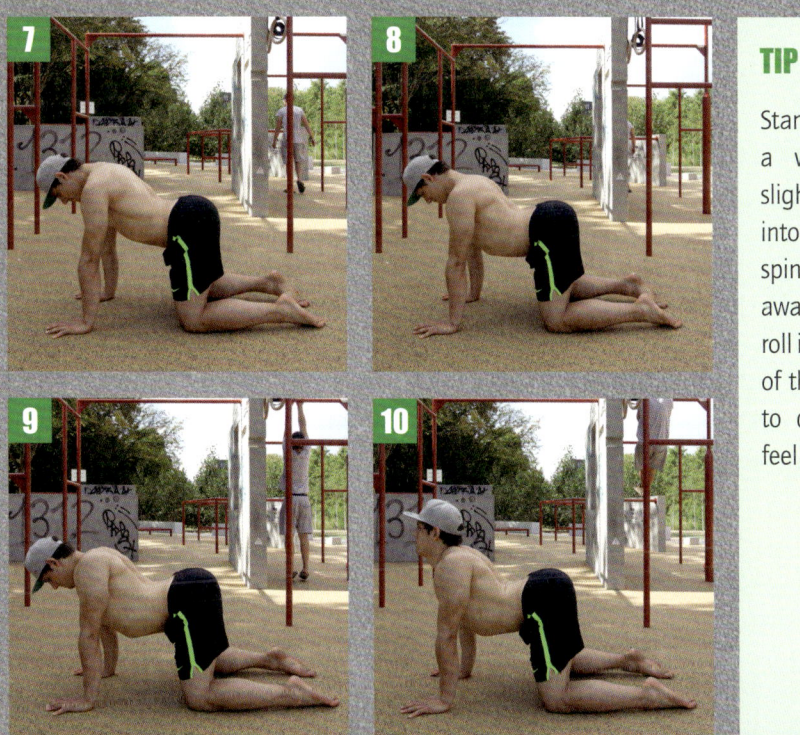

TIP

Stand with your back against a wall, bend your knees slightly, and press your spine into the wall. Now roll your spine, vertebra by vertebra, away from the wall and then roll it back again. The pressure of the wall allows you to develop a better feel for your back.

7.2.3 SPINAL WAVE 2 🍌🍌🍌

1. Stand a forearm's length from a wall. You'll move your spine in a wave-like motion.

2. One after the other, touch your nose, chin, chest, stomach, and pelvis to the wall.

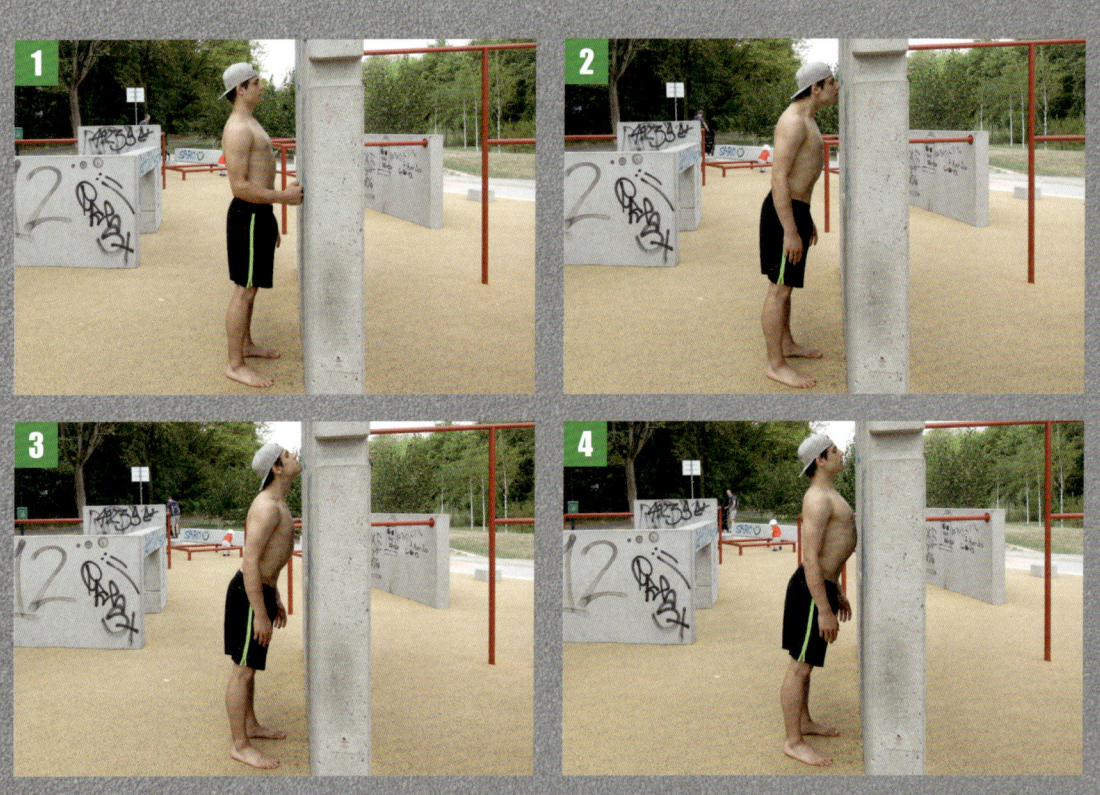

Mobility Exercises 103

3. Between stations, release the previous point (e.g., as you move your chin to the wall, simultaneously release your nose).

4. Before you try to smoothly link all the listed points, practice the order of the individual points.

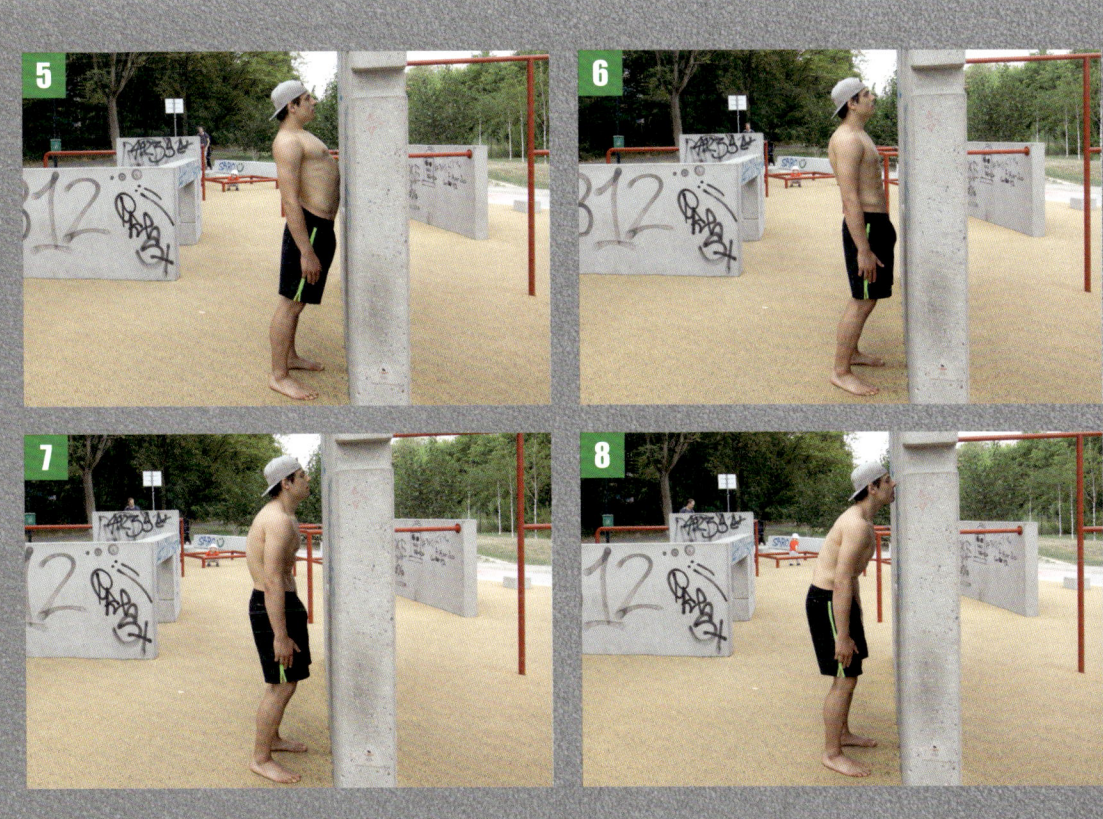

7.2.4 NECK MOBILIZATION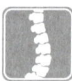

1. Move your neck in all directions and back to the center.

2. Rotate your head to the right and the left (looking over your shoulder).

3. Nod (as if saying yes).

4. Tilt your head to each side (resting your ear close to your shoulder, without raising your shoulder).

5. Push your head forward (without nodding) and backward (making a double chin).

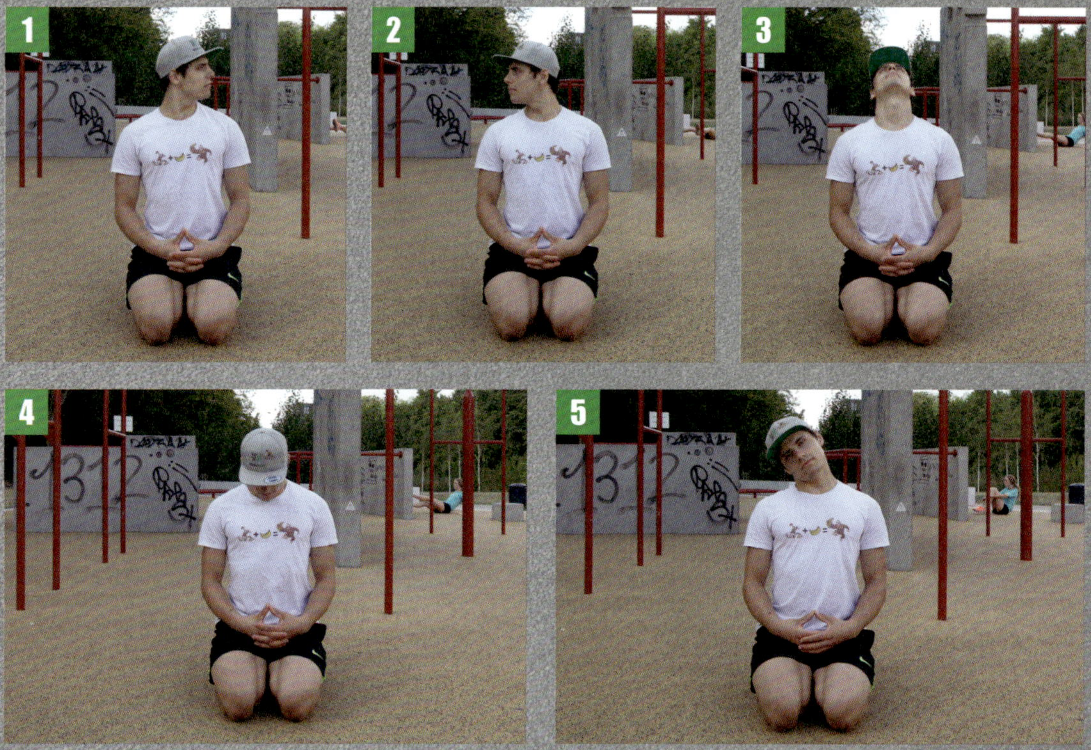

Mobility Exercises 105

6. Do a side-to-side translation, shifting your neck sideways. Imagine your head sits on a track that's attached to your shoulders and moves to the left and right without you getting in one of the aforementioned positions. Keep in mind that this movement is considerably more difficult, and most people aren't able to do it.

TIP

Practice the movements in front of a mirror so you can closely observe your compensating movements.

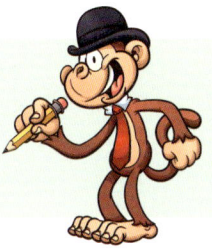

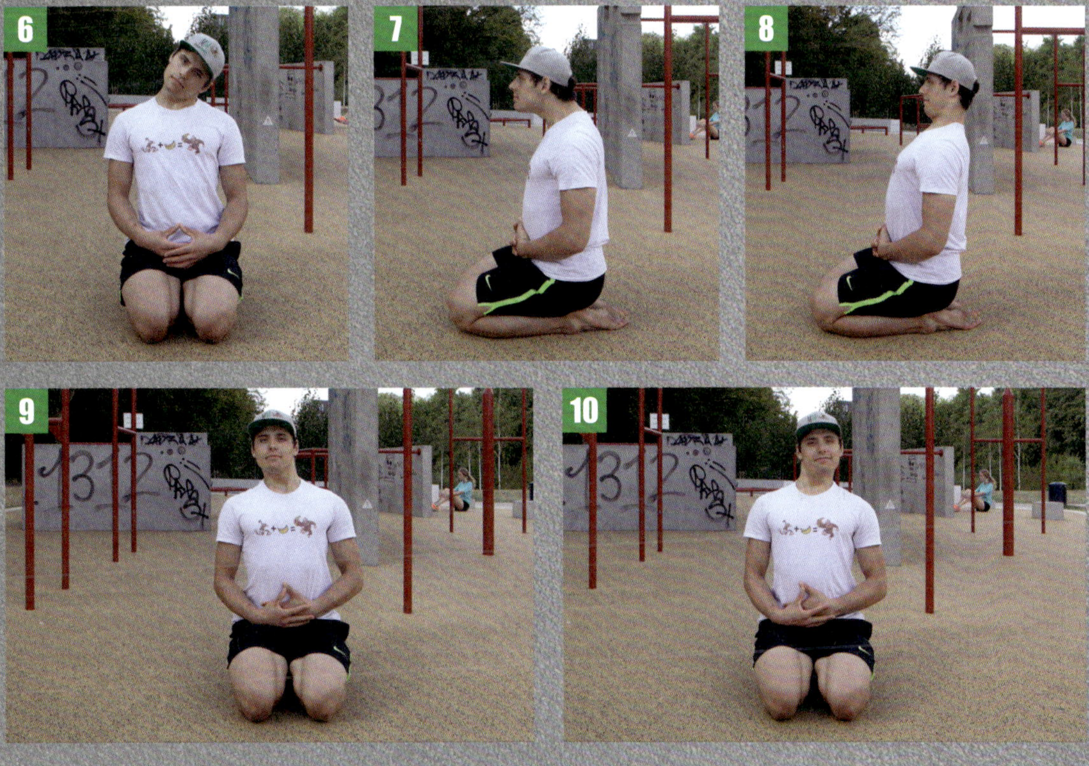

7.2.5 THREE-POINT THORACIC-SPINE ROTATION

1. Lying on your back, bend one knee 90 degrees and rest it on the ground on the opposite side of your body.

2. Hold on to the bent leg with the arm that's on the side you're resting your leg on. You now have six points you can link in one movement . . .

3. . . . three on the side on which the leg is resting and three behind your back. Imagine stretching a rope between the opposing points.

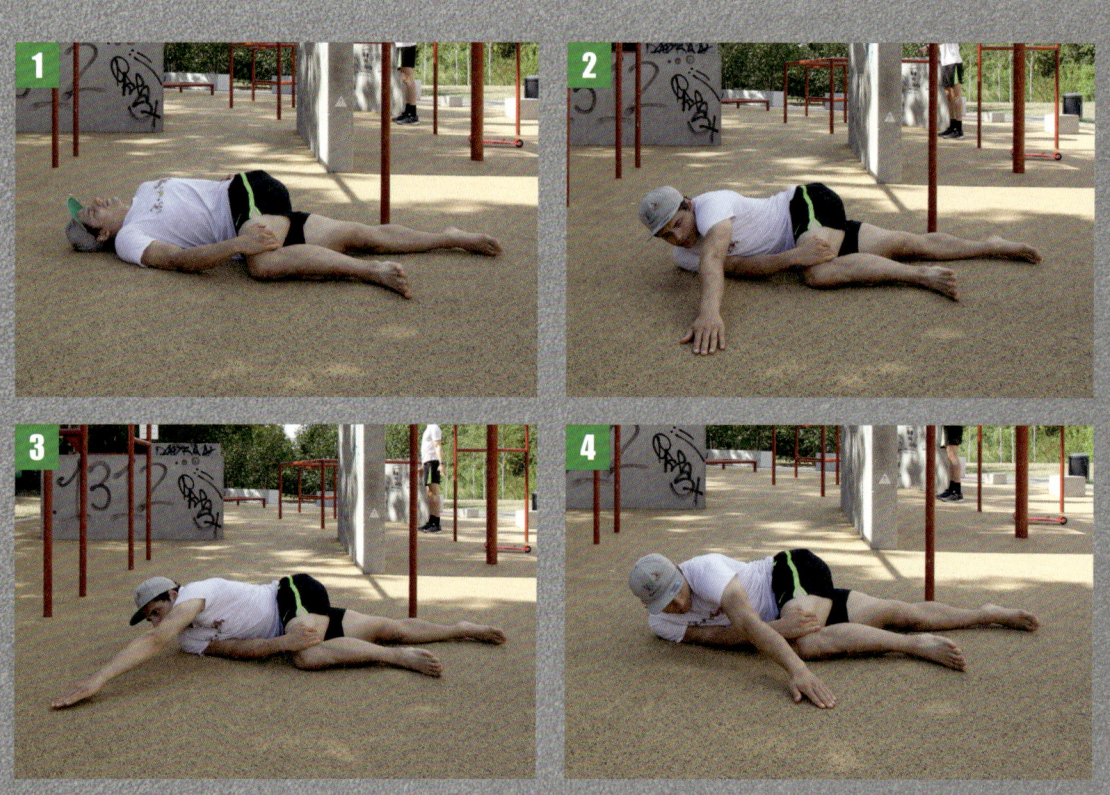

4. The movements all start on the side the leg rests on.

5. Use your other arm to stretch the imaginary rope on the diagonals: top front to bottom rear, middle front to middle rear, and bottom front to top rear. Stretch these three diagonals on both sides of your body using the same arm.

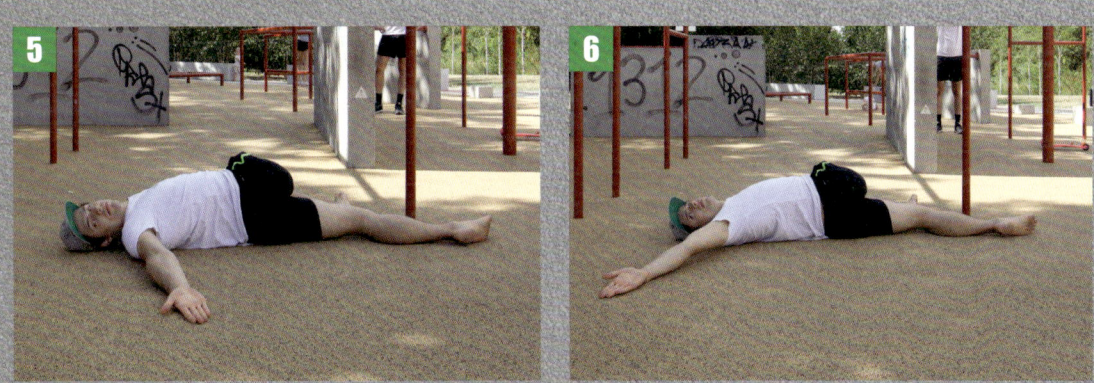

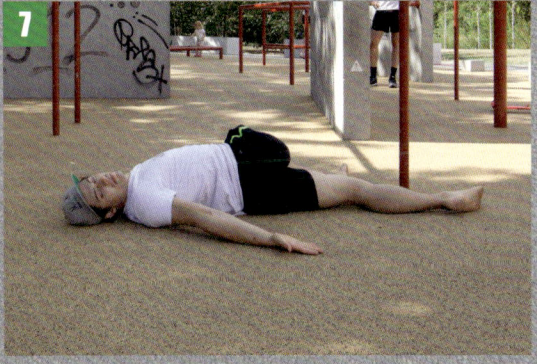

7.2.6 ALL-FOURS ROTATION 🍌🍌

1. Start in an all-fours position.

2. Take a breath, push the ground away from you, release one arm, and extend it to the sky.

3. Rotate your spine as far as you can without letting your hip move in the opposite direction. Keep holding your breath so you're rotating against a filled ribcage.

4. Now exhale and rotate a little bit farther.

5. Inhale and exhale in the highest position . . .

6. and then return to the starting position. Of course, you can vary your breathing at will. I do recommend you try breathing as described before changing it.

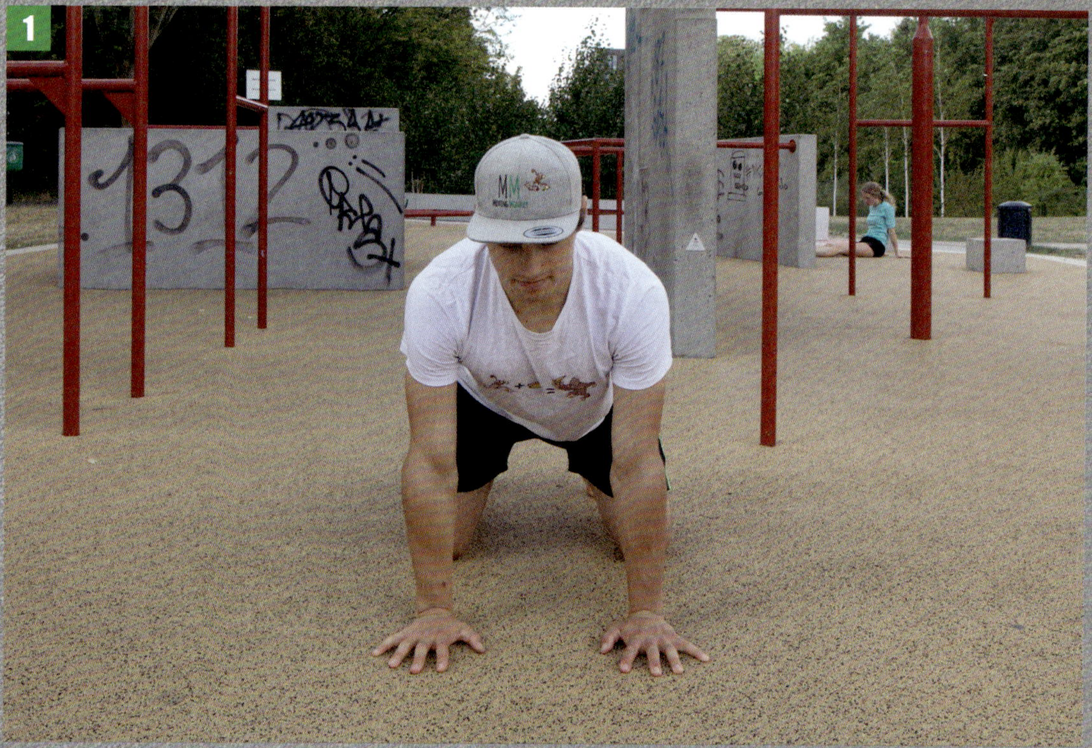

Mobility Exercises

> **TIP**
>
> You can place your hip against a box or a wall to prevent major compensating movements.
>
> You can use the breathing technique for all spinal rotations.

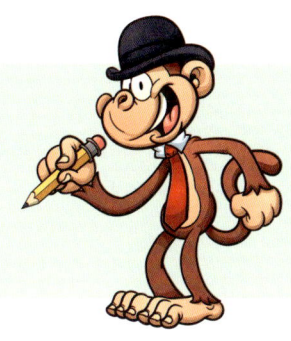

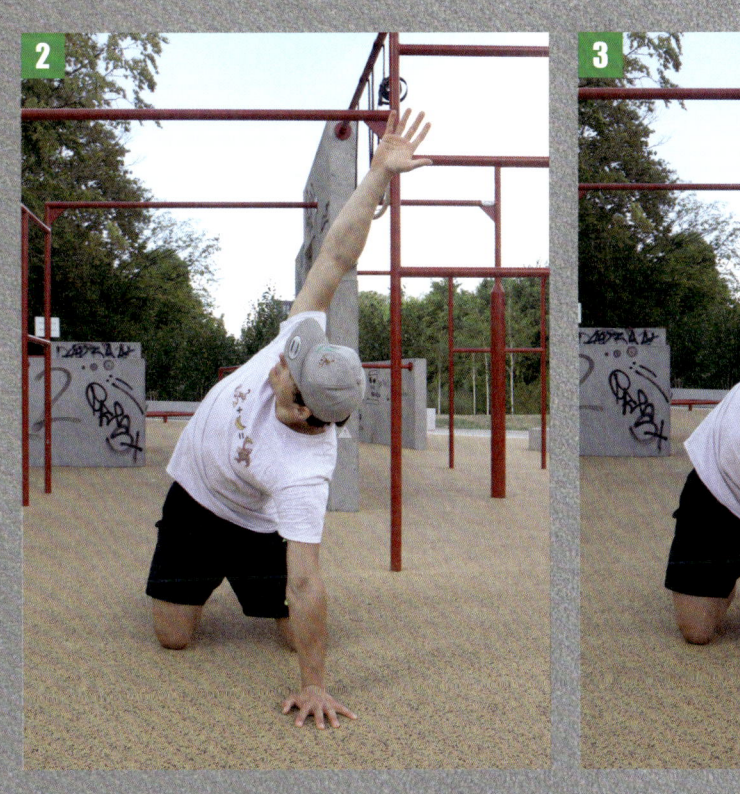

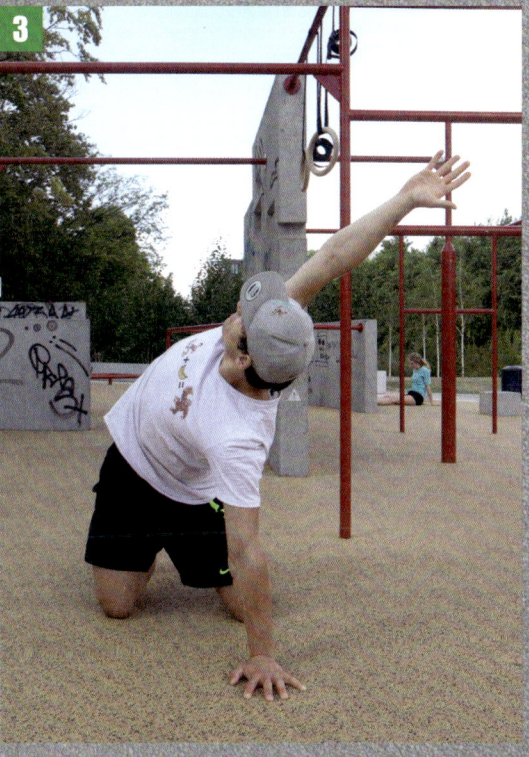

VARIATION 1 🍌🍌🍌

1. To intensify the exercise, rest one arm on the ground.

2. Press the lower part of the arm into the ground while you extend the other arm to the sky and rotate.

3. Look toward your raised arm and try to rotate more.

> **IMPORTANT**
>
> If you simply throw your arm back, you won't achieve a rotation in the thoracic spine. It might look like you're rotating, but if you feel it only in your shoulder, this variation is still too difficult for you.

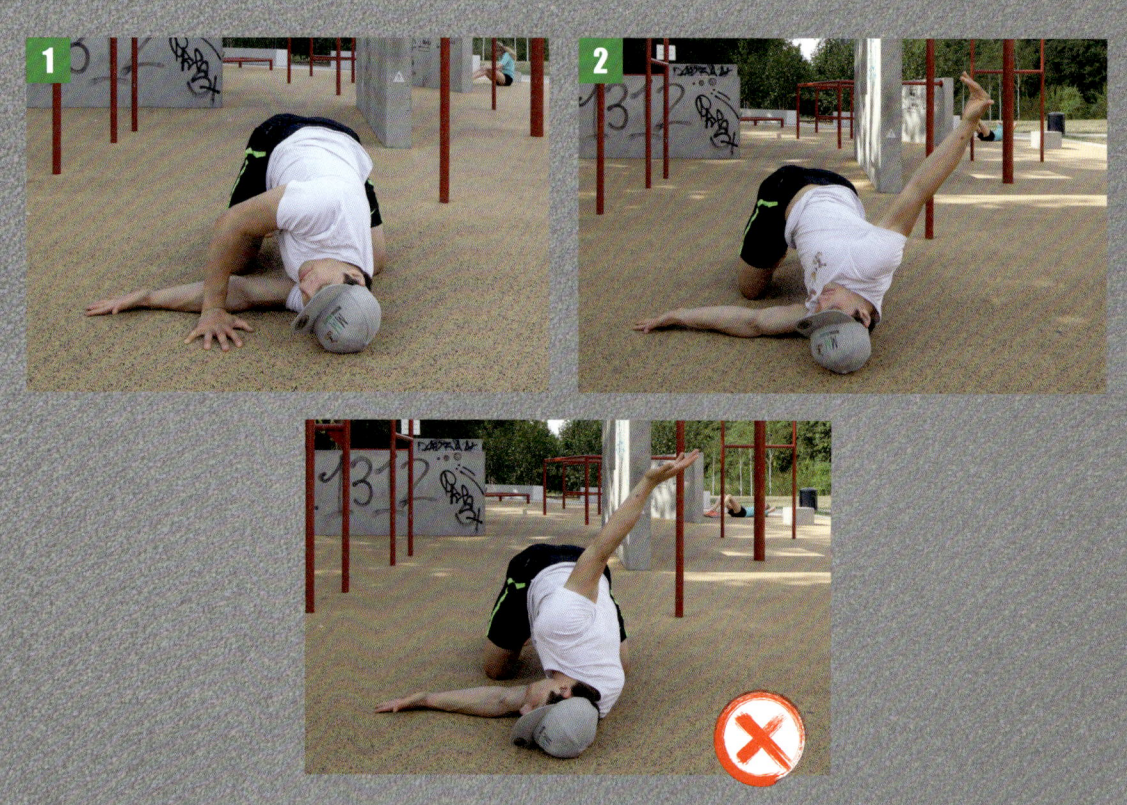

Mobility Exercises

VARIATION 2

1. Combine the basic position and the first variation by lifting your lower arm off the ground and continuing to rotate in the direction in which your fingers point.

2. Next, extend your arm overhead by rotating your torso. Then move back into the basic position.

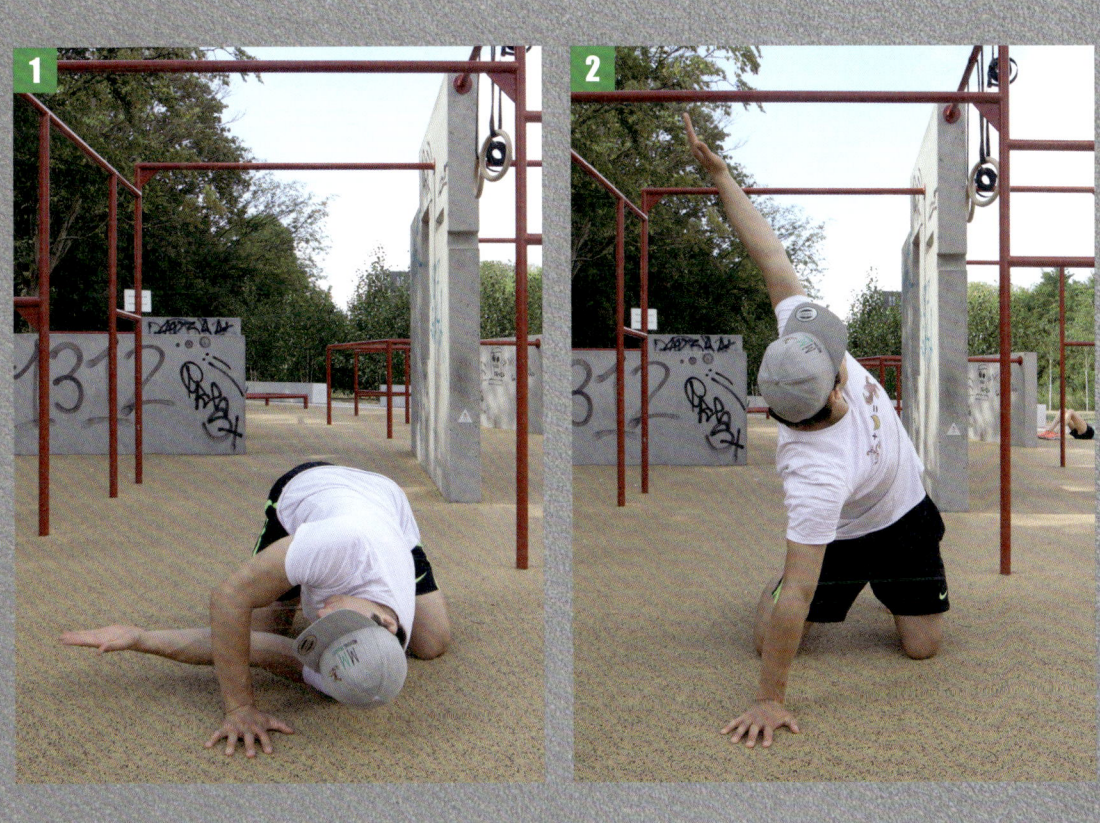

7.2.7 BALL 🍌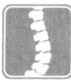

1. Sit up straight and pull your knees in to your chest as close as you can.

2. Hug your shins and hold on to one wrist.

3. Take a breath, pull your knees in even closer, and move your shoulders back and down.

4. As you exhale, round your back and press your legs against your closed arms (maintain your grip).

5. Pull your shoulder blades even farther apart.

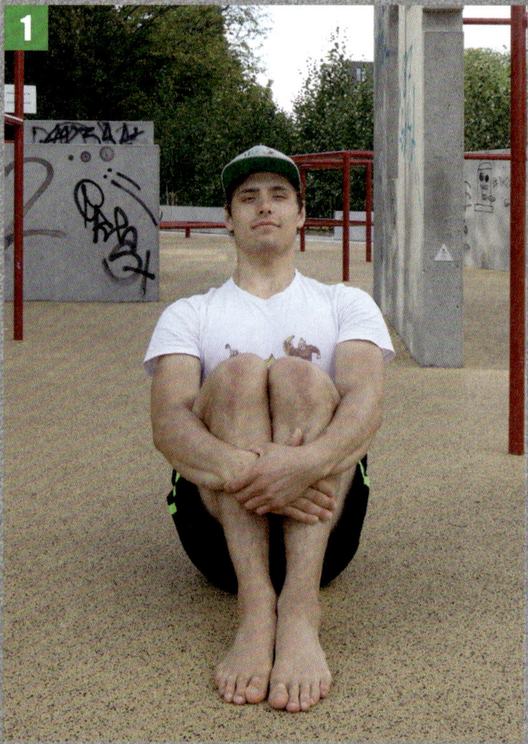

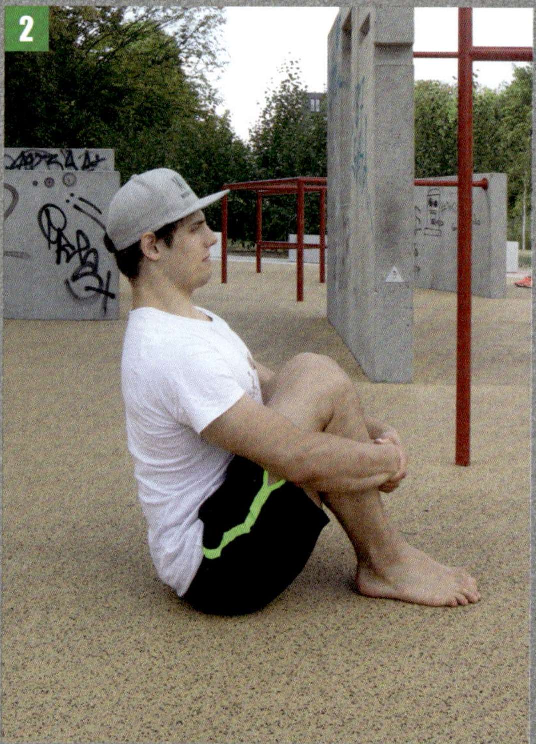

Mobility Exercises

6. Once you've rounded as much as you can, lean slightly to the right and left to shift the built-up tension.

7. Return to the center, take a breath, and pull back up into the starting position.

> **TIP**
>
> If hugging your shins is awkward, you can instead hold on to your thighs.

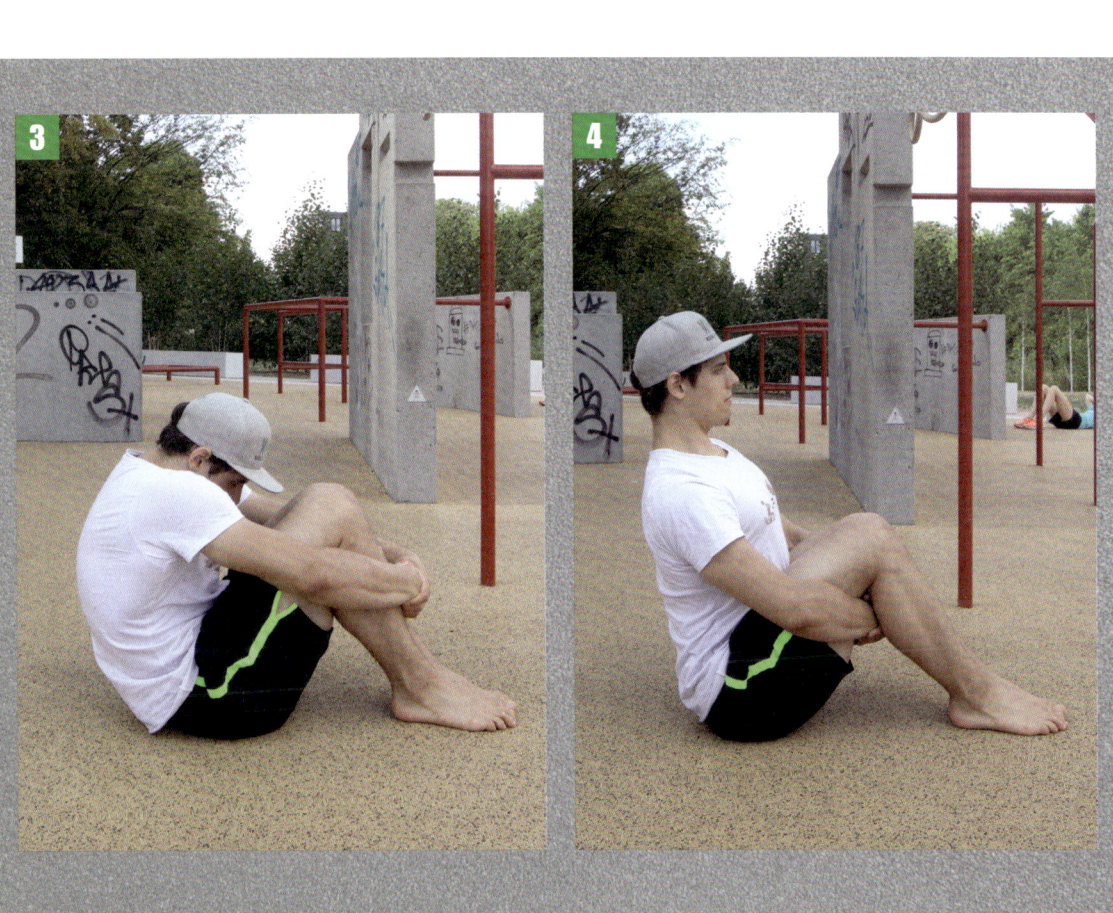

7.2.8 PRONE THORACIC-SPINE ROTATION 🍌

1. Lie on your stomach, with your arms against the ground and extended above your head.

2. Press one arm into the ground and raise the other arm so it's at a 90-degree angle to your body.

3. Repeat with your other arm.

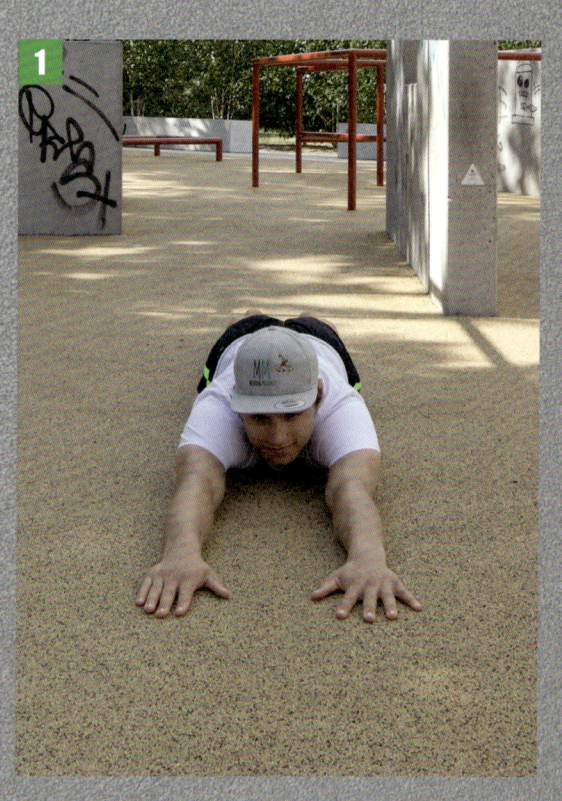
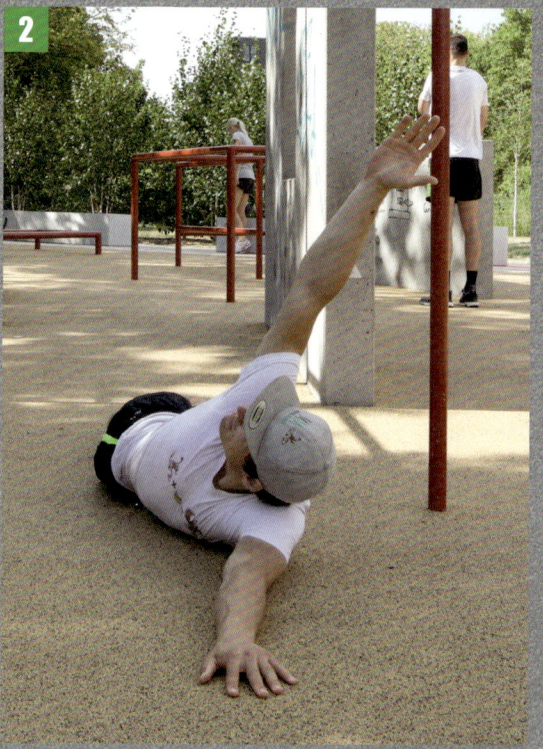

7.2.9 WRESTLER ROTATION 🍌🍌

1. Lie on your back and bend your knees.

2. Lift your pelvis toward the sky and build up tension.

3. Roll diagonally onto your shoulder by lifting your pelvis higher and pushing it back.

4. Reach behind you with your arm extended (reach to the right and back with your left arm or vice versa).

5. Return to the starting position, rest your pelvis on the ground, and then rotate over onto the other shoulder.

6. **Important:** keep your eyes on your hand as you move and also lift your chest off the ground so you're resting on only the side of your shoulder.

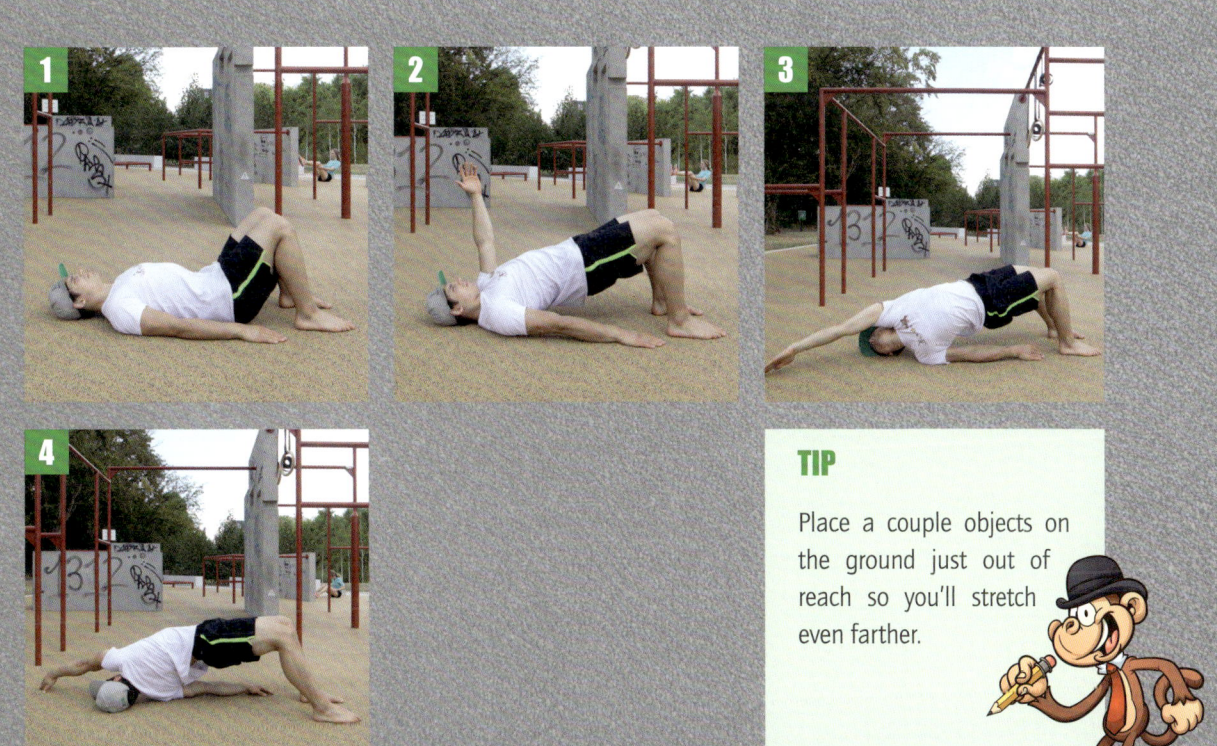

TIP

Place a couple objects on the ground just out of reach so you'll stretch even farther.

7.2.10 TABLE ROTATION 🍌🍌🍌

1. Start in a seated posture.

2. Support yourself with your hands on the ground just behind your hips (fingertips pointing away from your body).

3. Press your heels into the ground.

4. Lift your pelvis into table pose.

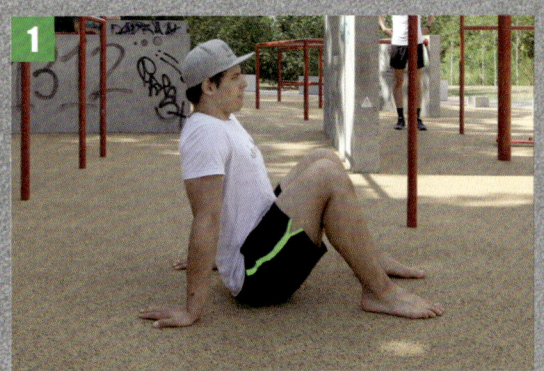

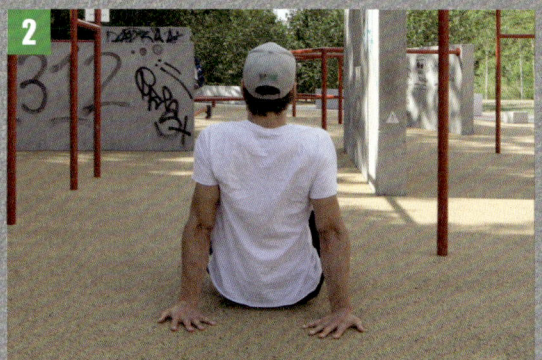

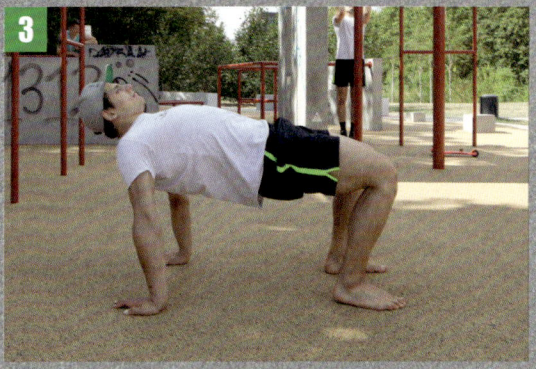

Mobility Exercises

5. Release one arm from the ground, pushing out of that shoulder, rotate to the other side over the supporting arm, and try to touch the ground.

6. Rotate back to table pose and repeat step 5 on the other side.

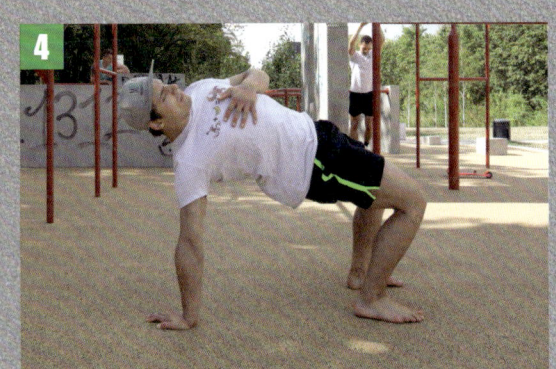
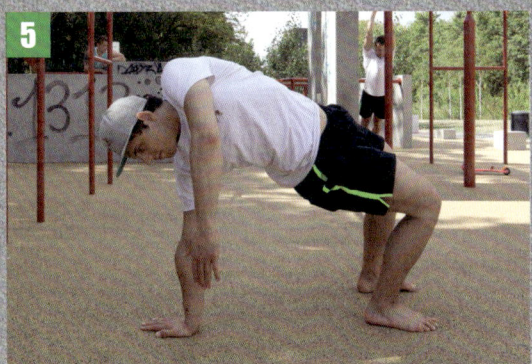
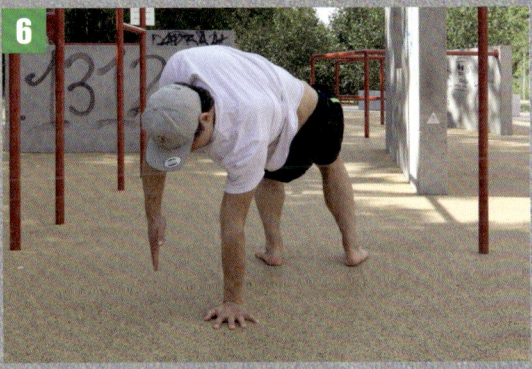

7.2.11 HEEL-SITTING ROTATION

As the name suggests, this exercise requires you to sit on your heels. If you're not yet able to do so, you should first practice getting into this position.

1. Place one hand on the ground in line with the foot on the same side.

2. Push your pelvis forward by pressing your shins into the ground, lifting your posterior off your heels and tightening it.

3. Now rest your forearm on the ground too.

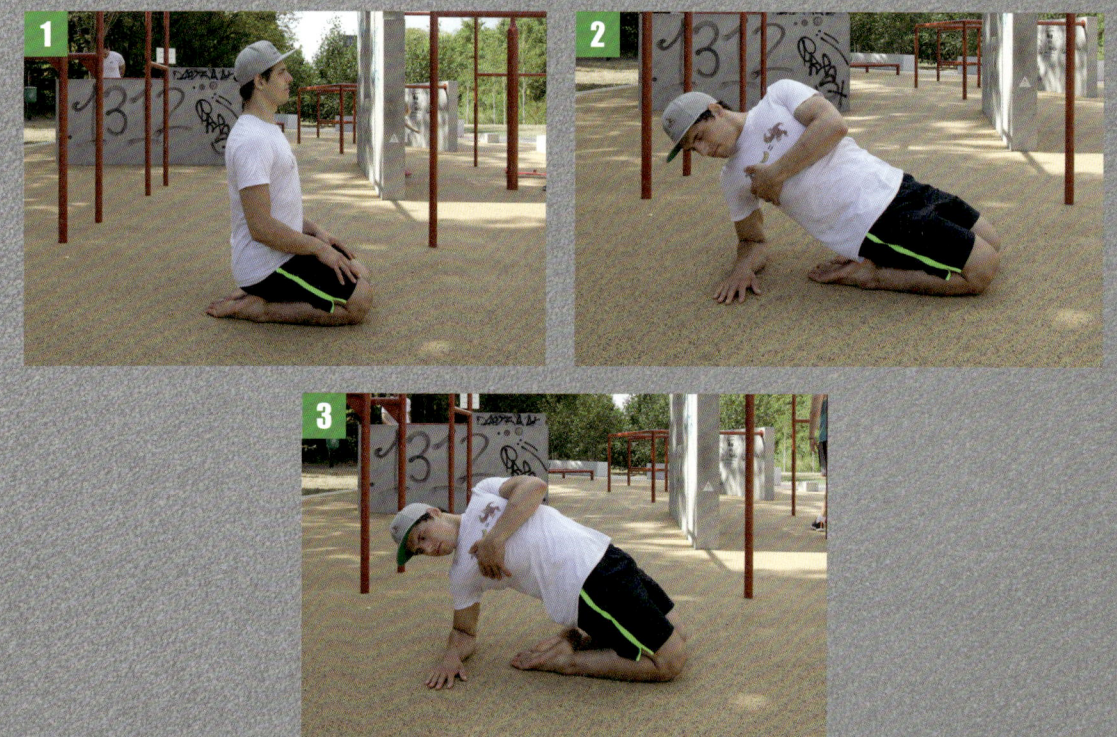

4. Pull yourself deeper into the rotation.

5. **Important:** Maintain muscle tension in your posterior and your abdominals. You don't want to twist your lower back without muscle tension in your core (see section 2.3, "Not Every Joint Should Be Mobilized").

6. Rotate back to the starting position and repeat steps 2–4.

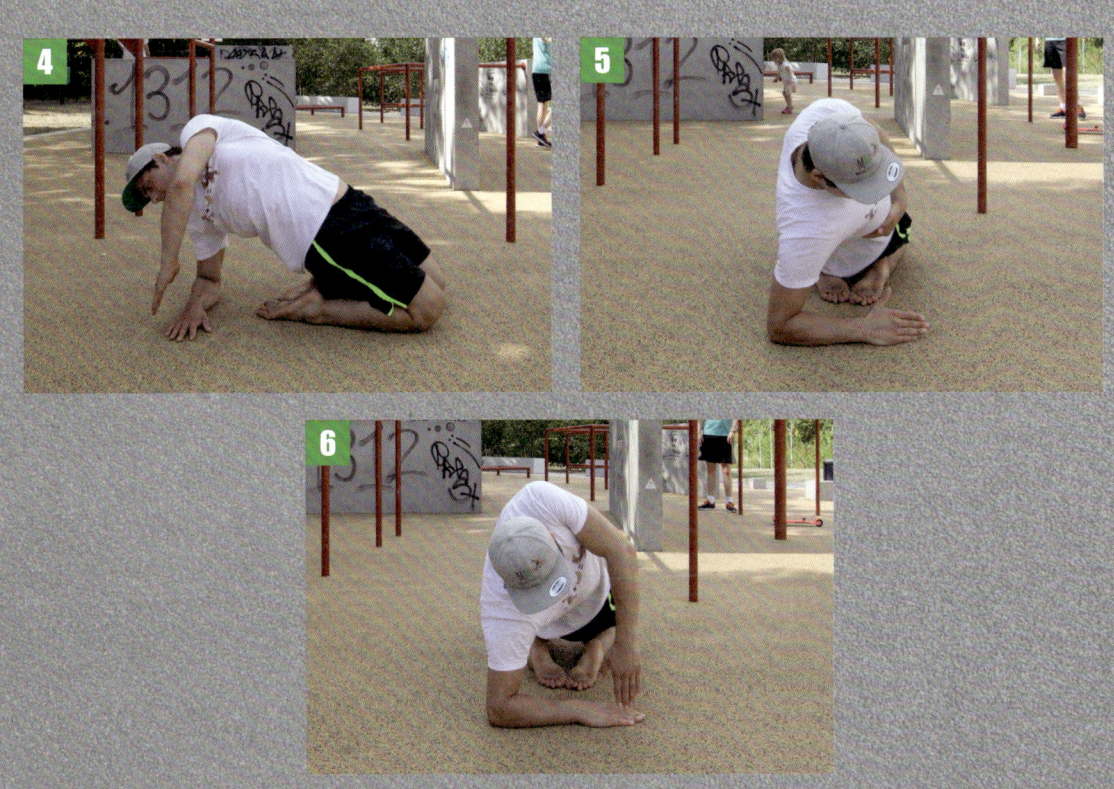

7.2.12 CROSS-LEGGED ROTATION

I include the cross-legged rotation primarily to show you how many possible variations there are for spinal rotations. As I mention in section 2.7, "How Mobility Makes You Stronger," and chapter 5, "Mobility Lifestyle Hacks," variety is the key to success.

1. Begin in a seated cross-legged posture.

2. Bend forward and rest one forearm on the ground.

3. Externally rotate, leading with your free arm, and face that hand.

4. Twist farther and think about your breathing.

5. Repeat steps 3 and 4 or make a smooth transition to the forward bend and switch arms.

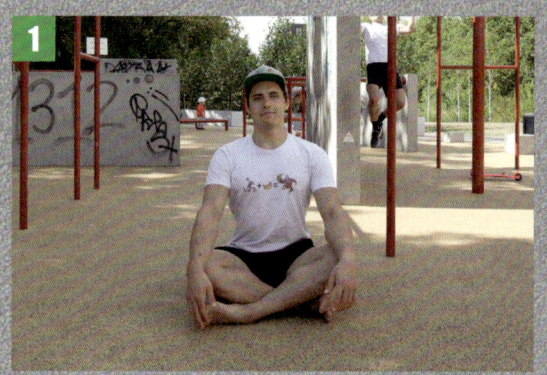
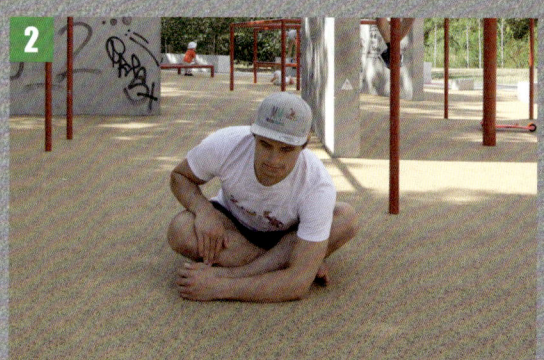
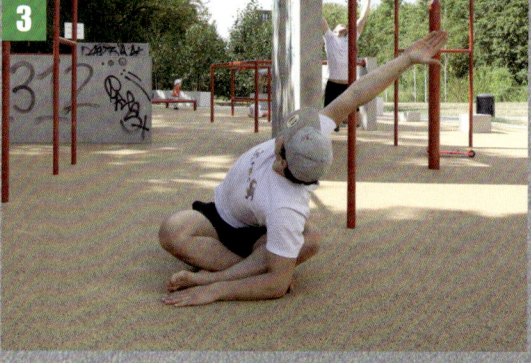

Mobility Exercises | **121**

7.2.13 COBRA

1. Kneel in front of two rings that are attached at standing hip level.

2. Grip the rings, lift your posterior off your heels, and lean forward into the rings.

3. Actively pull yourself into an extension of the spine while simultaneously pulling your shoulder blades together ("crack a walnut").

VARIATION

To intensify the exercise, extend your legs and rotate left and right around your body's axis.
Important: maintain core tension throughout this advanced variation.

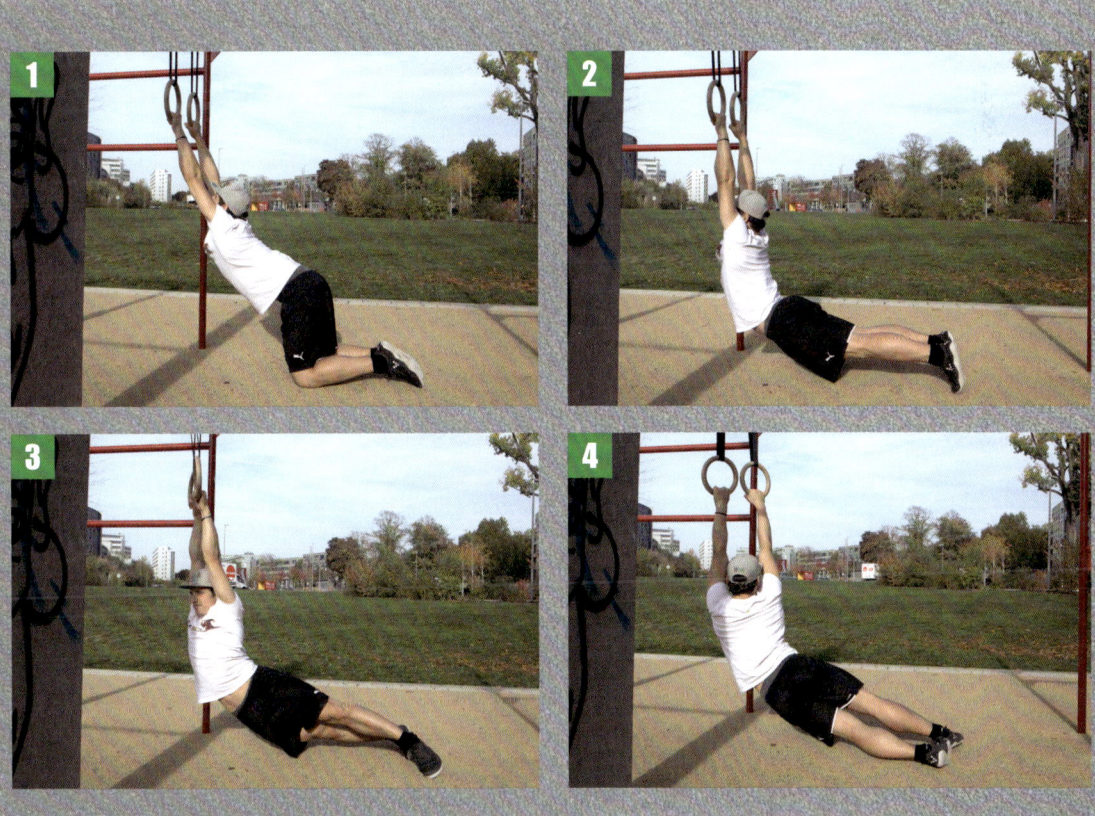

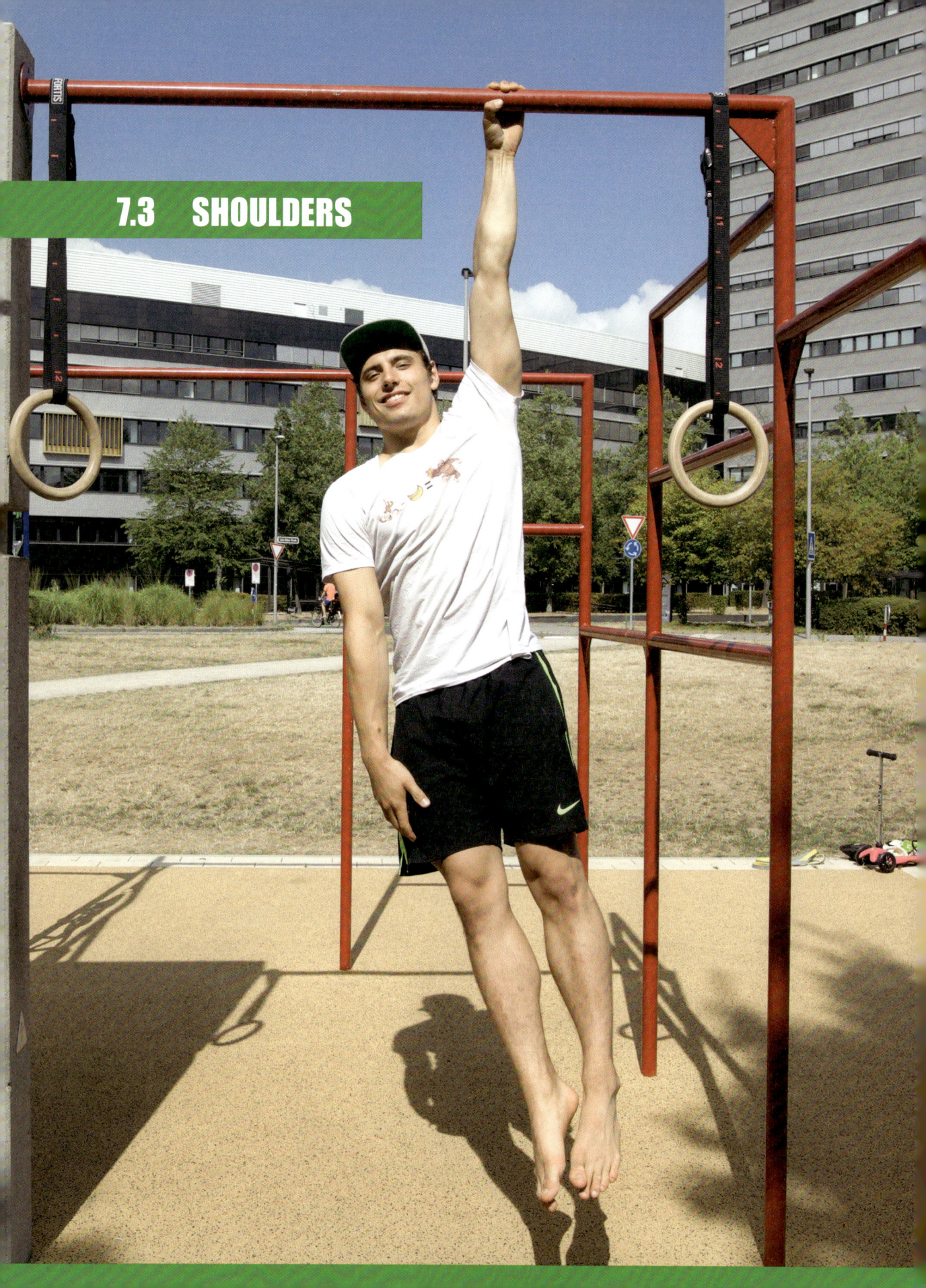

7.3 SHOULDERS

Mobility Exercises

7.3.1 SHOULDER ROTATIONS (CARS)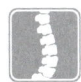

1. Stand tall and extend one arm parallel to the ground.

2. Trace a circle with your shoulder by moving the shoulder blade from **protraction** to **elevation** to **retraction** and finally to **depression** in one fluid motion (see section 10.9, "Shoulder-Blade Positions" for definitions of these terms).

3. Keep your arm extended throughout and maintain core tension.

> **TIP**
>
> To make control easier, first practice the individual phases of the movement before linking them in a circle. For the circular motion, visualize how the wheels on a locomotive move.

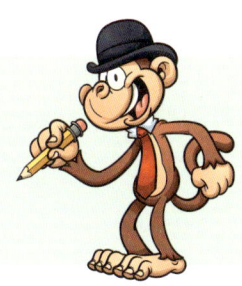

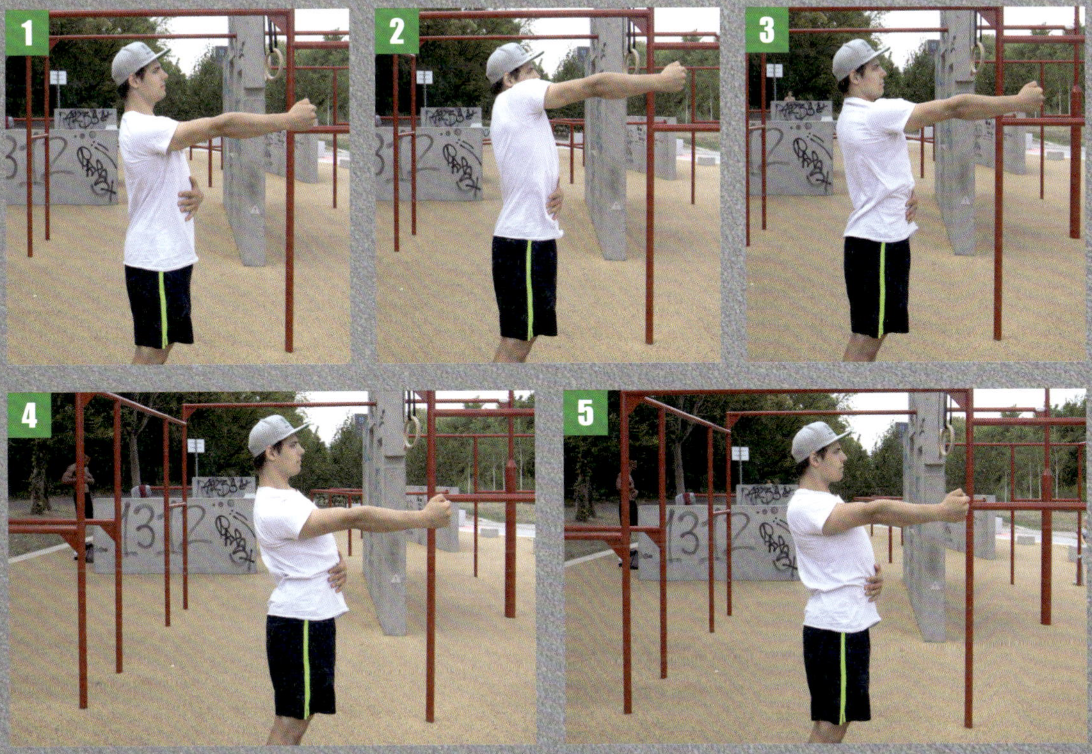

7.3.2 SHOULDER ROTATIONS (AGAINST THE WALL)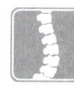

1. Stand with your side facing a wall.

2. Position the back of your hand to face the wall.

3. Raise your arm overhead as high as you can.

4. Internally rotate your arm and shoulder. Your thumb will first point forward, then to the wall, and finally behind you as you move your arm farther behind your body.

5. On your arm and shoulder's way back, keep your shoulder internally rotated until you can go no farther, and then slowly open your arm as you move it back into the starting position.

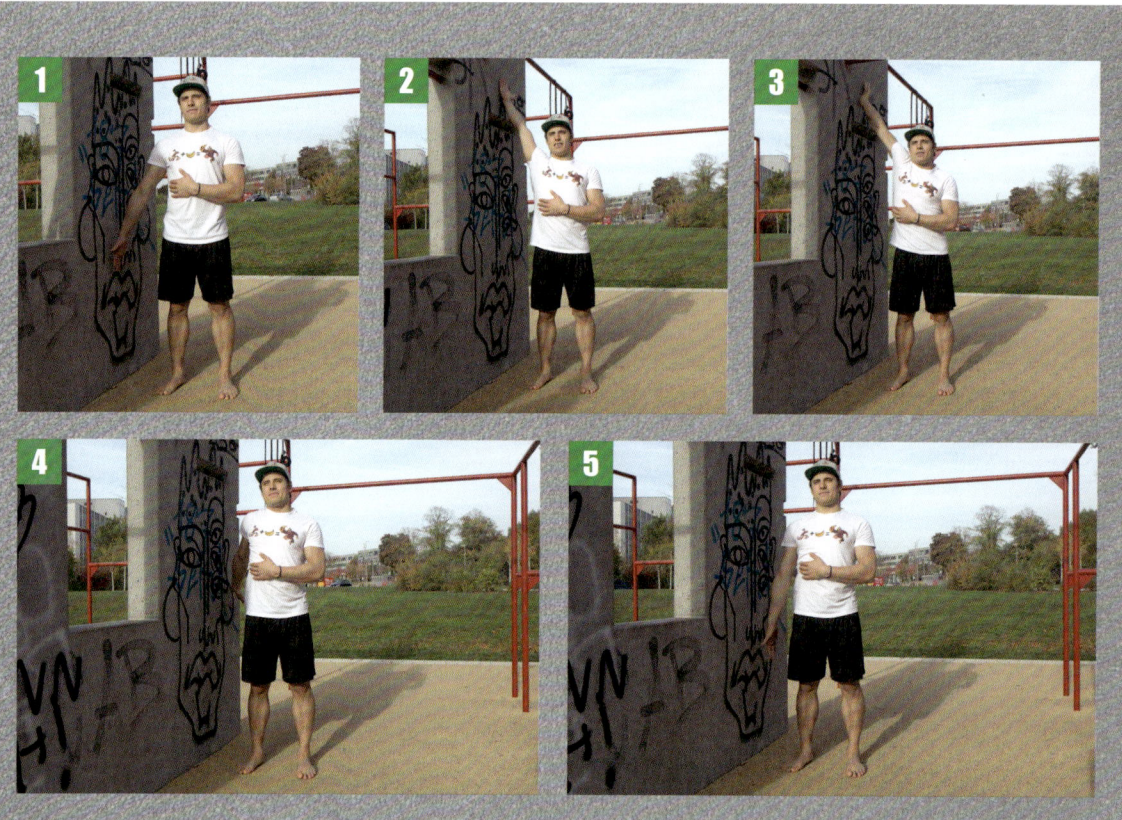

Mobility Exercises

7.3.3 HANGING

Passively hang from a bar (more on passive and active hanging in section 11.2, "Activation Exercises").

> **TIP**
>
> If you have trouble hanging for more than ten seconds, start by letting your feet touch the ground.

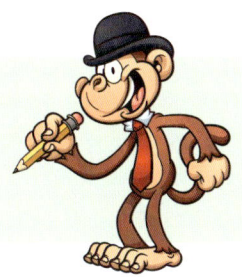

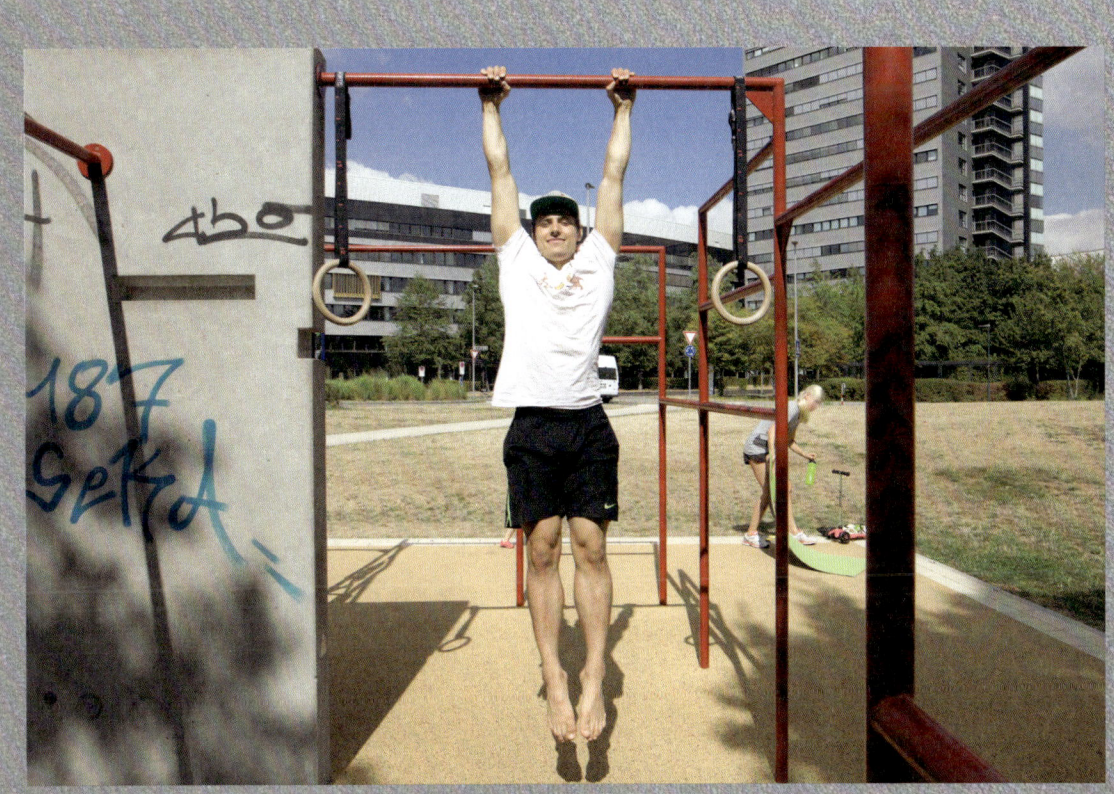

7.3.4 SINGLE-ARM HANGING

Just like hanging but with only one arm.

TIP

To learn hanging by one arm, practice hanging from the bar for sixty seconds with both arms. Then move on to hanging with one arm with your feet touching the ground, thereby practicing hanging by one arm with less than your entire bodyweight.

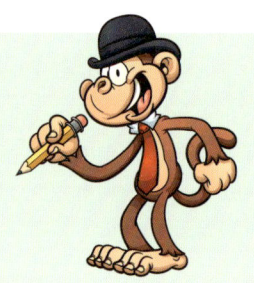

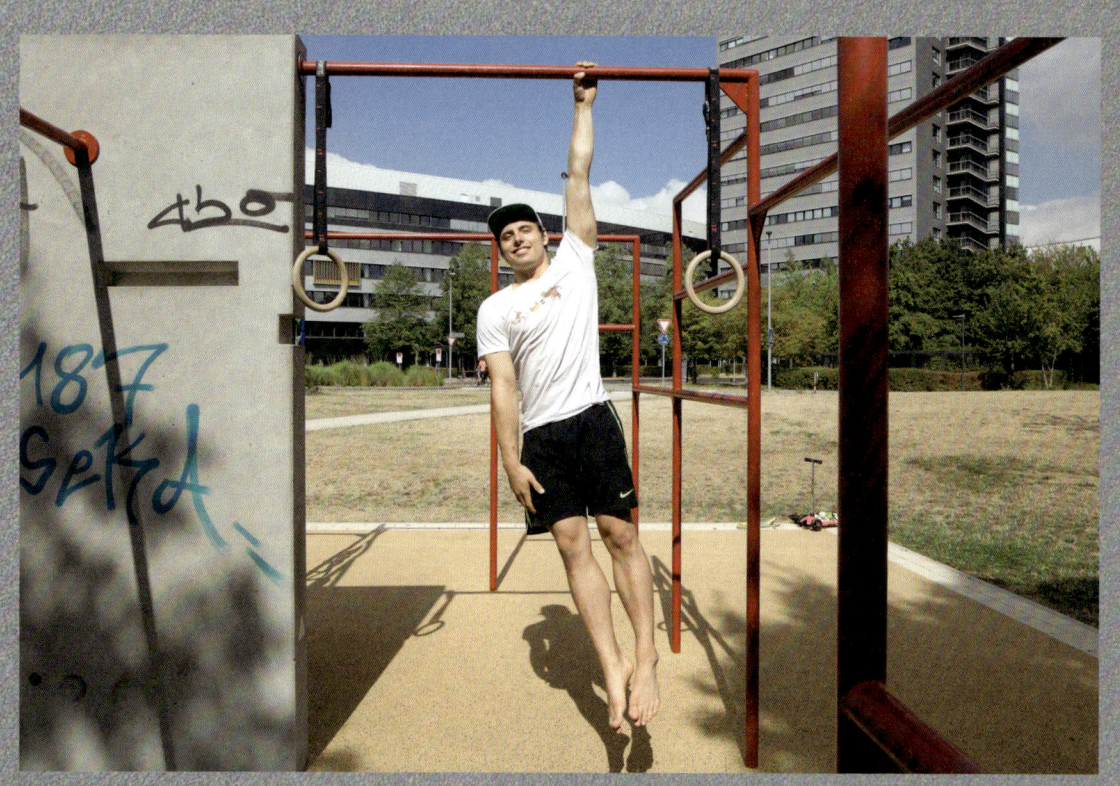

Mobility Exercises 127

7.3.5 WALL SLIDES

1. Sit against a wall with your legs extended forward.

2. Place your arms against the wall with your elbows bent at a 90-degree angle (upper arm to trunk at 90 degrees and forearm to upper arm at 90 degrees).

3. Keep the backs your hands against the wall as you extend your arms overhead.

4. Return your arms to the 90-degree positions.

TIP

If you aren't able to place your hands against the wall, increase practicing hanging (7.3.3), swimmer (7.3.7), and side bends (7.3.11).

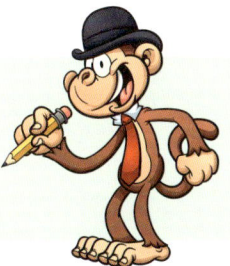

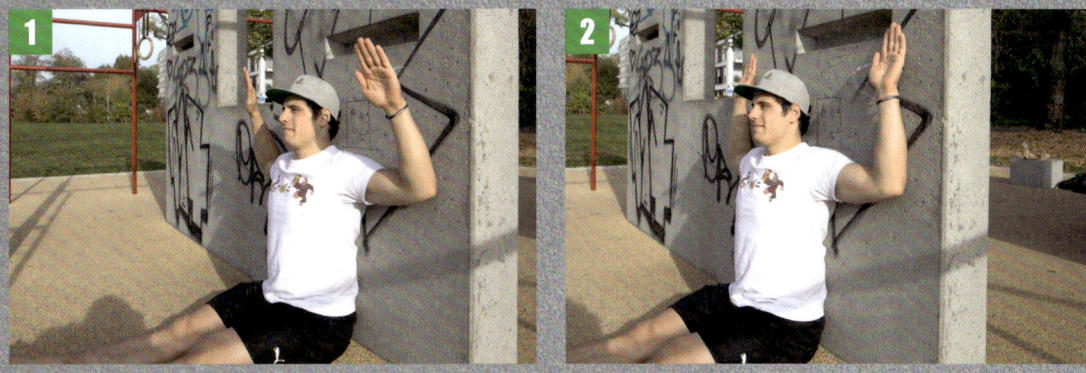

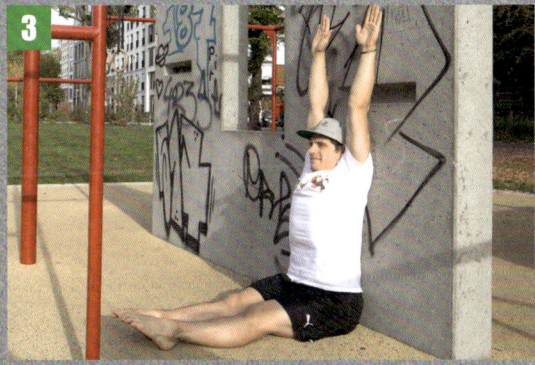

7.3.6 SHOULDER CRAWL 🍌🍌🍌

1. Start in a seated posture with your hands propped behind you, shoulder-distance apart and fingers spread.

2. Let your fingers crawl farther behind you until they can go no farther and until you can feel a stretch in your chest and the front of your shoulders. Keep your arms straight throughout.

3. When your arms are extended backward as far as possible, lean and try to touch your shoulders to the ground (or at least lean right and left)

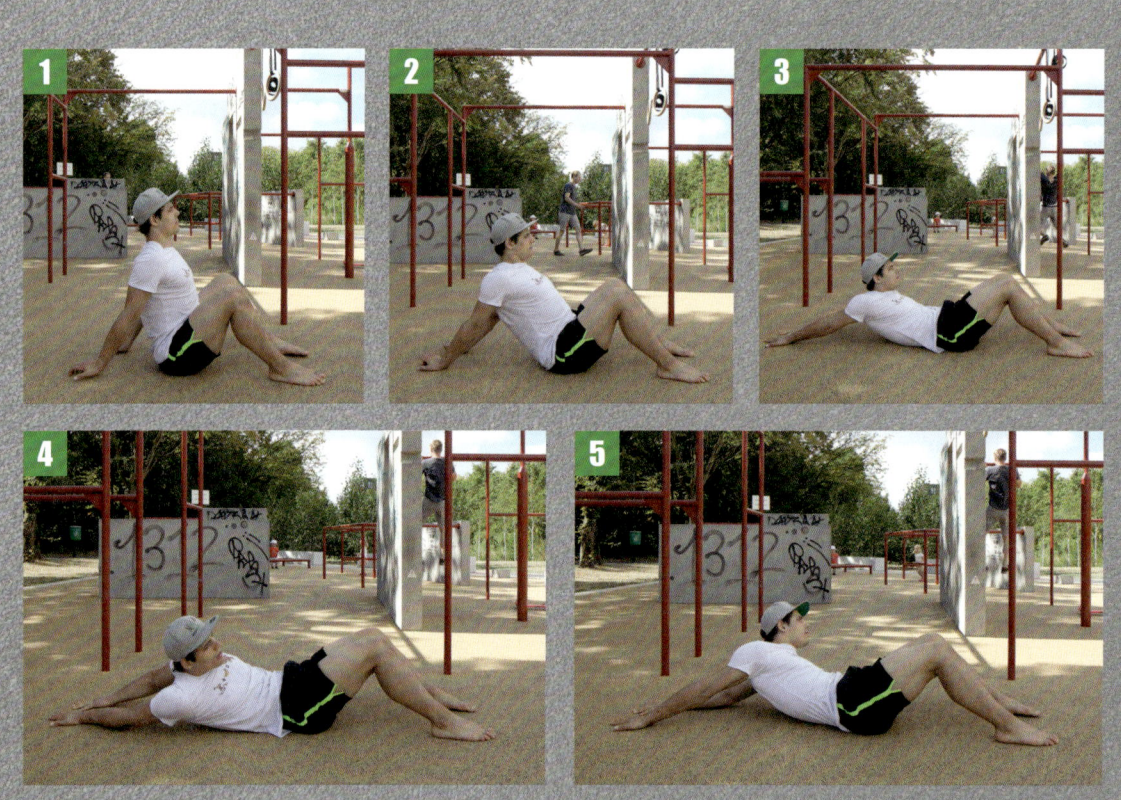

4. Crawl your hands approximately two to three hand-lengths back toward your body and circle your shoulders forward and backward.

5. As a final variation, you can also bend and straighten your arms.

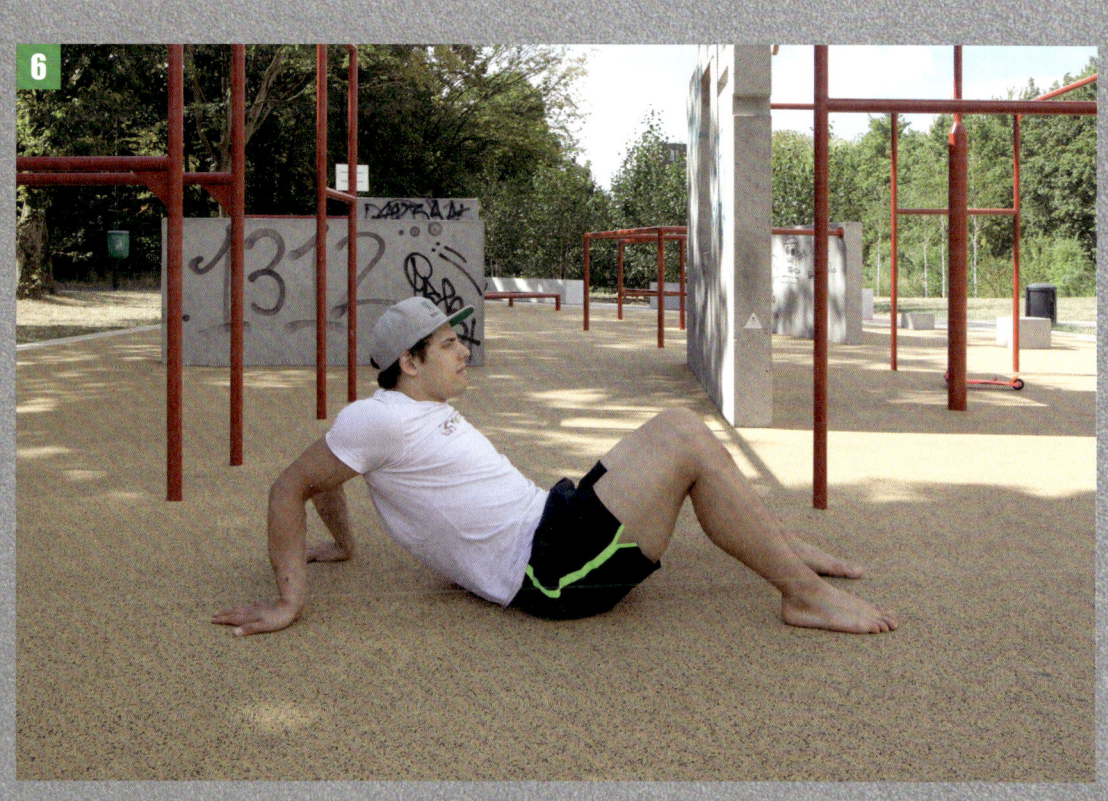

7.3.7 SWIMMER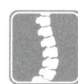

1. Lie on your stomach (with your forehead resting on the ground).

2. Rest your hands on your low back with your shoulders rotated inward.

3. Lift your arms away from your back.

4. Straighten your arms. As you move your arms (extended) overhead, rotate your arms outward (external shoulder rotation—see 10.9).

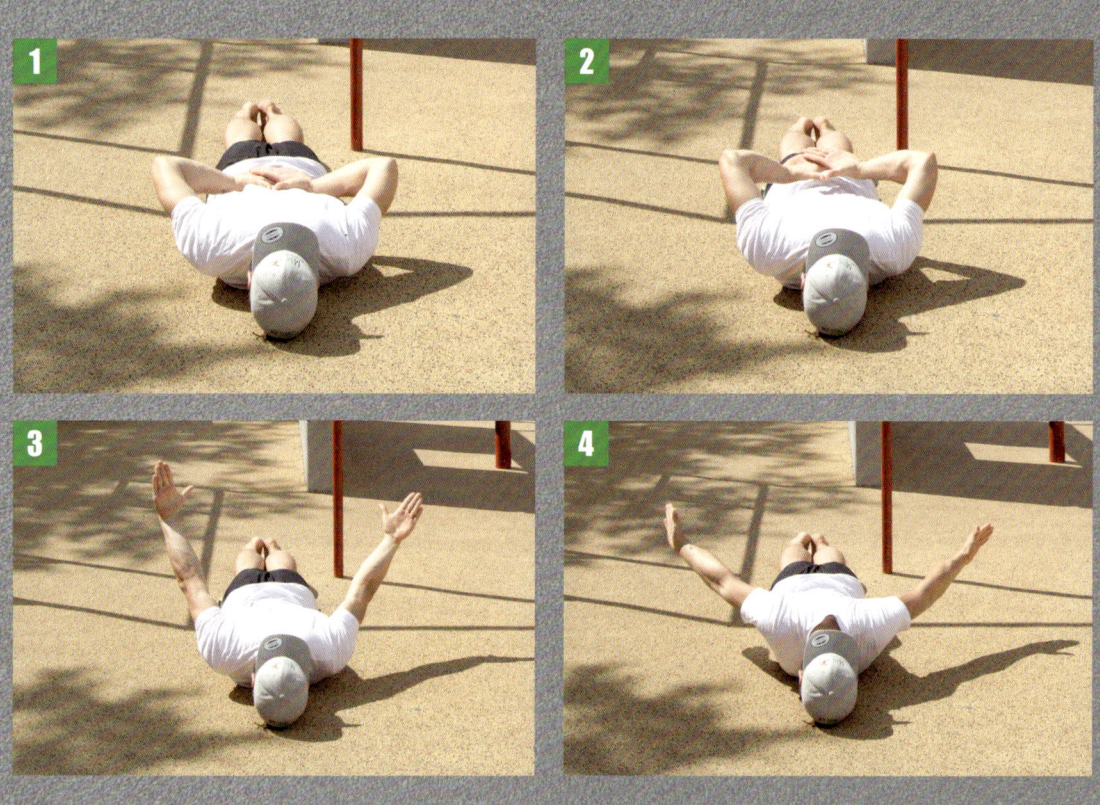

Mobility Exercises

5. In their uppermost position, your arms should be parallel and still extended. (Also pull your shoulders up toward your ears—a shoulder elevation).

6. Bend your elbows, rest your hands on your head, and then relax your arms for a brief moment.

7. When returning to the starting position, make sure to rotate your arms inward from the overhead position.

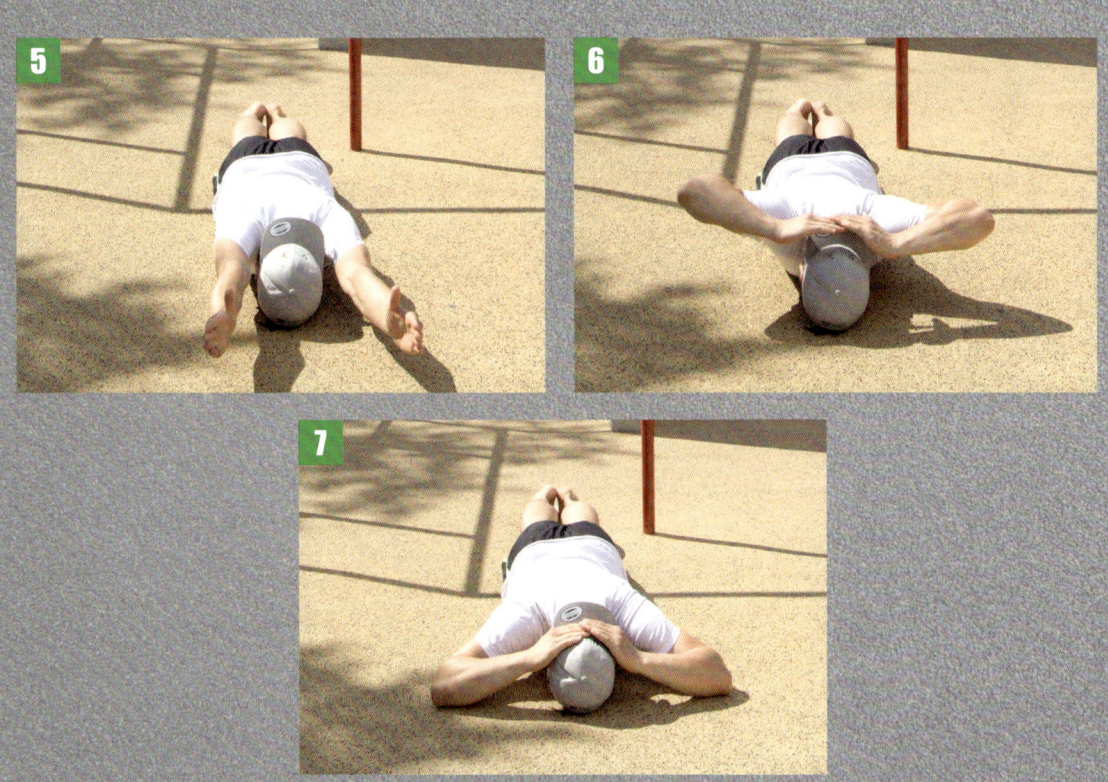

7.3.8 PROTRACTION AND RETRACTION DRILL 🍌🍌🍌

1. Stand facing a wall, your arms extended forward.

2. Pull your fingertips toward you, flexing your wrists, and lean forward against the wall.

3. Begin the exercise by protracting your shoulder blades (and depressing your shoulders).

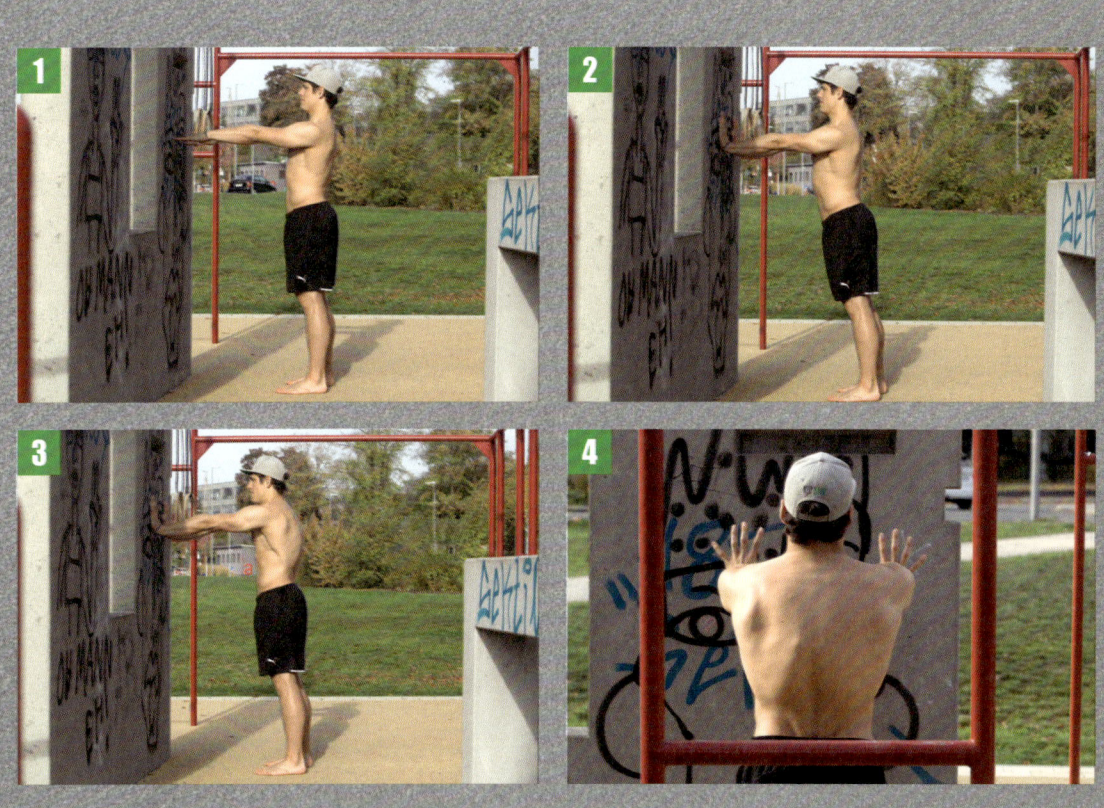

4. Remove your arms (still extended) from the wall and push your shoulders out a little farther.

5. Lean forward against the wall once more and retract your shoulders.

6. Repeat step 4, but this time, retract your shoulders even more.

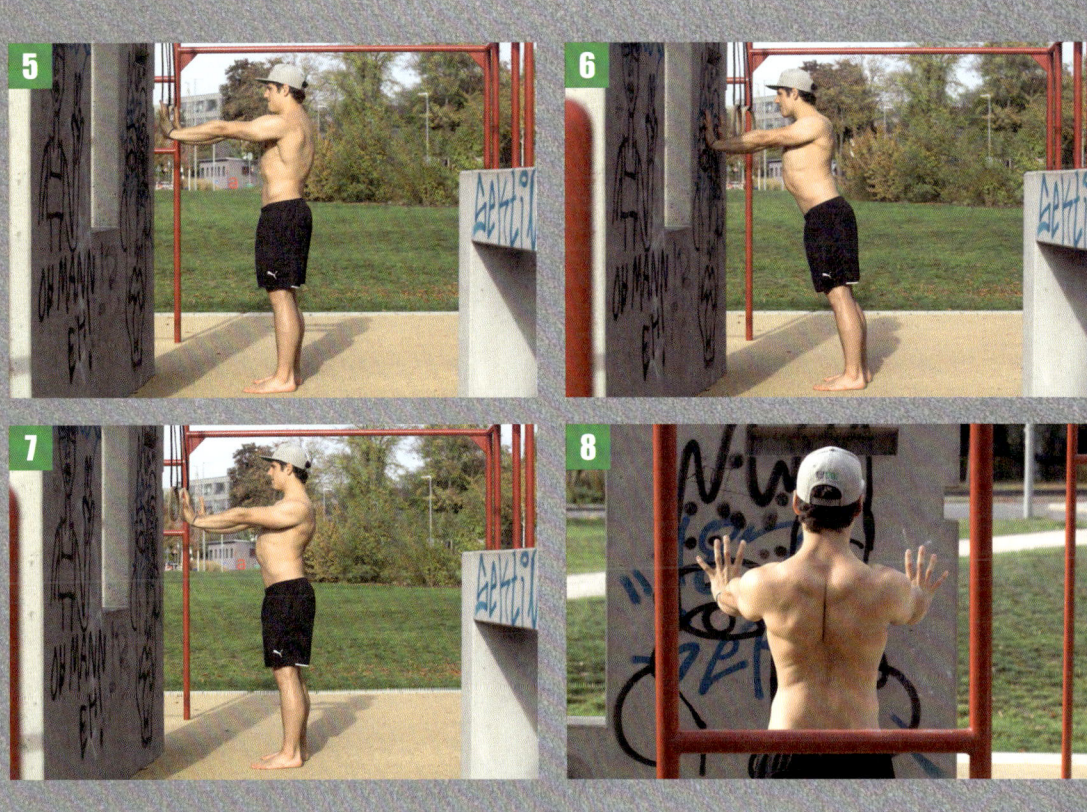

7.3.9 SHOULDER DISLOCATOR (WITH A BAND)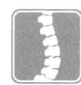

The name *shoulder dislocator* is a little misleading, since your shoulders don't actually dislocate during this exercise.

You may already be familiar with this exercise from your fitness facility, but at such facilities, it's usually performed with a bar. I prefer a band because it provides steady resistance and mobilizes your shoulders much more.

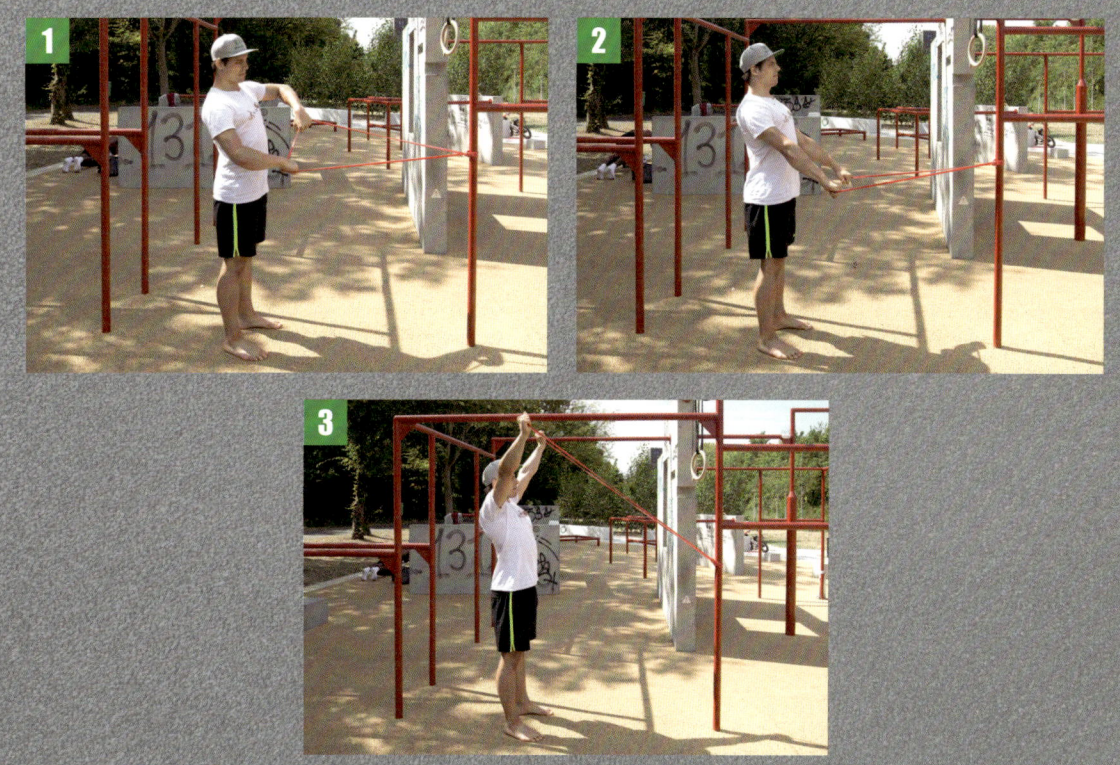

Mobility Exercises

1. Use a lightweight, looped resistance band and attach it at hip level to a pole.

2. With both hands, hold the band from the inside and stand tall in front of it.

3. Pull it overhead, and when you can't go any farther, pull it apart and move your arms behind you until you've closed the circle.

4. As you return to the starting position, make sure to maintain tension on the band.

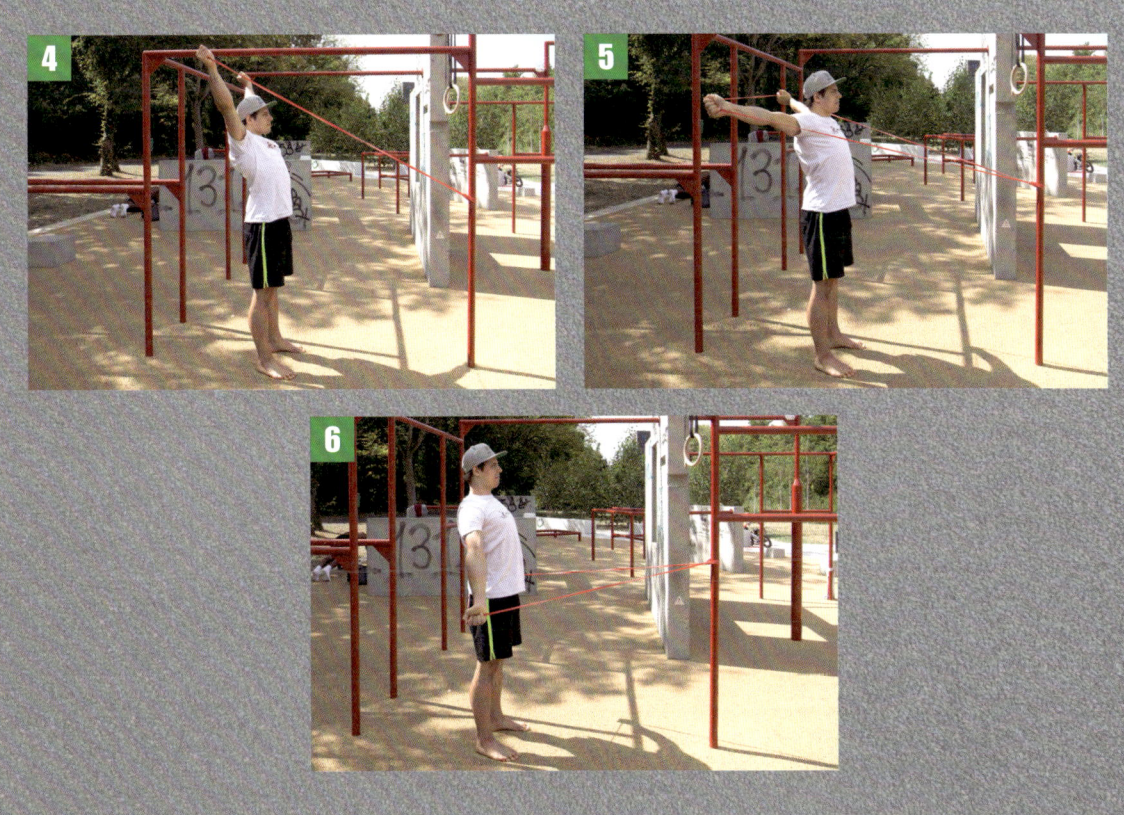

7.3.10 SHOULDER ROTATION WITH A BAND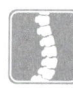

1. Grip the band and stand so that it is behind you.

2. Rest your arm against your back (internal shoulder rotation).

3. Extend and externally rotate the arm (external shoulder rotation—see 10.9).

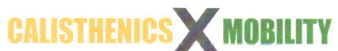

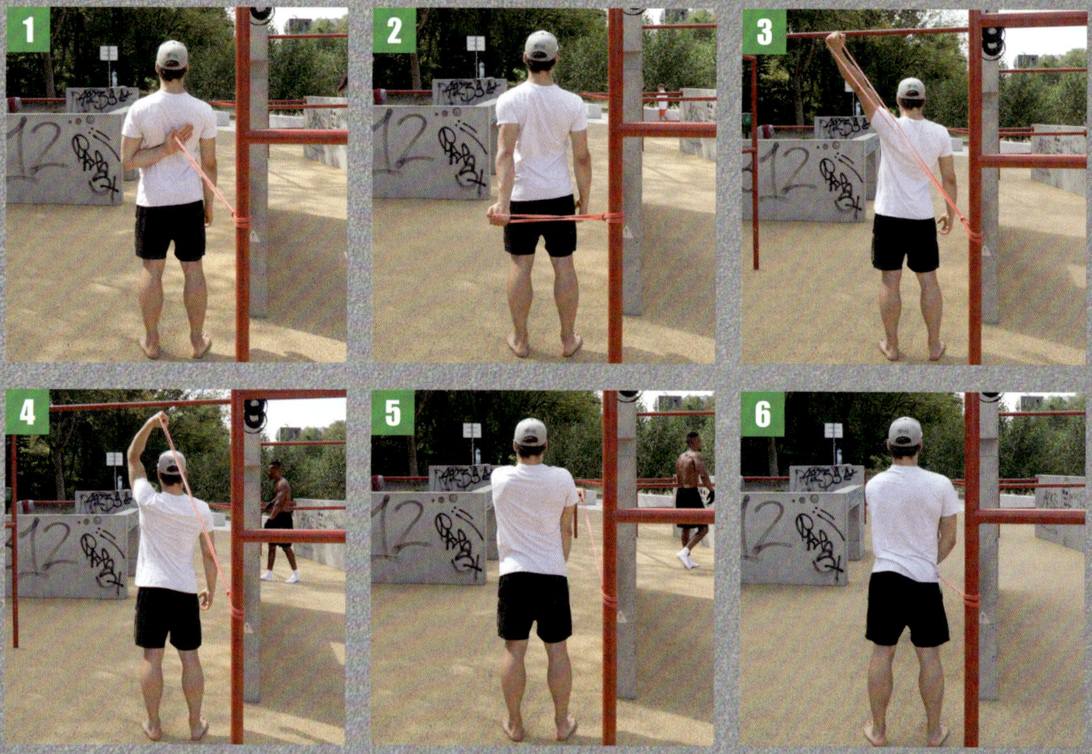

Mobility Exercises 137

4. With your elbow slightly bent, move the band overhead and on toward the opposite hip.

5. In its highest position, internally rotate your arm again as you return it to the starting position.

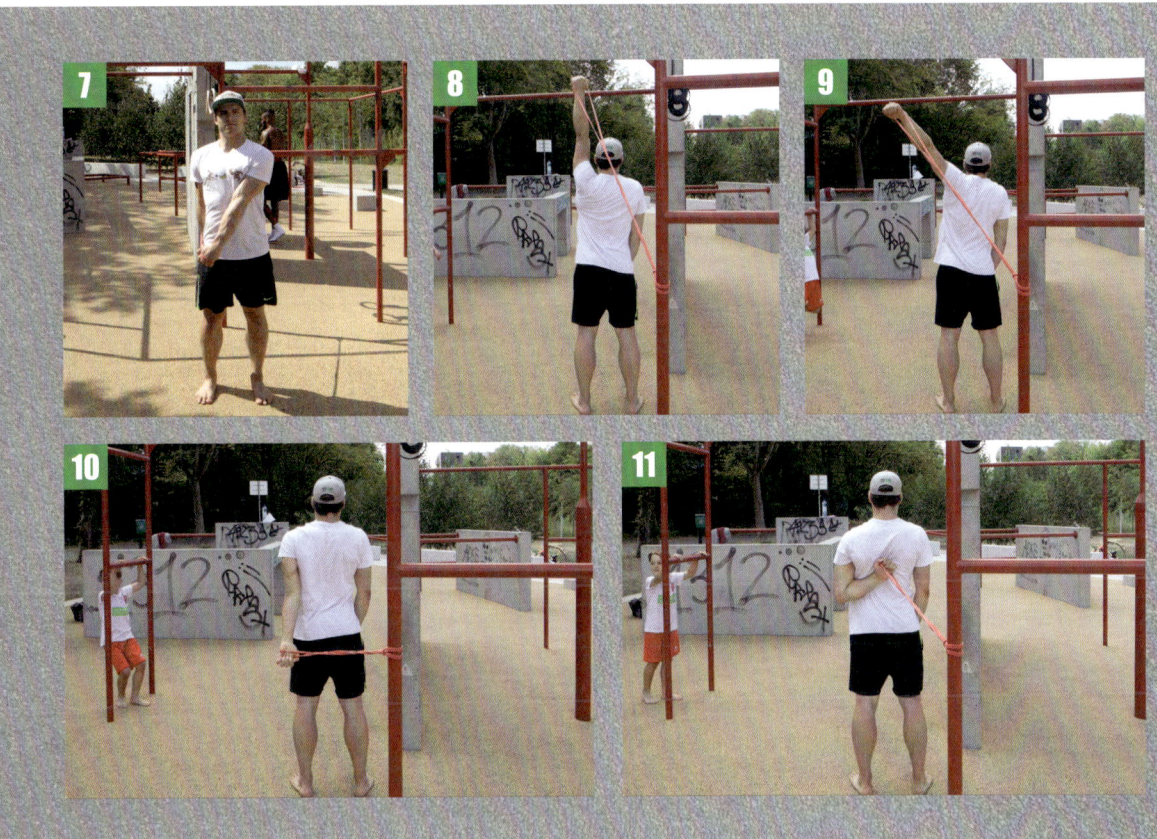

7.3.11 SIDE BEND 🍌

1. The basic setup is the same as that of the more-difficult variation of cobra (see 7.2.13).

2. Open your body to one side and cross the top leg in front of the leg resting on the ground and plant the top foot on the ground.

3. Lean into the ring and alternate between active and passive hanging and leaning in.

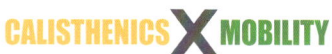

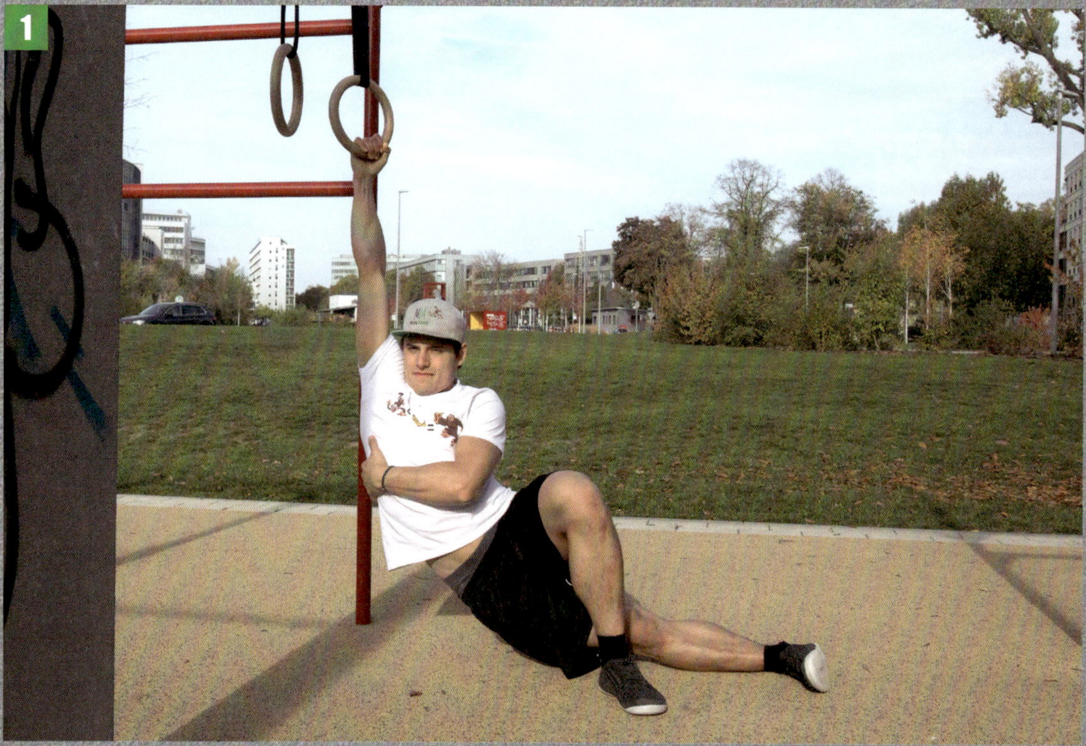

Mobility Exercises

TIP

If lifting your arm is still too difficult, keep your arm in the lower position and move away from the attachment point in order to increase tension on the band. This will allow you to work your rotator cuff isometrically so you can subsequently learn the elevation.

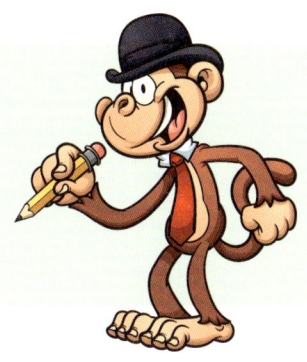

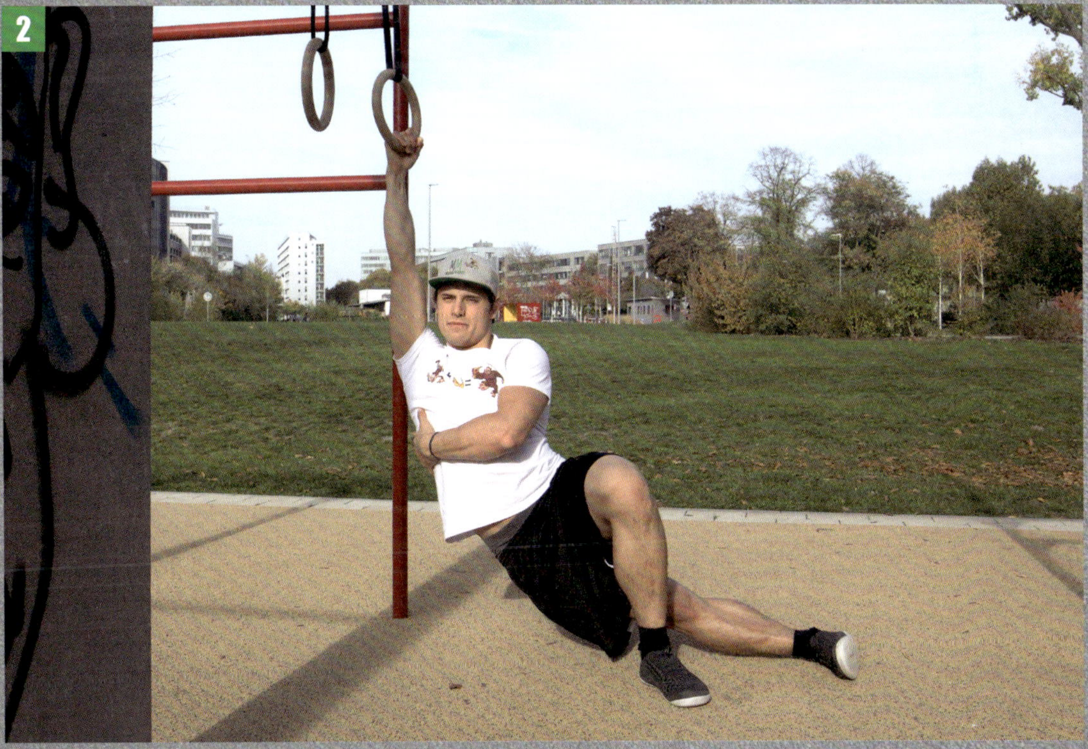

7.3.12 SKIN THE CAT (REGRESSION)

1. Find a low bar.

2. With your legs together, squat below the bar and grip the bar firmly.

3. Lift one leg ("free leg") and move it toward the bar.

4. Push off with the other leg ("takeoff leg") while your free leg finds the bar.

5. With your free leg, pull yourself around the bar. Let your takeoff leg follow and search for the ground to absorb your momentum.

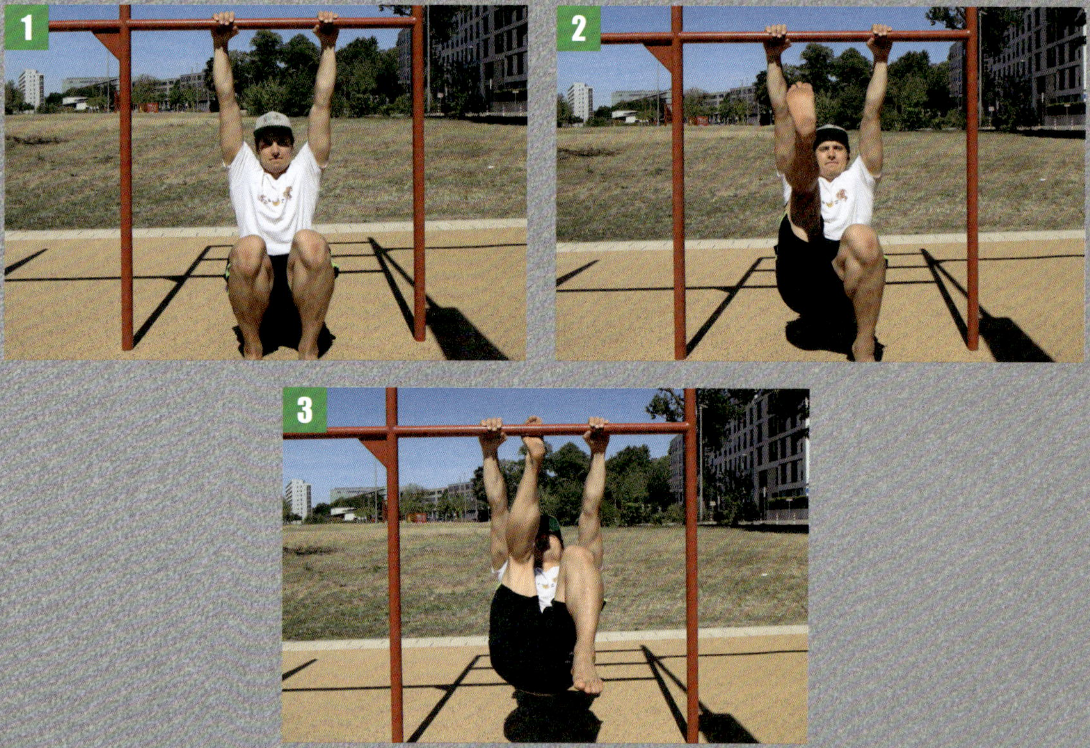

Mobility Exercises 141

6. On the way back to the starting position, use your takeoff leg again to get your legs up in the air while simultaneously pulling yourself back into the starting position with your arms.

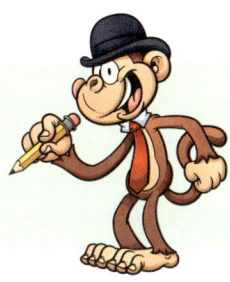

TIP

If you find this exercise too difficult, begin by practicing the shoulder crawl.

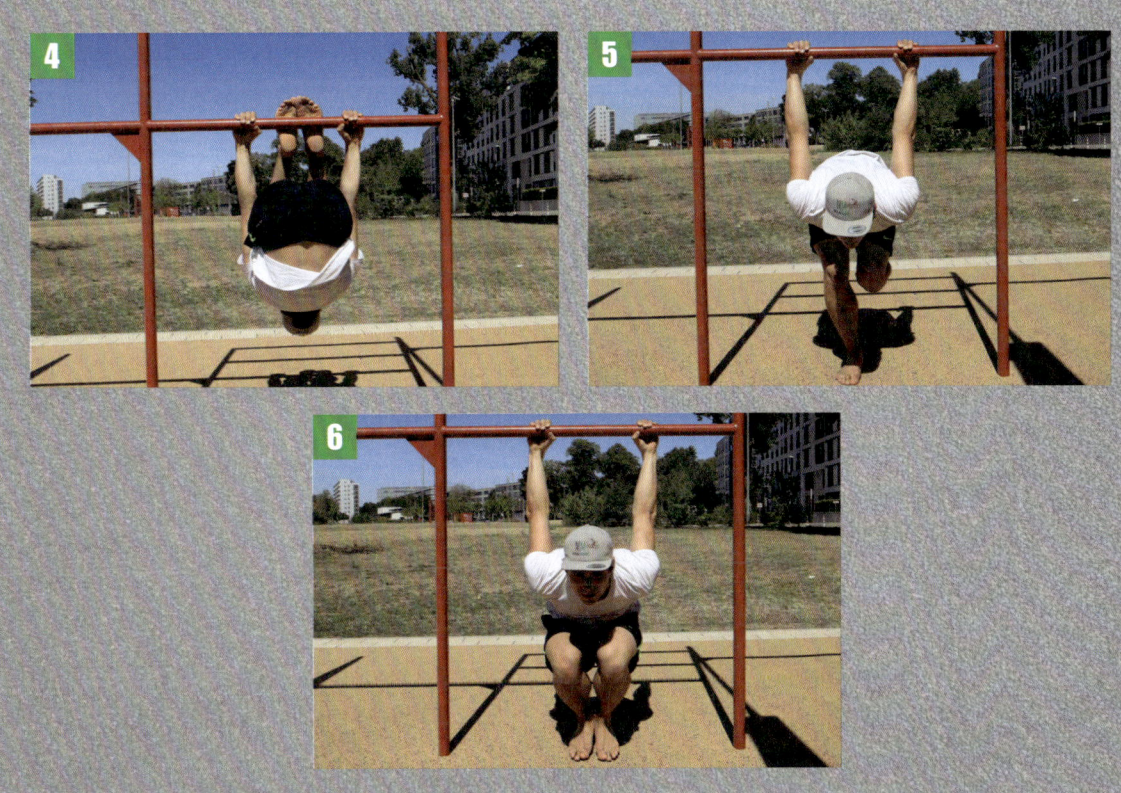

7.3.13 SKIN THE CAT

1. While hanging from the bar, perform a leg raise (see subsection 11.7.3 "Assisting Exercises").

2. You can do this with your elbows bent, although it doesn't look as good and doesn't automatically strengthen your abs.

3. Use your arm strength and shoulder strength to pull yourself around the bar (your legs slip through your arms).

4. Slowly lower your legs until you've reached the limit of your range of motion (end range).

5. Then begin to make your way back to the starting position.

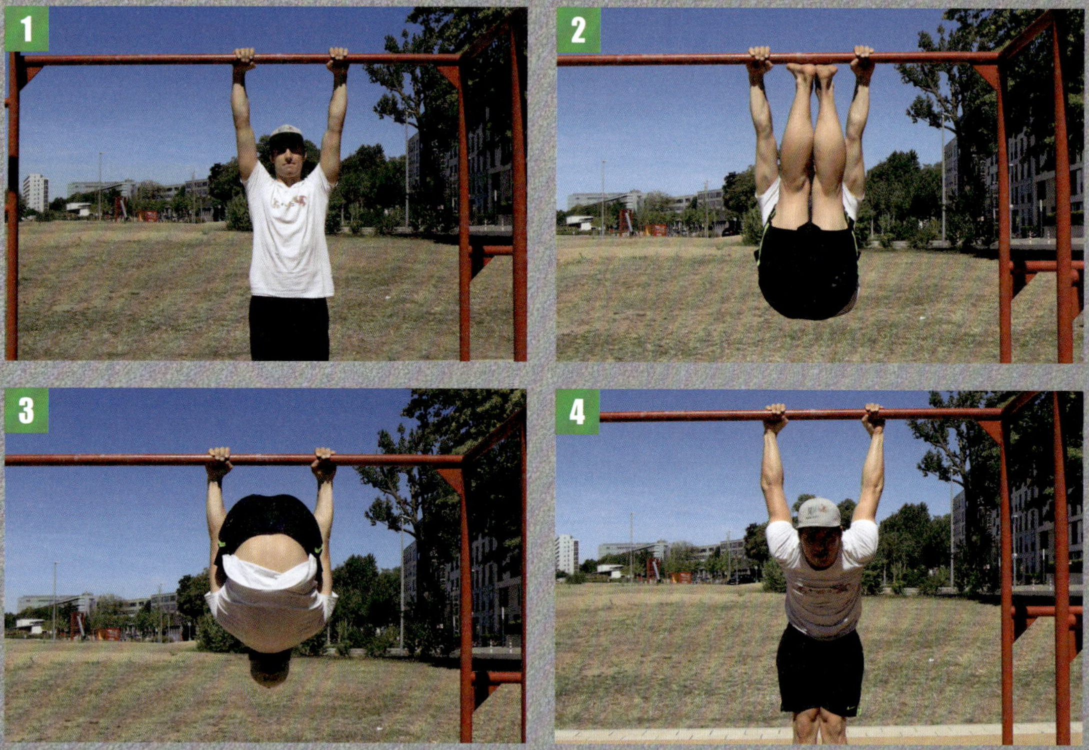

Mobility Exercises

7.3.14 SCAPULA PUSH-UP ROTATION 🍌🍌🍌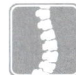

1. Begin in a plank position with your legs shoulder-width apart. (If you're unfamiliar with the basic plank position, read about it in section 11.4, "Push-ups and Possible Progressions.")

2. Lift one arm off the ground and rest it on the other shoulder.

3. Rotate toward your open side by using your shoulder strength to push yourself up.

4. Hold the position at the highest point and then let yourself sink slowly back into the neutral position so your shoulders are lined up once more.

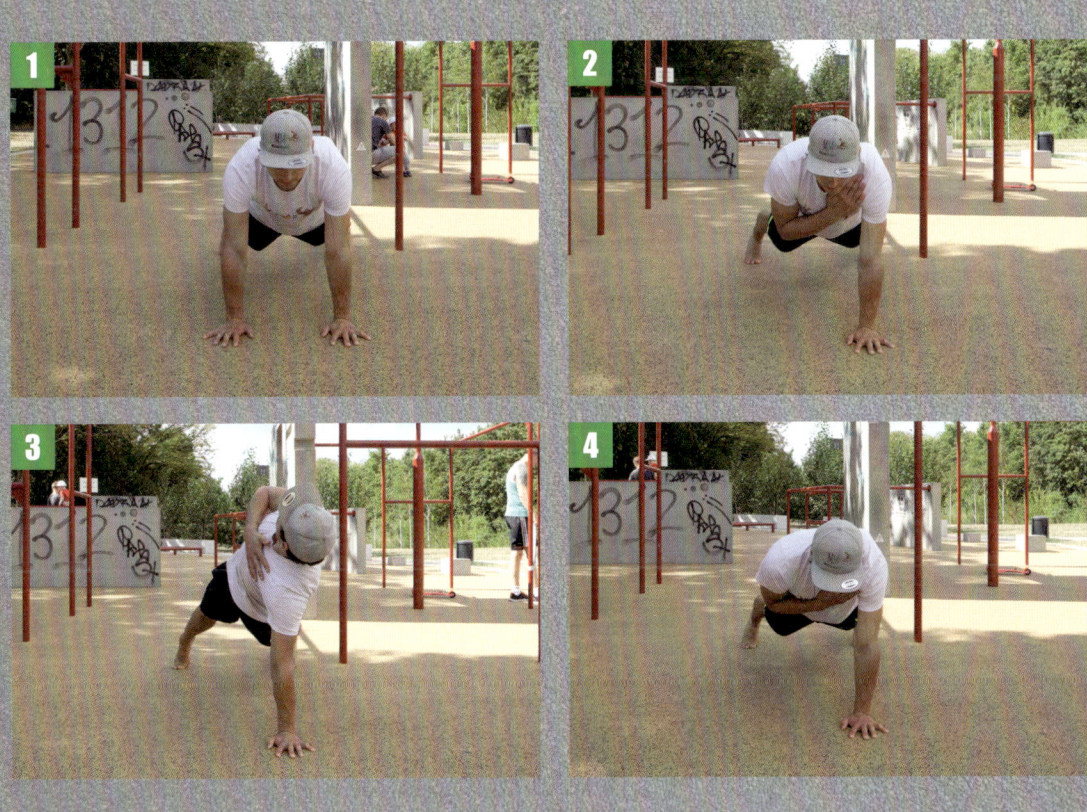

7.3.15 ARCHED-BACK PULLS

1. Hang from a bar.

2. Bend your knees to allow better activation of your posterior chain.

3. Pull yourself into an active hanging position.

4. While actively hanging, imagine screwing your arms into the bar (internal shoulder rotation) while simultaneously pulling your body farther back and up without bending your elbows.

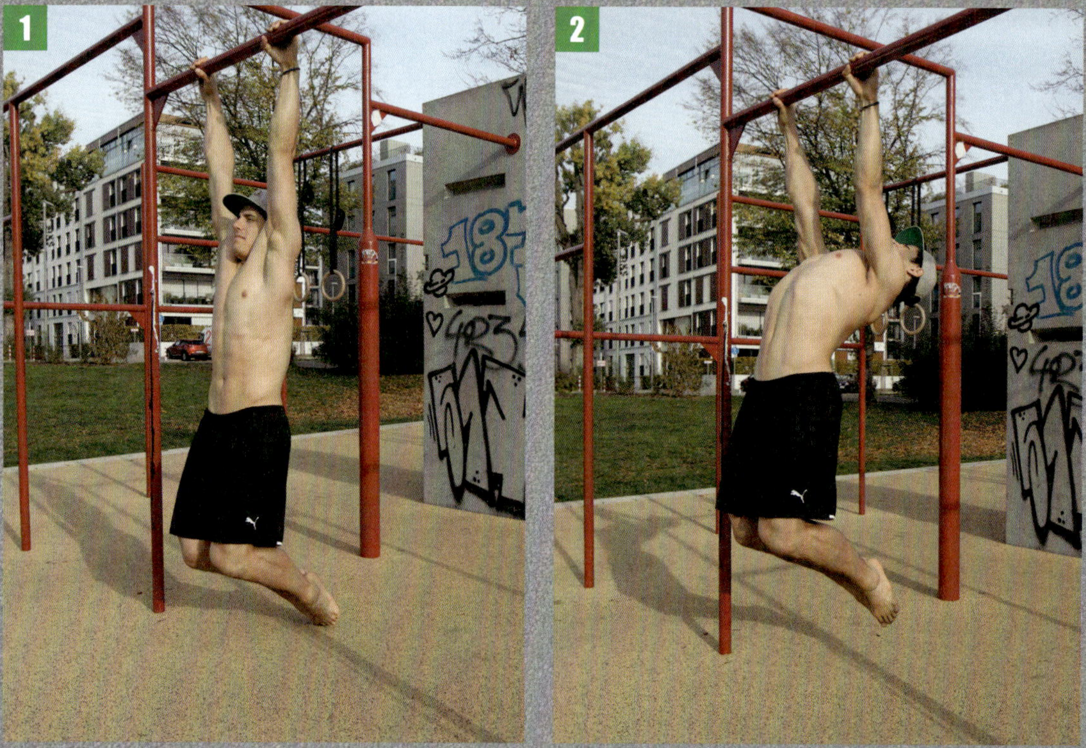

Mobility Exercises 145

5. Effectively, push the bar away from you while trying to pull farther into the active hanging position and squeezing your shoulder blades together in the uppermost position.

6. This exercise is an ideal preparatory exercise for arched-back pull-ups (see Monique's subsection 11.3.6, "Arched-Back Pull-ups").

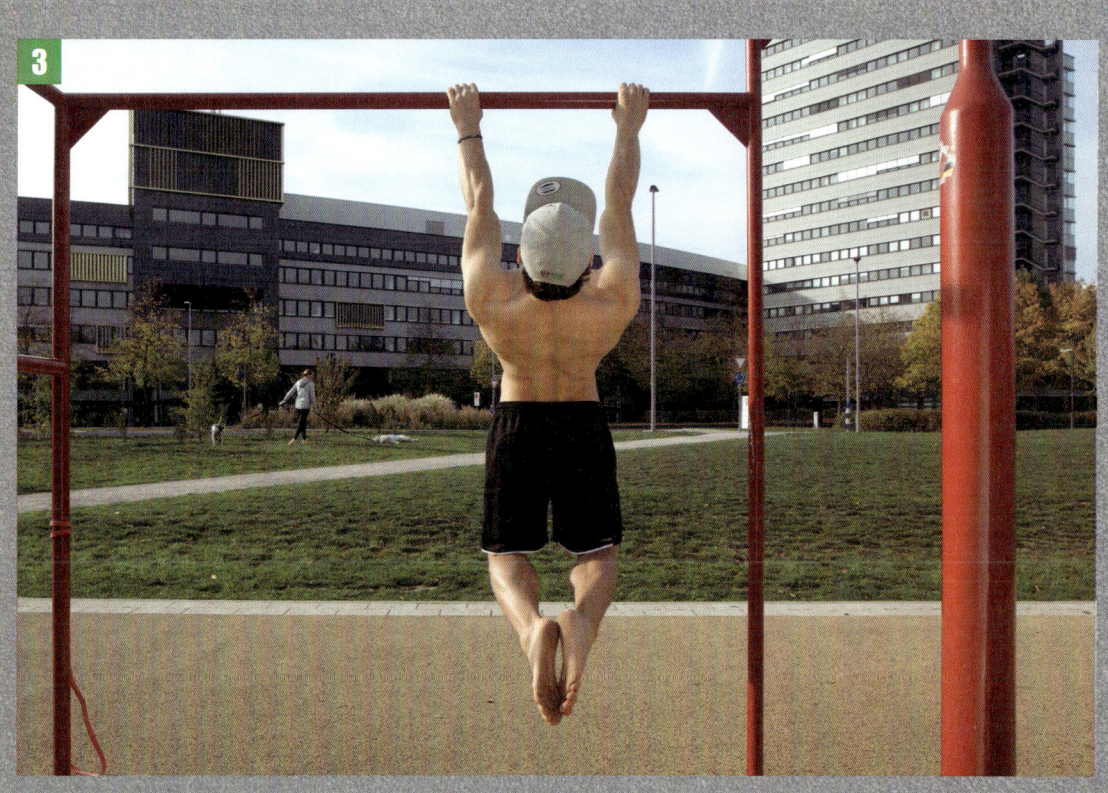

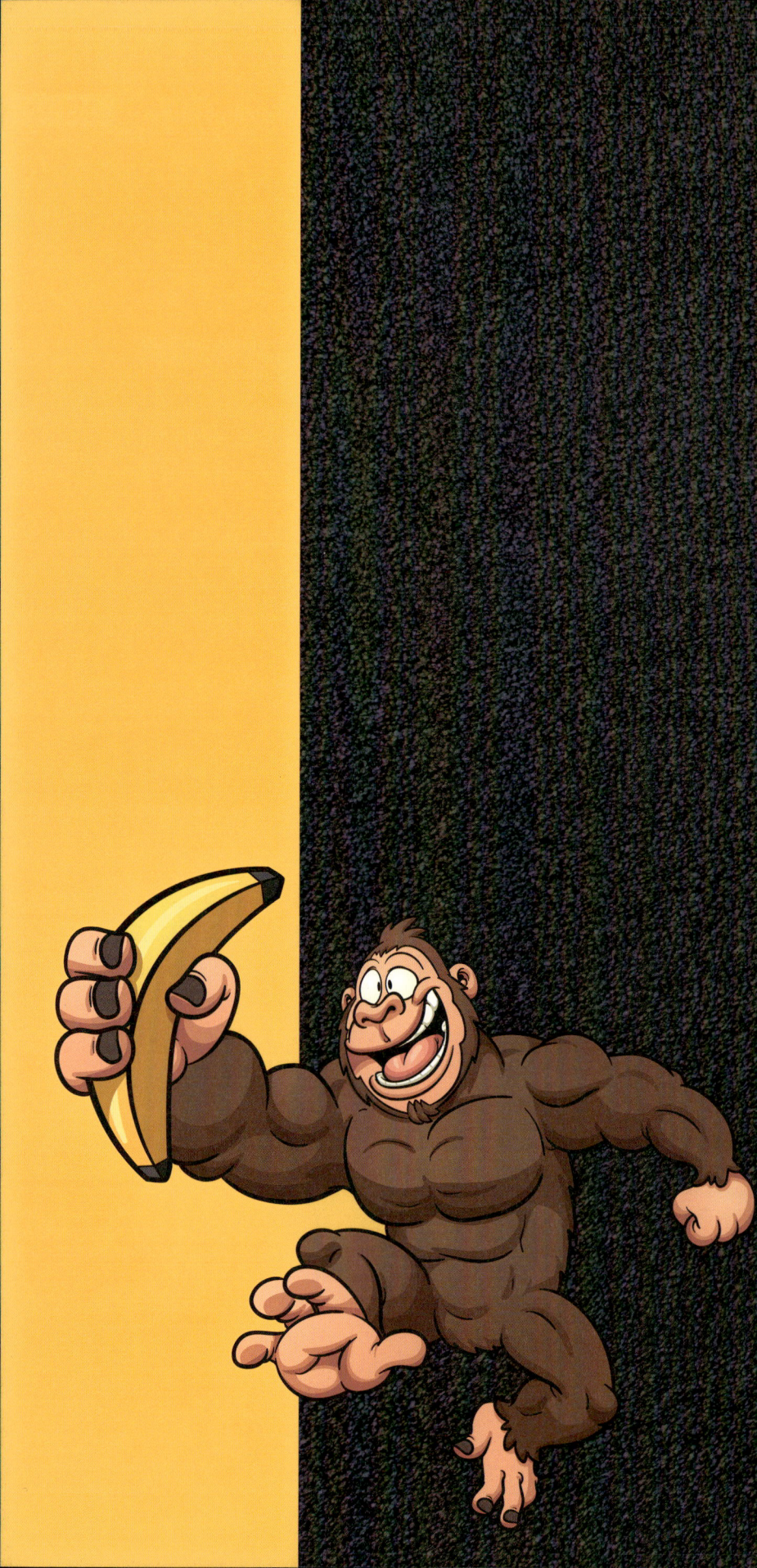

CALISTHENICS

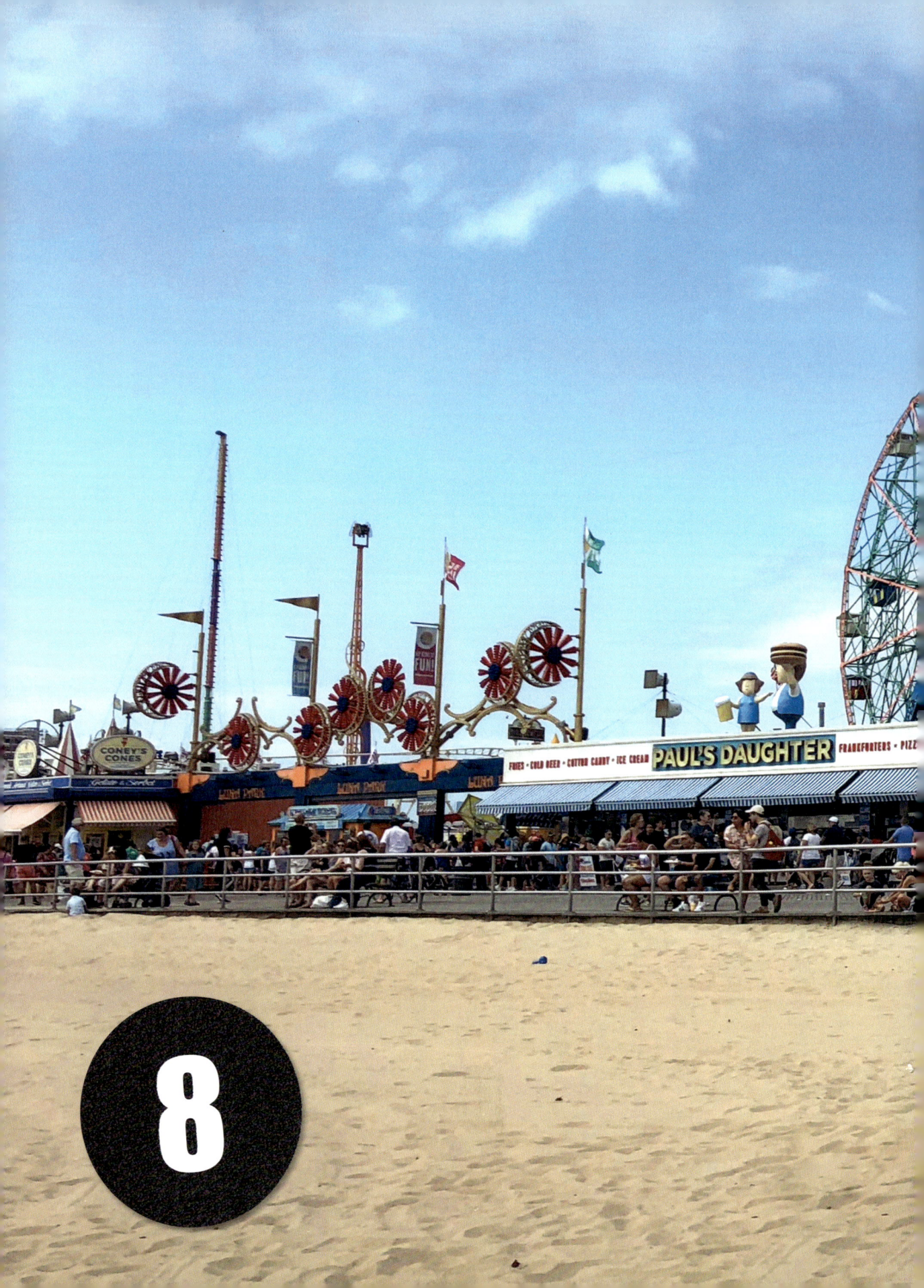

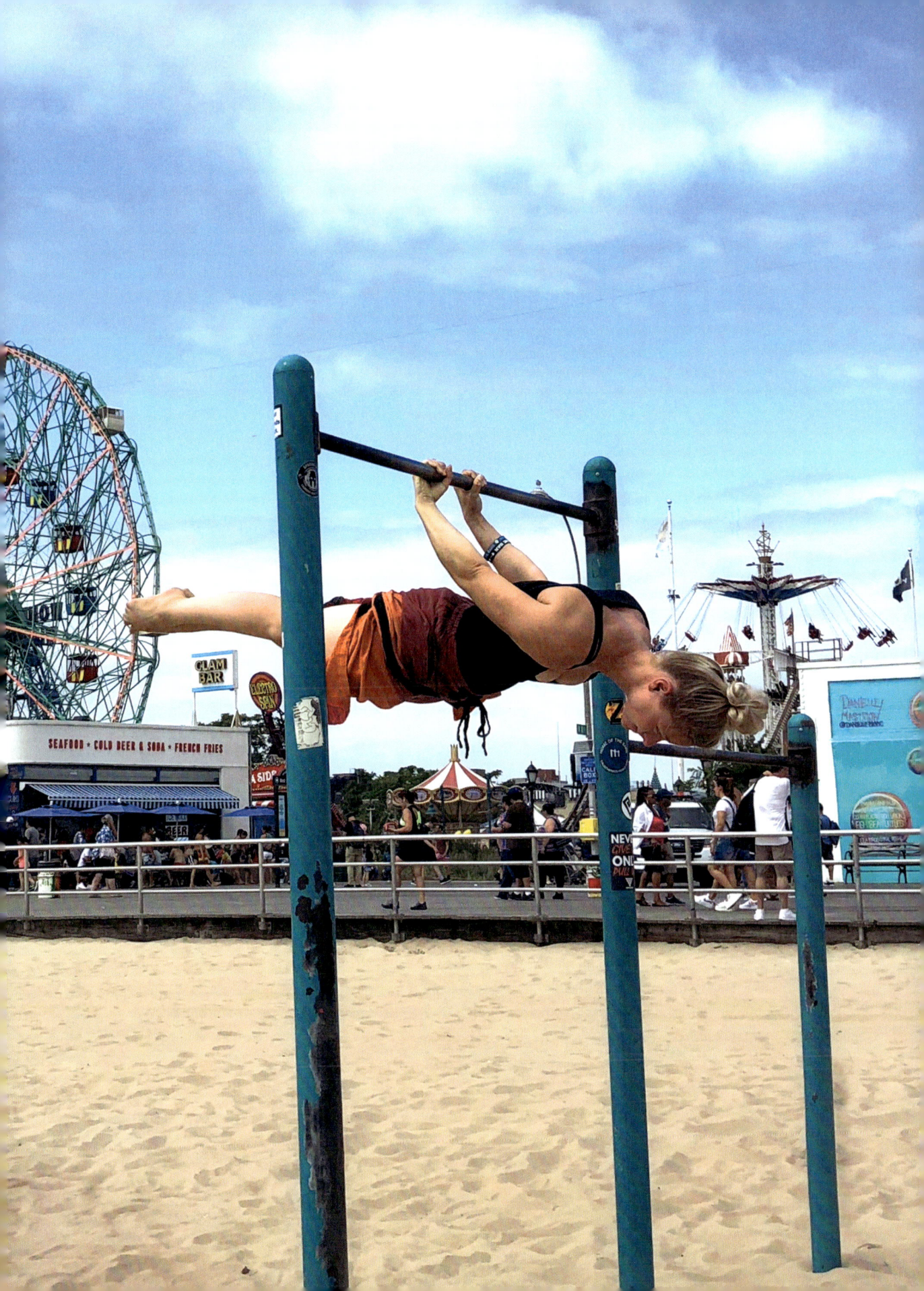

8   My Path to the Pull-up Bar

Calisthenics is a sport that's dominated my life since the winter of 2014. I'd started to train in the fall of 2013, mostly on some construction scaffolding at University of Düsseldorf. I credit my partner at the time, Paul Böhme (cofounder of **Calisthenics Parks**), with my passion and present vocation. He'd already been practicing this sport for some time and gave me my first instructions and exercises.

It wasn't long before I managed to do my first pull-up, which I thought would be easy due to my athletic career in my youth (see chapter 15, "The Authors"). Wrong! Although I was able to perform the other basics quite well at that point, pull-ups weren't part of my skill set. So I was really proud when my repetition numbers went up. My training occasionally stagnated, so I made changes to provide new stimuli and take my performance to a higher level.

In addition to my minor in sports studies, I trained four to five times a week, initially by myself—until I learned about an interest group in Erfurt, Germany, which (thanks to my contacts in the athletic department of University of Erfurt) subsequently established itself as an athletic club, under the name of **EFC Calisthenics**. My position there was quickly established, which certainly was also a result of my expertise in the sports industry. I'd been serving as a trainer before joining the club and taught regular units in any kind of weather. I saw lots of people come and go, get stronger, and miss workouts due to injuries. I received lots of positive feedback for my commitment and the time I invested on top of my studies and part-time jobs. By contrast, other classmates didn't seem to understand what I was doing and either admired or derided my time-intensive hobby during my university studies.

Subsequently, as the assistant department head, I made plans with the department management and the board of the university's sports association for our own calisthenics park in Erfurt because such a facility didn't exist at that time. We practiced pull-ups on the four-sided fence at the Brühl gardens out of necessity and later rented a space in a hall in a nearby village for the winter. Since, by then, some cities were already equipped with such parks, we also wanted one for our city and our club.

We all helped dig passages for the power and lighting system, drilled holes in the concrete foundations with specialty tools, used screws to anchor the posts for pull-up bars and parallel bars, and froze our tails off in the frigid temperatures of November 2016. The building project took three years and, in April 2017, our facility opened on the university campus in Erfurt. From then on, there were no longer any makeshift bars mounted to a wall of the university's athletic building.

It was the beginning of a proper training site, with enough space for all the club's members, and the end of the desperate search for suitable locations and round bars.

During the time we were building the training site, I was also quickly becoming pretty good at calisthenics and made my mark as the first woman in Germany to make a name for herself in calisthenics. I needed some persuading to use social media to motivate others and offer tips. Bernhard from Wieden in Austria quickly recognized my talent and insisted I attend his annual athletic event and hold a workshop on calisthenics.

No sooner said than done. In August 2015, Bernhard paid for my flight to Austria and hosted me there. The era of calisthenics workshops had begun. I held my first workshop, Only for Girls, in Germany in May 2016 (in Bebra near Bad Hersfeld). I wanted to get more women excited about the sport and get them on the bar. Unfortunately, this concept wasn't very popular, which is why I expanded it to include men and offered calisthenics for all. During the workshops, I taught the basics, both practical and theoretical, and a few advanced skills. But the highest priority was—and is—always a technically clean execution along the lines of this principle: **quality beats quantity**.

In addition to the workshops, I participated in competitions and was able to score some wins. Power competitions consisted of the basics, like pull-ups, dips, and push-ups. Since I started calisthenics training with sets and reps (other types are covered in section 9.3, "The Four Types of Calisthenics"), doing lots of repetitions was something I was used to. I realized fairly early on that I no longer enjoyed preparing for competitions strictly by increasing the number of repetitions. Calisthenics has so much more to offer, which is why I stopped competing and restructured my training. I focused more on skills like the handstand and the back lever but still liked to integrate different sets and reps into my training. I became more versatile and stronger than ever.

In February 2017, I completed my master's thesis on the topic "The Positive Effects of Calisthenics on the Physical Perception of Elementary School Children: A Plea for the Introduction of Calisthenics in Physical Education." It was a project close to my heart, which I still promote today under the slogan "Calisthenics catches on—ditch the TV and get on the bar!" and for which I'm currently still seeking volunteer PE instructors to generate evidence-based studies to be used in a new book project.

I met Leon Staege of Moving Monkey in early 2017. He introduced me to mobility, and I showed him the most-important tools of the trade for calisthenics. But before I had a chance to combine the two, my training schedule was blown up by a shoulder injury. From that moment on, I could no longer do pushing and pulling motions the way I was used to. Instead, I did lots of mobility and stability exercises around the shoulder girdle. My eighteen-month break from calisthenics training showed me how valuable these exercises would have been at the beginning of my calisthenics career and how they might have been able to prevent me from getting injured. But mobility training had been popular since 2016.

The injury caused me to think even further outside the box, and as a result, I gained quite a bit of knowledge about healthy training. Leon and I now collaborate to share our knowledge at workshops named Calisthenics X Mobility, showing people how to stay healthy while training.

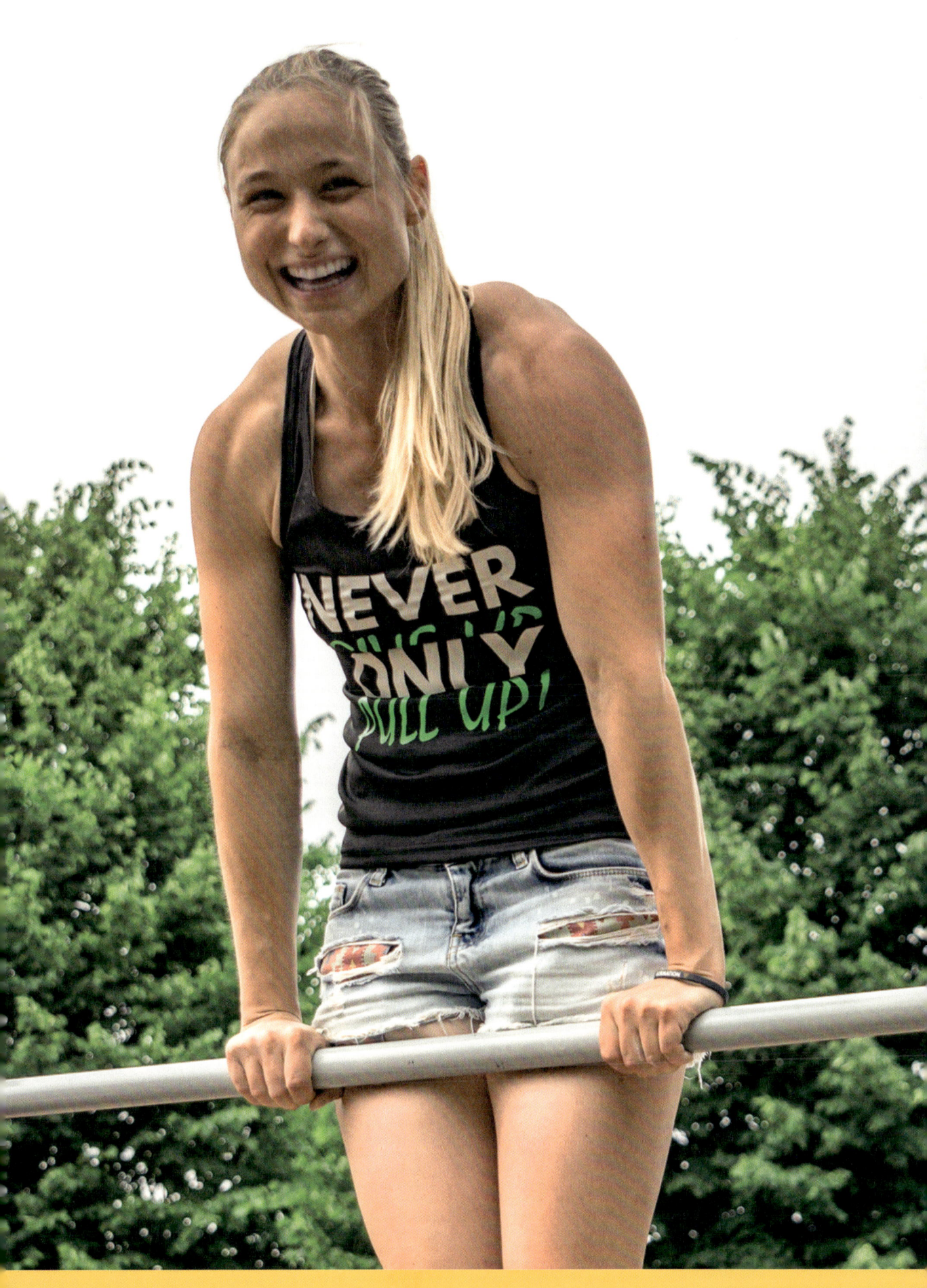

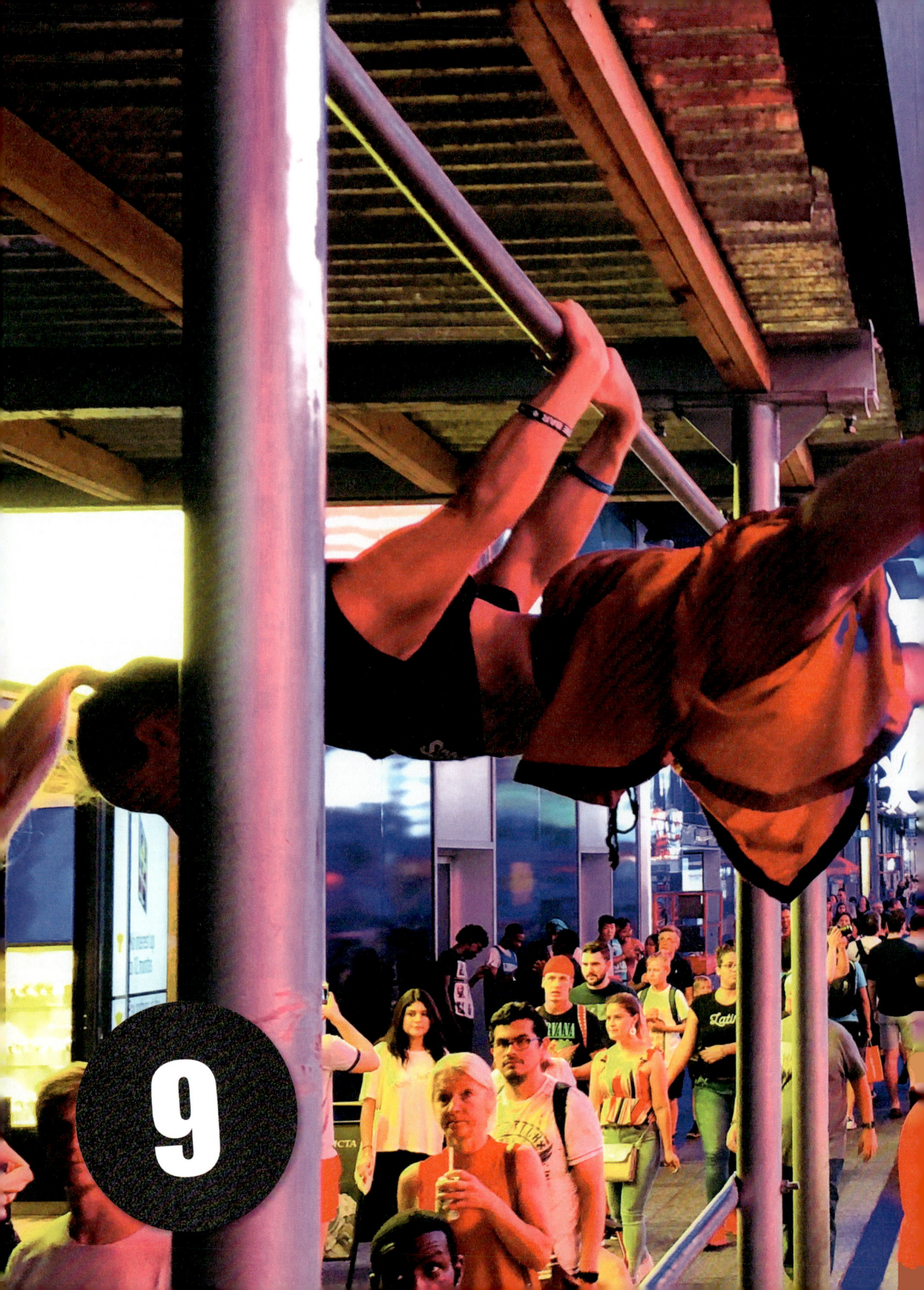

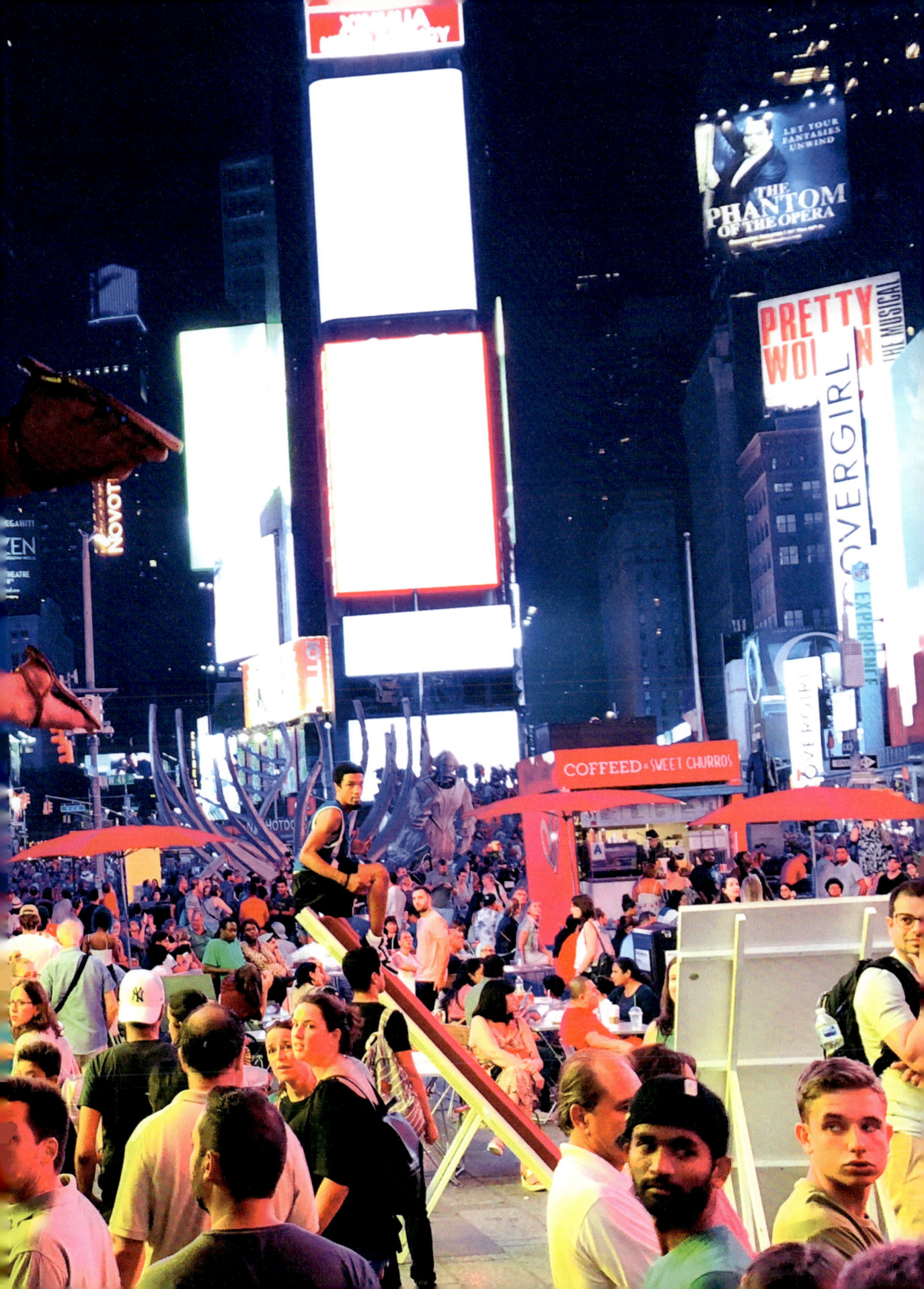

9 Calisthenics

So often I hear absolute newbies to calisthenics say, "I want to be able to do the human flag. Where do I start?" OK, before you even begin to worry about that, stop copying exercises you've seen other people perform, and ask yourself if you can meet the physical requirements for that advanced exercise.

Truly, anyone can start doing calisthenics, but please do so based on your current performance level. Anything else will inevitably, sooner or later, lead to injuries. Start at your fitness level and perfect the basics (pull-ups, push-ups, dips, and squats) before you start to dream. I say this not to discourage you but explicitly to save you from making mistakes many others have already made and most likely could have avoided had they known what we know today.

9.1 ROOTS OF CALISTHENICS

Calisthenics, also called *street workouts*, consists of physical exercises based on simple and basic movement patterns. In the 19th century, American educator Catharine Beecher introduced calisthenics as a form of physical education, particularly for women. Around this time, those who practiced the gymnastic exercises developed by Friedrich Ludwig Jahn, the father of German gymnastics, brought these training concepts to the US. There, his classic bodyweight exercises were modified and combined with elements from calisthenics and other sports, like breakdancing, parkour, and freerunning. The new, modern calisthenics, with its typical elements, was created. Here, I'm referring to a newly coined name for an age-old type of physical exercise that uses one's own body (bodyweight training) without adding external weights. As the popularity of calisthenics grew, it was ultimately the calisthenics program of the Royal Canadian Air Force in the 1960s that helped secure its place in modern fitness culture. Calisthenics is still used today as baseline physical evaluations for the military (e.g., U.S. Army Physical Fitness Test and the U.S.M.C. Physical Fitnes Test).

Calisthenics

If people ask you what calisthenics is, simply tell them this:

> Calisthenics is nothing more than strength training with one's own body against gravity and with the use of levers (arms and legs), which allow you to vary the degree of difficulty. Calisthenics combines static and dynamic exercises primarily from gymnastics, which is why we say calisthenics is street gymnastics.

This sport uses apparatuses like pull-up bars for a variety of pulling exercises, parallel bars for pushing exercises, and monkey bars and wall bars that were freely accessible in many places in America. Because Catharine Beecher was from New York, it is considered the birthplace. There, sports parks allowed young people to train outside without a fitness facility.

The method's objective is to achieve overall fitness and resilience based on the resistance one's own bodyweight generates without isolated training of muscle groups. But in the course of this book, we clarify why isolated training of certain muscle groups is still important (see section 10.5, "Assistance Exercises").

Originally, a person used whatever his environment had to offer—be it vertical streetlights, scaffolding, or the like—to build strength with his own body. Over the years, outdoor facilities were built specifically for calisthenics, so now there are public or limited-use parks that can be used for training. Section 9.9, "Calisthenics Parks: The Best Spots for Your Training," will tell you where and how to find suitable places.

The wishful thinking that calisthenics is a sport that's independent of time, place, and equipment is only partly true and, even so, under only certain conditions. In section 9.8, "Useful Equipment," you'll learn which equipment makes sense to use. Ultimately, your surroundings will determine if, where, and how you can train.

9.2 THE RAIN-OR-SHINE TRAINING MENTALITY

Cold weather entices a growing number of athletes to resort to a weatherproof and independent indoor alternative, which is the why the original concept of "training out on the street," independent of fitness studio memberships, has dwindled away. But you can hardly blame many advanced athletes. That "I train outside rain or shine, during every season" mentality is the wrong approach and points to some not very intelligent training.

Sure, it might make you less susceptible to illness, because you're strengthening your immune system, but it won't make you better at the sport. Preventing hypothermia during wintery temperatures necessitates HIIT (high-intensity interval training) units, which makes little sense at an advanced stage. This is also true with respect to regular breaks, which can be up to three minutes long in the maximum-strength area in order to regenerate participating muscles as well as the nervous system for the next set.

An optimal training environment is priceless and will help you make more training progress than cold hands and slick surfaces. So if you really want to get strong, you should set aside your "only the strong survive" airs, don't even consider gloves, and train sensibly without trudging through the winter season. I also enjoy training outside and use every opportunity to do so. It's just a different feeling. You're in the fresh air, have lots of open space to let off steam. But every once in a while, you need equipment that isn't available out in nature. When it gets too cold, I do my training indoors so I can stay focused.

9.3 THE FOUR TYPES OF CALISTHENICS

Calisthenics, as I understand it, should be divided into four categories.

CATEGORY ONE: SETS AND REPS

There are the classic sets-and-reps advocates who practice calisthenics primarily in the area of strength endurance. Depending on performance level, they do lots of sets with lots of repetitions of the basics. They usually combine different exercises in a circuit (push-ups, pull-ups, dips). Such a set might look like this: ten reps of bar muscle-ups (advanced skill combo of a pull-up and a dip), ten reps of dips, and ten reps of pull-ups, without leaving the bar.

CATEGORY TWO: WEIGHTED CALISTHENICS

Proponents of the sets-and-reps category usually also train with additional weights, doing *weighted calisthenics*, primarily to provide new stimuli and to take their training to a new performance level.

CATEGORY THREE: FREESTYLE (OR BARHOPPING)

Then there are freestylers, also called barhoppers. They prefer dynamic elements and, in doing so, perform spectacular rolls, jumps, and the like as a combo on the bar. They combine exercises, creating choreography.

CATEGORY FOUR: SKILL-FOCUSED

The fourth category includes calisthenics athletes who learn elements (skills) beyond the basics, which they practice with a focus on technique and perfect over their years of training.

Time and experience have shown that *hybrid workouts,* meaning a combination of multiple types of training and sports, are absolutely recommended to keep the body healthy. Mobility as a combination of mobility training and calisthenics supply the necessary balance between agility and stability. Beyond that, you can integrate any other sport into your daily workout, be it weightlifting, yoga, or dance. The more versatile, the better. You can find more on this in section 2.7, "How Mobility Makes You Stronger."

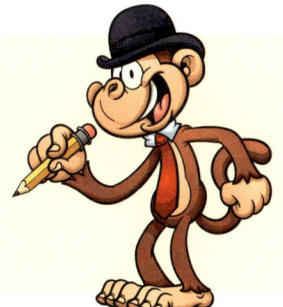

TIPS

To help you supplement mobility and calisthenics training, we recommend integrating something like kettlebells or hand weights for preventative or rehabilitative exercises. And finally, it's important to determine individual weak spots and imbalances and take the appropriate measures.

In all the possible calisthenics variations, fanatical calisthenics athletes aren't primarily focused on visual improvements but, rather, on controlling the body during the elements, with the goal of making them look as easy as possible. But you can't avoid the basics with any of these approaches (see section 10.1, "Overview of Basic Exercises").

9.4 FROM TREND SPORT TO BUSINESS: CALISTHENICS IN GERMANY

Calisthenics has changed over the years. Since I began practicing the sport in 2013, I've been able to observe this development. Back when I started with calisthenics, the scene in Germany was still very manageable. There were a few people here and there practicing the same sport. But the sport as it's practiced in America had not yet arrived in Germany. Even today, lots of people have no idea what calisthenics is. I learned from my former partner, who got inspiration for his own training from YouTube.

It was difficult to get information about the correct execution of the exercises. These days, the different social-media platforms on the internet, such as Facebook and YouTube, are overflowing with tutorials that provide beginners with tips on how to learn the different exercises. Lots of people who think they can impart knowledge try to give instructions. But these also include less-well-researched and less-well-edited tutorials, which is why it's difficult for a layperson to choose truly helpful and informative content. If you're really interested in the sport, you should delve deeper into the subject so you can differentiate the quality of the presentations.

As the only woman in Germany in the social-media public eye who practices the sport of calisthenics the way I do, I experience the trend's progression every day. After my entry into the sport, more and more interest groups were created in different cities, with their own names to differentiate them from others and make them more visible locally.

Their individual logos also had recognition value. They gathered at scene meetups, met at suitable locations in Germany with enough space for everyone, and trained together.

Athletes generally met at competitions that had been established over the years. Currently, we differentiate between *power competitions*, a competition in which men and women compete for the most repetitions of an exercise with and without additional weight, and *freestyle*. In section 9.3, "The Four Types of Calisthenics," these are divided into categories. The **WSWCF (World Street Workout and Calisthenics Foundation)** holds championships in all participating countries and invites the best athletes to the world championships, which are usually in Moscow.

This sense of community and the passion for the sport connected the community and created a regular exchange. In retrospect, these community meetups offered exactly what distinguished the calisthenics sport: helping, strengthening, and motivating each other.

Since 2017, anyone calling herself or himself a calisthenics athlete has wanted to profit from the sport. These athletes call themselves calisthenics trainers, sell training programs, and coach as personal trainers or online. While the sport is trendy and has potential, calisthenics is now commercialized. Money and sponsors play a major role and determine success or failure. Of course, other athletes in other European countries and beyond have already figured this out and approach it that way. In Germany, the formerly collaborative scene disappeared, and a chasm opened.

And with commercialization, competitiveness arose. As one of the calisthenic pioneers in Germany, I also felt the effects. People often forget that we all have the same goal: to get more people excited about calisthenics as a sport and to help them in word and deed. I learned to continue to pursue my mission, by myself and in cooperation with Leon, our "Calisthenics X Mobility" project, and other concepts. At the same time, I remain open to anything that's authentic and that I can represent to the best of my knowledge and belief.

9.5 CALISTHENICS VERSUS CROSSFIT VERSUS FREELETICS

In my opinion, calisthenics is different from other sports like CrossFit or Freeletics, which often are erroneously equated with calisthenics due to the clean execution of the exercises. The basic exercises are the same in all three sports. Pull-ups, dips, push-ups, and squats are part of any sport that focuses on using one's own bodyweight. Beyond that, there are basic exercises that are also part of endurance training for basketball players, soccer players, and triathletes. Thus, they're not new and aren't specific to calisthenics.

In calisthenics, the difference in these exercises is that the focus is on a technically clean execution. Time isn't your enemy, and it isn't about chasing certain records. If that's your only goal, you're exposing yourself to an increased risk of injury, particularly as an inexperienced beginner who hasn't mastered the basics. And there are skills that tend to be more gymnastic in nature and are considered advanced elements. CrossFit also includes gymnastic elements, but they're diverted, via *kipping*, to be completed as quickly as possible.

Ultimately, if you practice calisthenics noncompetitively, you're your own opponent. The focus is on learning a diverse spectrum of skills and body control. And besides, you'll make an impression and cause quite a stir in public if that's what you're after or if you train in public places. But if you just want to do it for physical fitness, stick to the basics and make sure your training is balanced.

9.6 WHY EVERYONE BENEFITS FROM BODYWEIGHT TRAINING

As I mention elsewhere, finances and location are important factors, depending on the goal you're pursuing. For someone starting with a bodyweight home workout, that's better than nothing. But if you want to use all the options to bring out the best in you, a willingness to accept change is essential. This often requires leaving the house unless you have a home gym. There is a lot of value in having your own home gym, as we do. Though it's small, so due to a lack of equipment, we sometimes go to a fitness center for squats and deadlifts. But when you have little time, a home gym is perfect for getting a short workout in.

At best, you invest in your health and find capable trainers to accompany you on your journey. Although, with too little prior knowledge, failure can come when choosing a suitable trainer. Listen to the experiences of others and ask to be coached according to your own ideas.

If it's not a trainer, maybe you have a fitness facility that, along with capable trainers, has everything that might in some way influence your athletic ambition. An athletic environment often generates more motivation than one's own four walls. Besides, access to important and useful equipment is essential to comprehensive training.

In general, working out with the own body is practical because you always have it with you. You learn to control your body, to integrate movements into your system, and to make them retrievable via the body awareness you acquired.

From an anatomical perspective, calisthenics training activates and strengthens nearly all muscle groups during every exercise. By contrast, working out with weights often focuses on targeting isolated muscles. Both variations, of course, promote muscle growth, and as previously mentioned, training should, ideally, include multiple options. Free weights are perfectly suited for targeting some weak spots and thus should be part of all-around, holistic training.

One example is the push-up. It primarily works shoulders, triceps, and chest muscles. In addition, it also requires core tension to provide stability. By contrast, when we look at exercise machines, it becomes apparent that this stabilizing component is largely decreased, since the exercises focus primarily on isolated muscle groups. Shoulders, the chest, and the core are divided between multiple machines and thus worked separately from each other.

The misconception that it's not possible to increase performance capacity with bodyweight exercises because the exercises are prespecified and that it's not possible to add weight can be dispelled. Due to the many variations of a basic exercise, it's possible for the individual to increase his performance. When training goals aren't achieved, new ones are set that must be met at the next stage via targeted practice. Thus, calisthenics is in no way inferior to working out with weights. While, in weightlifting, the amount of weight is gradually increased to generate performance increases, calisthenics athletes resort to more-difficult variations and movement patterns.

Hence calisthenics is a sport consisting of few exercises and their variations to work the entire body simultaneously. It's a way to improve one's outward appearance at one's discretion and in accordance with one's goals.

9.7   YOUR PREREQUISITES

There are no specific basic physical requirements. Anyone can learn exercises like push-ups, pull-ups, dips, or squats, regardless of gender, age, or performance level. Training depends on your primary goal. If the goal is to build up basic fitness, it suffices to build these exercises into your workout regimen, to promote strength, **hypertrophy** (muscle-fiber thickening), and strength endurance. If you want more, you have to invest more time, and the basic exercises must be specific.

Every person should be able to complete the following movement patterns:

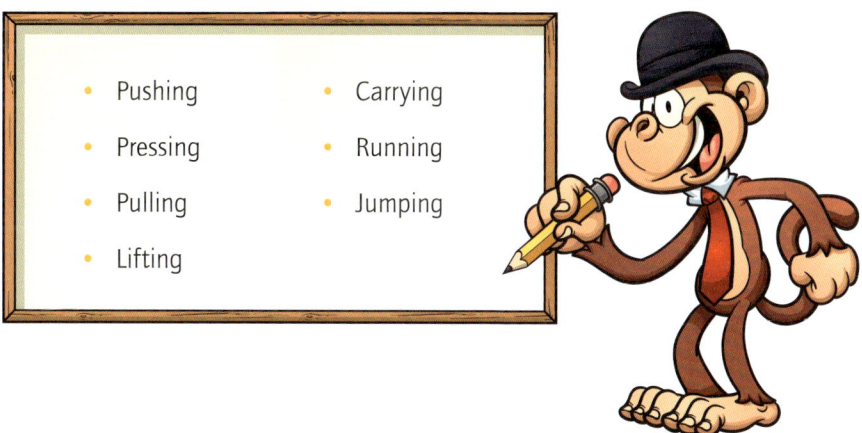

- Pushing
- Pressing
- Pulling
- Lifting
- Carrying
- Running
- Jumping

Many of our daily tasks require one of these physical abilities. Without them, we'd be incapable of putting a box on the top shelf of the storage room, lifting the just-purchased case of water into the car trunk, pushing the baby stroller, or carrying the baby in the baby wrap against our chest.

9.8 USEFUL EQUIPMENT

As the description of the sport of calisthenics indicates, you ideally don't need anything more than your body. But that's only conditionally true. You can do pushing exercises on the ground, and chairs or other pieces of furniture work well for dips. But when it comes to completing a balanced workout that requires different planes of movement, you need a pull-up bar or rings for pulling exercises. You can also row at a table or attach a towel to a door. Bodyweight training at home with such basic exercises is possible and certainly sufficient, particularly for beginners. But as soon as you progress and the exercises are getting easier, you're no longer providing stimuli that will move you forward.

So get the basic equipment. A *pull-up bar or rings* (or both) are a must. In terms of diameter, make sure the bar fits well in your hands and isn't too thin. We recommend a diameter of approximately 46 to 50 inches (33 mm). Polished stainless steel gets slippery in your hands. Sandblasted, rough varieties are the better choice.

Wooden rings offer a better and more-comfortable grip. Also, the buckles on the straps should be easy to operate, so you don't break your thumbs while attaching the rings. There are rings with numbered straps that make adjusting them to the same height much easier. You can attach the rings to lugs on the ceiling, but I think a width-adjustable version is better. You can set the rings wide or narrow on a bar.

I recommend *parallel bars* for doing proper dips. Since most homes don't have space for them, we need alternatives—either *dip bars* to mount on the wall, *wall* bars, or *equalizers*, two separate bar elements that can be used for dips when placed side by side. But there are two main disadvantages. They're usually not high enough to keep your legs straight, and they're often quite unstable. Besides, the width of the two bars must be adjusted to your personal needs. You can read more on this in section 11.5, "Dips and Possible Progressions." *Parallettes*, similar to equalizers but much smaller, are great for *L*-sits or handstands and take up very little space.

If, at some point, bodyweight pull-ups become too easy for you and you don't just want to train in the strength-endurance range with more than fifteen repetitions and want to add some difficulty, get a weighted belt or a weighted vest. If you're considering purchasing a weighted vest, consider possible restrictions to shoulder-blade movement, whereby keeping the center of gravity close to your body is better than externally placed added weight like with the belt. Ultimately, you need to decide what works better for you.

Also get some *resistance bands* of various strengths. I recommend getting a red and a black band. The exercises demonstrate how to use them.

Gym chalk is a must-have for better grip on the bar—something I consider essential. Yes, chalk dries out your hands, but here's a question: Do you want to be able to perform or to have silky-smooth hands? Callouses form as a protective mechanism in areas of the body that are less fleshy and are subjected to compressive loads. Thus, they have an important function and shouldn't be filed down to nothing because they don't conform to a beauty ideal. Gloves aren't a solution.

Remember, doing calisthenics alone isn't enough to strengthen all the body's required structures. I therefore also recommend the use of *kettlebells* and *dumbbells*. If you want to build visibly bulging muscles on your legs, you won't be able to do so without a *barbell* and the appropriate *plates*.

Sounds expensive and space-intensive? Indeed. So if you don't want to convert your home into a gym, you're probably better off at a fitness facility with all its equipment. Especially if you're really serious, can see the benefits, and don't want to go without anything that will make you stronger.

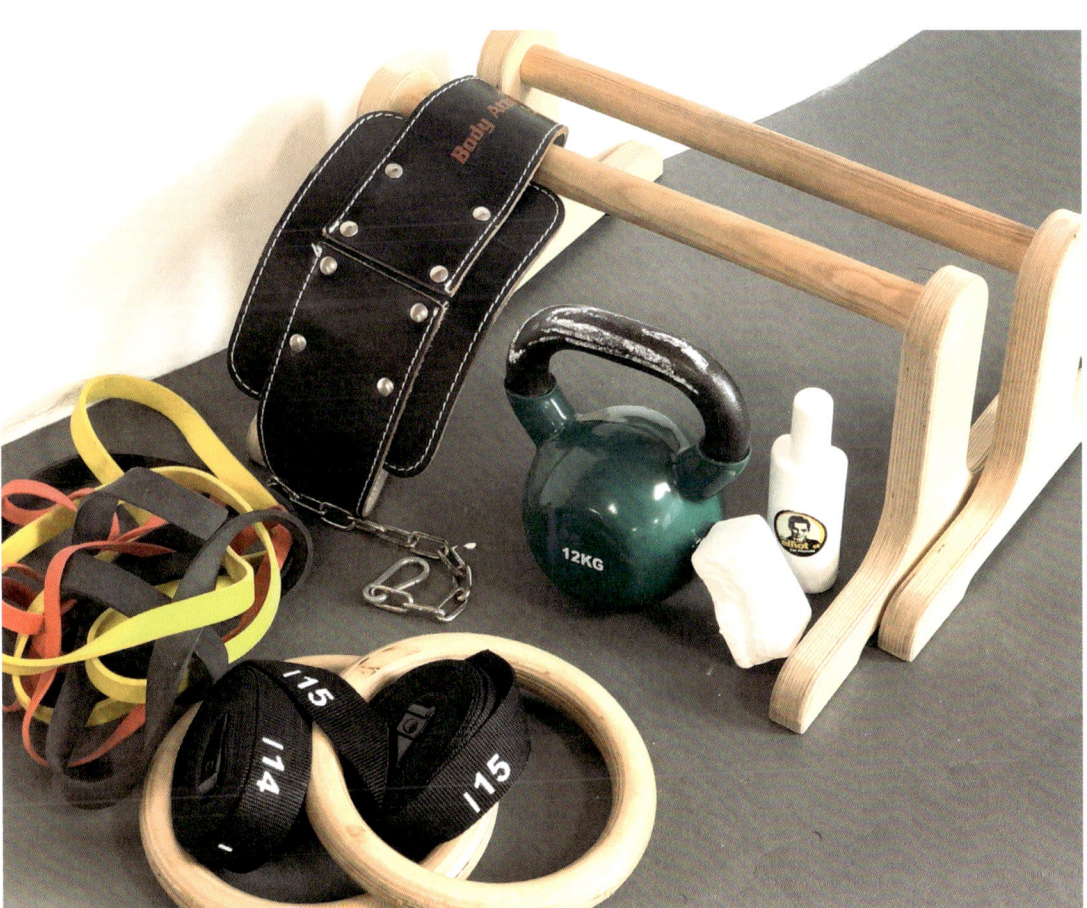

9.9 CALISTHENICS PARKS: THE BEST SPOTS FOR YOUR TRAINING

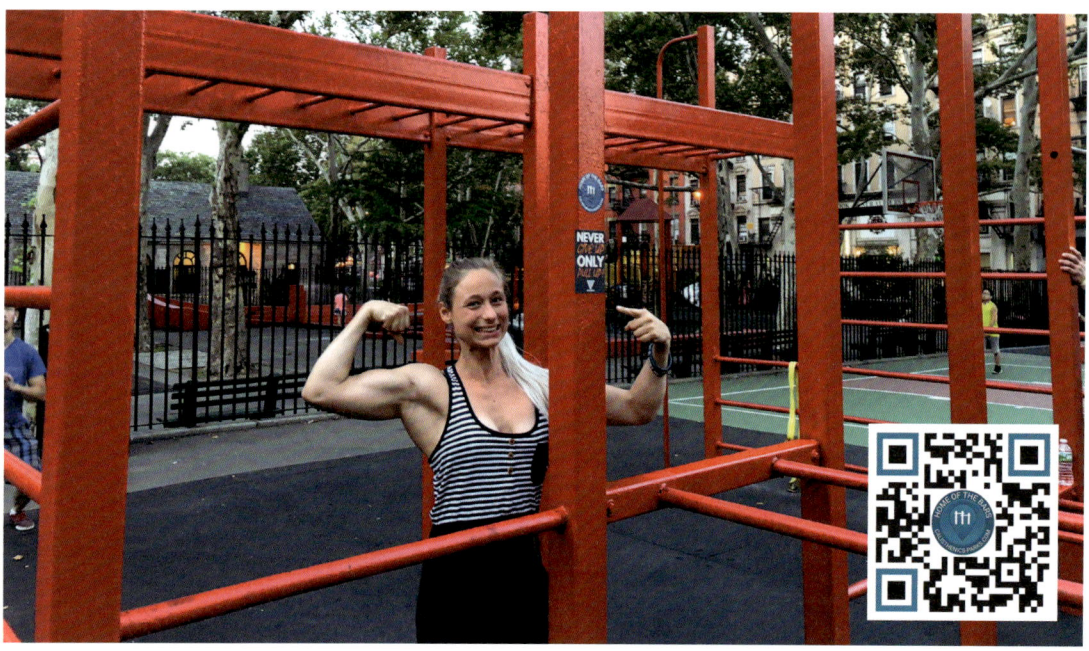

Finding suitable outdoor options is no longer a problem, thanks to Calisthenics Parks. There's no comparable or easier approach to finding a place near you, regardless of where you are in the world. On vacation, and in addition to that relaxing summer feeling, need some bars and more for your calisthenics training? Pick up your smartphone, visit the app, and find the training location nearest you. Sound easy? It is.

9.10 GUIDELINES FOR AMBITIOUS CALISTHENICS BEGINNERS

CHECKLIST

- Find a **training partner** and an outdoor training location for the summer.
- Set **measurable goals** for yourself but not too many at one time.
- Be **patient** with yourself and give your body time to adjust to the loads.
- Make sure your training is **versatile** rather than one particular focus (combine movement and strength).
- Allow your **body phases of rest** to regenerate.
- Work step-by-step with **progressions**.
- Start with the **basics** and master them before moving on to bigger things.
- **Don't** compare yourself to others. Role models are fine.
- **Have fun** with what you do and don't expect too much of yourself.
- Did I mention **quality beats quantity**?

9.11 DITCHING FAMILIAR MOVEMENT PATTERNS: EMBRACING THE UNUSUAL

I like to try new things. Especially when I know that my counterpart is familiar with the subject matter. And trying new things is important to our neuromuscular circuits, which get excited about every new movement experience and correspondingly create new connections with new stimuli.

Imagine a construction site. The workers are adept at their daily tasks at the site, and their hand movements are almost automatic. If you don't provide them with materials (new input), the construction project winds down and doesn't progress. But when the workers are given unfamiliar tasks, they must first consult each other, identify possible methods, and find solutions. The second or third time, everything already runs more smoothly until, ultimately, it becomes routine.

Thus, new stimuli challenge your brain and your body in a new way. The more diversity you provide, the more versatile you'll become (if you stick with it), and the more movement tasks you'll be able to solve.

Go outside, look for a challenging task, and tackle it. Wholeheartedly.

9.12 EXERTION TO THE POINT OF EXHAUSTION: THE 80-PERCENT RULE

Many athletes need to feel completely exhausted after a workout. Is that what it takes for you to feel like you're training properly?

It's such a misconception: keep going, keep going, and push to the limit until you're on the ground, on your back, like a bug, unable to go any further. And then there's the injury risk. Of course, we want to feel good after a training session and, ideally, already feel the effects during our workout.

But I'll tell you a secret. I hardly ever sweat during my calisthenics workouts except when I add some static core exercises, like dips, at the end. I remain in the dip position without exhausting myself. And after more than seven years in this sport, I don't have the feeling that my gains (building new muscle mass) and progress are lacking.

This piece of wisdom is another that's based on the 80-percent rule:

Don't train to your physical limit, but do allow yourself some room for improvement with the repetitions.

That means to do only as many repetitions as you can do cleanly. *But my trainer says I need to do x number of repetitions.* Stay two repetitions below what you think you can do. The most-important thing is that you stay clean. Split the sets so you end up with the total number of specified repetitions per exercise (cluster training). Then you've met your **volume**, even if you needed more attempts and time.

That doesn't automatically mean you'll stay below your performance. Heavy weights are allowed and must absolutely be moved. Advantage? You'll start your next training session much more rested. Your body is able to restore readiness for the loading processes more quickly, so your central nervous system is also ready for a workout.

To me, there's nothing worse than a trainer talking loudly and insistently at his already-exhausted client. Competitive settings that require you to give it your all are the exception.

But if you really need that worn-out feeling, let it not be the norm but the icing on the cake. Get your worn-out kick once a week.

Personally, I save that stuff for my free time, like when I have to rush on foot or by bike, because I didn't get my butt in gear. So, train smart and not like you're on the run or being chased by a herd of wildebeest.

9.13 SETTING GOALS THE RIGHT WAY

How you can set specific training goals and how you can continuously increase your performance can be easily explained using the **SMART principle**. The training method depends on your goals. Qualitative goals help you create a structured training plan and make sure you meet your goal. This method doesn't account for mistakes that can creep in and cause your progress to stagnate, which may prompt you to choose other methods in order to keep moving forward. But mistakes, too, are an important process on the training path. We all know that we learn from our mistakes.

Calisthenics is primarily about optimizing your strength performance. Here, strength isn't defined as how much weight one can move but in what way and how versatilely the athlete can execute the sport's different elements. Since many strength exercises require a certain amount of mobility, you must also take that into consideration when setting goals. Without a certain amount of basic strength, you could find yourself quickly at your limit in terms of technical execution and coordination.

The letters in the acronym *SMART* indicate the requirements a goal should meet.

S: *specific*

M: *measurable*—for example, the goal can be tracked via the increasing number of repetitions

A: *achievable*—the goal is achievable

R: *realistic*—whether a goal is realistic depends on your current fitness level, how much time you can invest in your training in addition to your workday, and if you have access to the necessary equipment

T: *time-phased*—depending on your training progress, you can set a time frame within which you want to achieve your goal

The following are examples of SMART goals:

- decreasing body fat by 10 percent in three months
- doing ten pull-ups in a row with FROM having had a fitness level of zero five months earlier
- holding a handstand for ten seconds without stopping or without walking on your hands

By contrast, ineffective goals can be completely nonspecific:

- Losing weight
- Building muscle mass
- Getting more fit

It's like making a resolution at the beginning of the year to quit smoking. Either you're not tough enough, you forget, or due to the long time period, you put it off until the end of the year. Having a limited time span, such as a deadline for turning in a paper that will be graded, creates pressure to tackle the goal.

If your goals include strength and endurance, prioritize them or accept that you'll make slower progress in both. If you want more of one, it necessitates doing less of the other. Endurance and strength have different stimuli. While endurance-oriented athletes, like marathon runners, have **slow-twitch muscle fibers** (type 1 muscle fiber equals slow-twitch), meaning muscles that fatigue more slowly, sports that require strength or power, like sprinting, use primarily **fast-twitch muscle fibers** (type 2 muscle fiber equals fast-twitch). They're capable of generating lots of strength quickly but also fatigue correspondingly fast because the strength reserves are completely exhausted at the beginning of the preliminary movement.

Thus, 150 consecutive push-ups aren't an indication of strength but, rather, endurance and therefore aren't a good goal for increasing strength.

> **TIP**
>
> Write down your goals so you can always look at them and feel a sense of obligation before you fall victim to the daily grind or follow familiar workout routines without adhering to the actual goal.

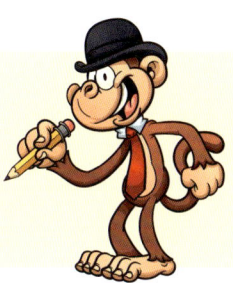

Go easy with the number of goals you set. Set two to three goals and pursue them. Once you reach them, set new ones.

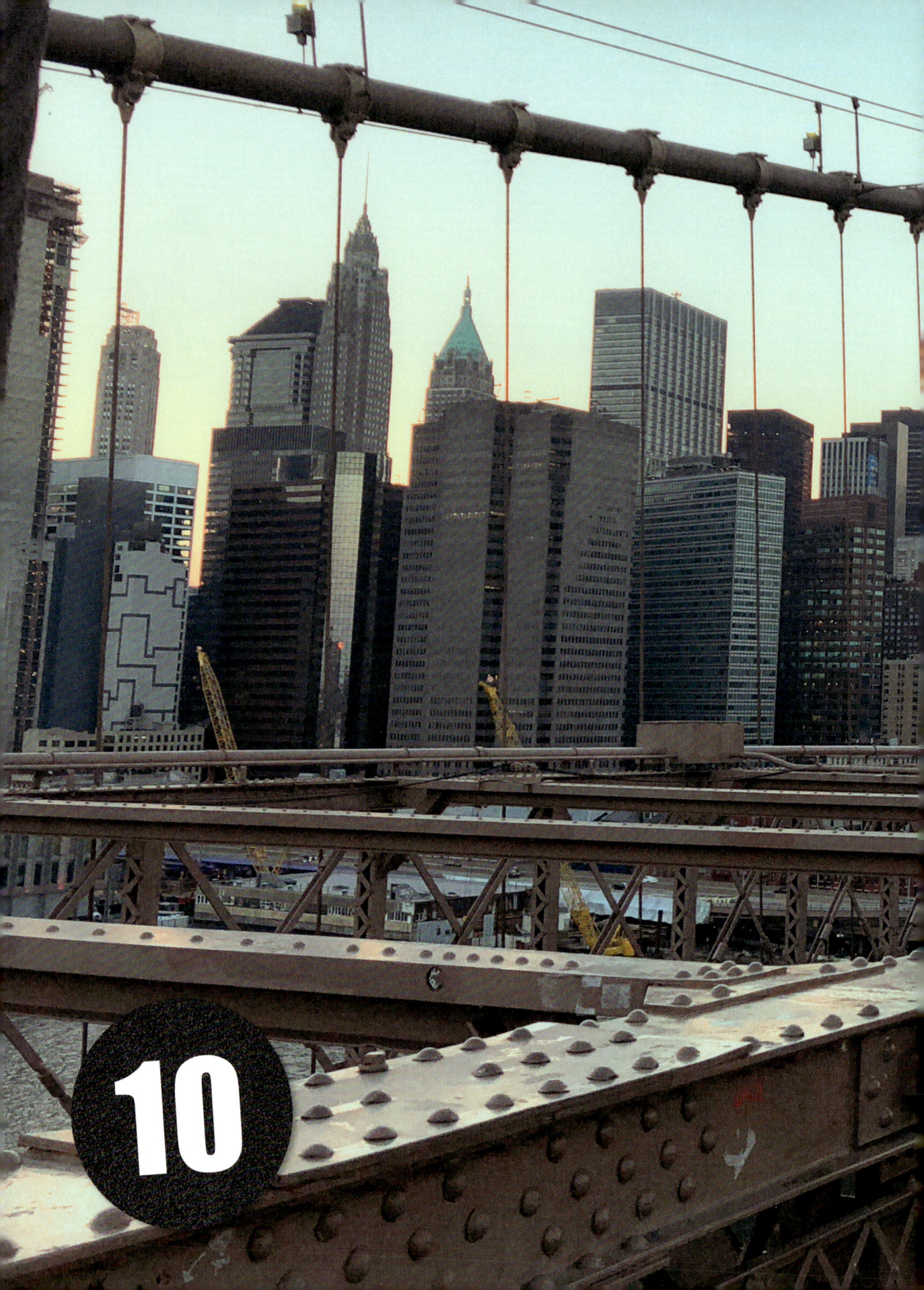

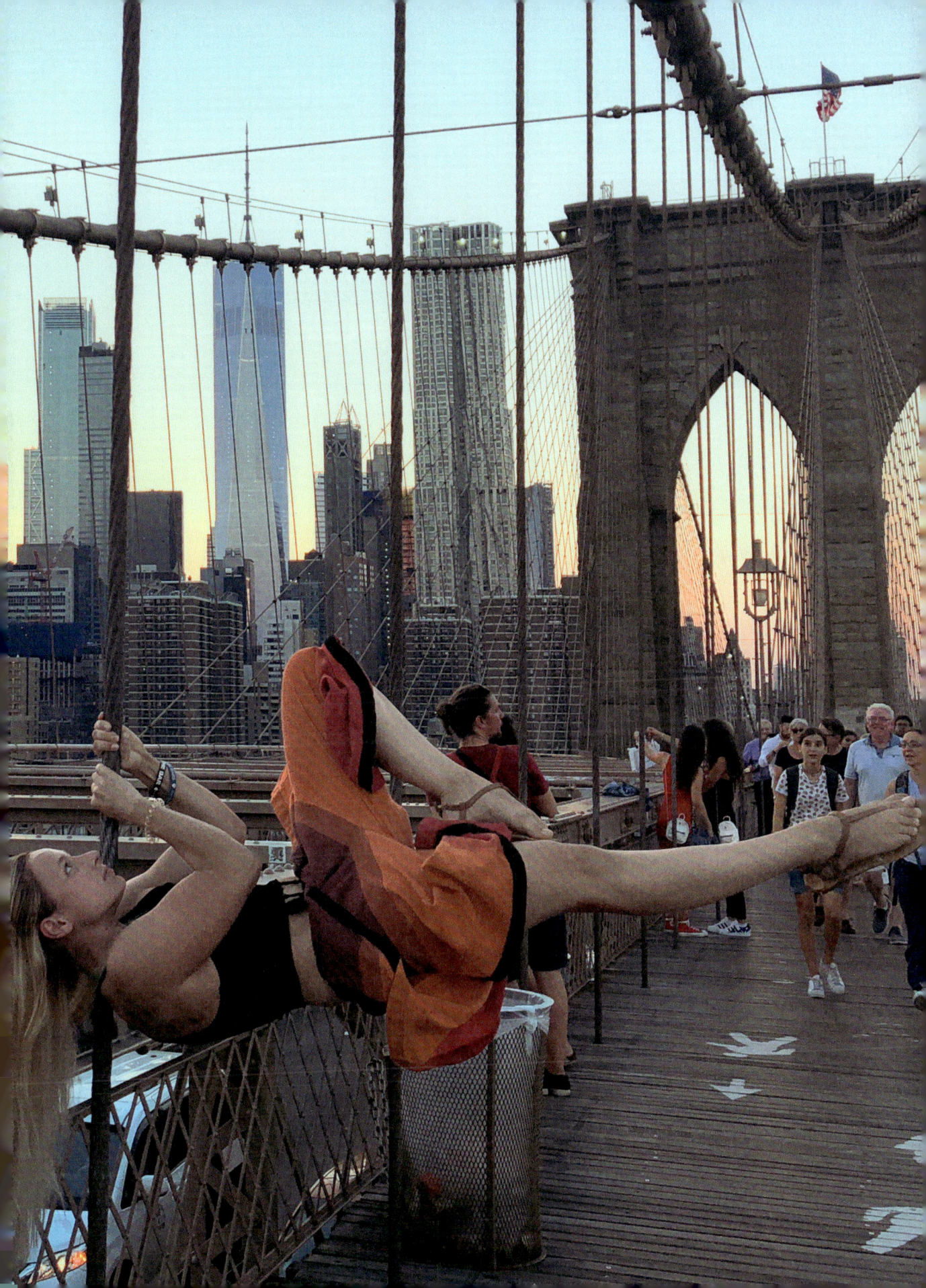

10 Calisthenics Fundamentals: What You Need to Know

10.1 OVERVIEW OF BASIC EXERCISES

This list offers a general overview of the planes of movement in which calisthenics athletes operate to create balanced workouts.

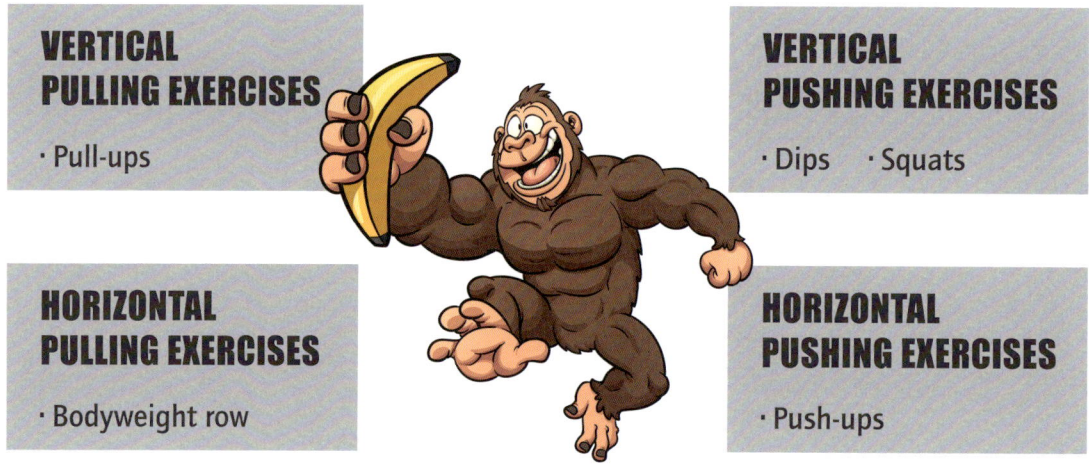

VERTICAL PULLING EXERCISES
- Pull-ups

VERTICAL PUSHING EXERCISES
- Dips
- Squats

HORIZONTAL PULLING EXERCISES
- Bodyweight row

HORIZONTAL PUSHING EXERCISES
- Push-ups

The following diagram shows the standard exercises (basics) and training units, along with their **regressions** (easier variations), that make up the initial foundation of the calisthenics sport.

Calisthenics Fundamentals: What You Need to Know

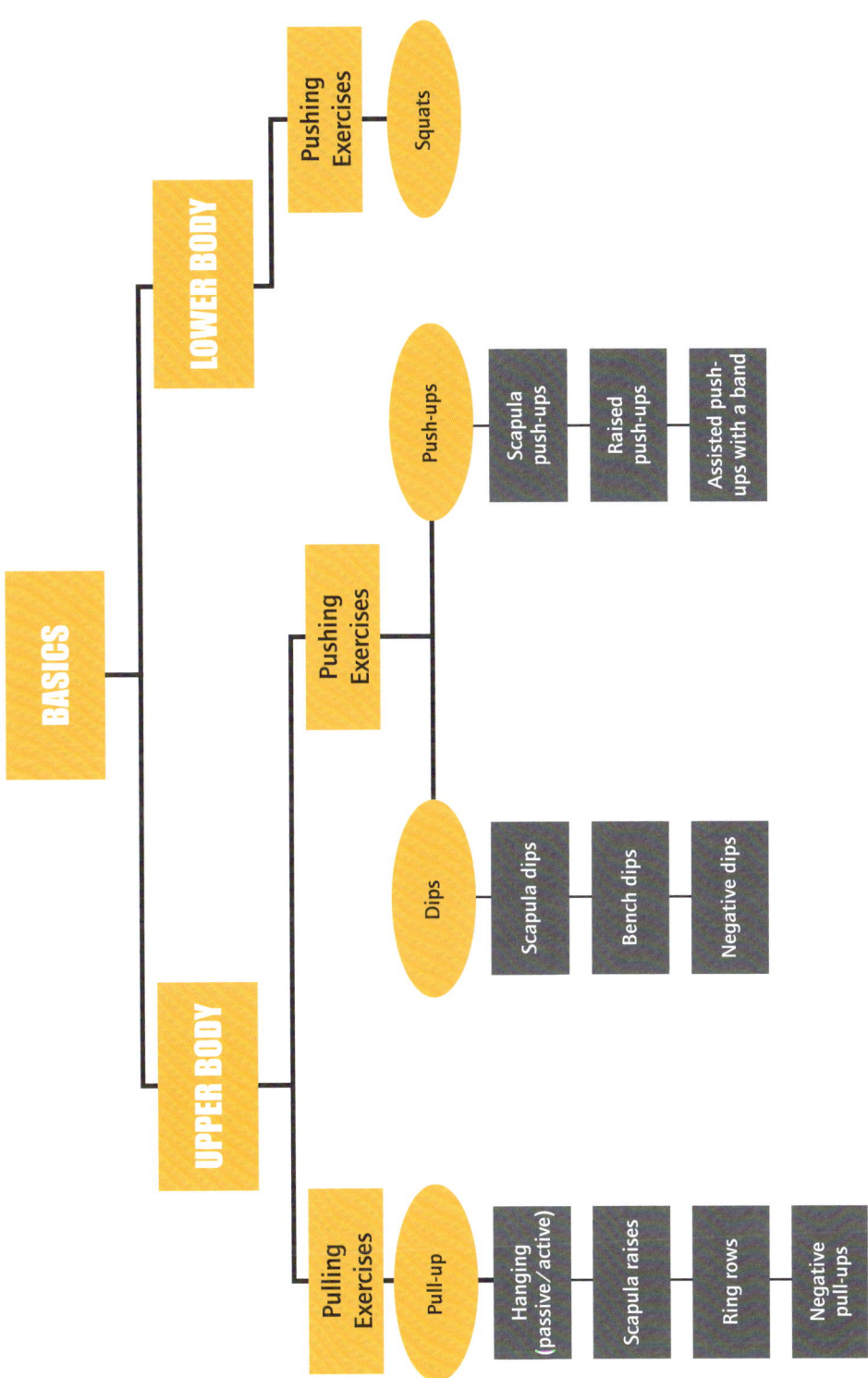

In chapter 11, "Beginner Basics and Their Possible Progressions," you can see detailed images and descriptions of the individual exercises and their variations.

Of course, there are additional exercises beyond this presentation, but they're more complex and aren't considered basics but, rather, skills. Such exercises should be divided into pushing (push-ups, dips, squats) and pulling exercises (pull-ups).

No one is anatomically or biomechanically able to do the chapter 11 exercises without a certain amount of mobility and strength, which is why I include easier variations (regressions) along with the target exercises. The regressions of these exercises are performed vertically as well as horizontally. As basics, these exercises represent the core of calisthenics training and contribute to building the basic strength necessary to master skills like muscle-ups, the human flag, a back lever (from gymnastics), a handstand, or a planche.

Since calisthenics is very upper-body intensive, the squat is the only leg exercise. There are hardly any meaningful regressions for the knee bend as it's the simplest form of the squat. Limited mobility and lack of strength in the lower extremities can by limiting factors when performing squats. Pistol squats, single-leg squats, are good exercises and include various pre-exercises for performing them correctly.

Heavy squats, knee bends (vertical pushing exercise), and deadlifts (vertical pulling exercise) are other basic movements that should be part of your training plan.

Thus, the basics strengthen the muscles, tendons, and ligaments that participate in exercise execution, and they provide many adaptation mechanisms for a stable active and passive locomotor system. The pulling and pushing exercises are balanced and should be alternated when integrated into training, to prevent imbalances and possible pain.

Sections 10.9, "Shoulder-Blade Positions," and 10.11, "Hollow-Body Position," also show essential positions that provide stable body tension during the execution of all basics and skills and benefit shoulder health.

Once the foundation, in the form of basics, has been laid and the described foundational positions are considered, you're able to choose from a large number of exercises to combine them into expanded skills. The following applies while doing any of the exercises: **quality beats quantity**, whereby the physiologically correct joint position must also be taken into consideration to stay healthy in the long term.

10.2 BALANCING STABILITY AND MOBILITY

Often, sports are practiced too one-sided. It's important to be flexible and open when designing your training and to use the tools that can eliminate weak spots, in order to maintain good health while training. Prevention is the best way to do this rather than waiting until an injury has occurred. And I'm not just talking about different training methods or special exercises but about sports that, to provide some balance, can be integrated into your training.

An intensive yoga workout can safely make you mobile but also takes away the basic tension that's just as important, not only for you to be able to execute certain exercises correctly but also for health reasons. You can read more about the importance of a balance between stability and mobility in chapter 1, "Mobility—Modern Mobility Training."

10.3 MOVEMENT VARIATIONS

The purpose of this book isn't to tell you which muscles achieve maximum hypertrophy with which exercises. It's about perception of movement, learning movement, and mastering the basics and the subsequent skills. But please note that different planes (horizontal and vertical) and different grip variations work different parts of the muscles.

Combine. Be flexible. Find a recreational sport you enjoy. Strike a balance between strength and mobility training. Train preventatively and with common sense. Only then can you avoid shelving your athletic career prematurely while you're busy doing physical rehab exercises.

Mix it up occasionally and offer your body and your neural connections new ranges of motion that can help you create lots of new connections and branching. Ultimately, this means a division of labor within your locomotor system and will let you perform physical actions in a more efficient and more versatile way.

Cell regeneration takes place in regular cycles. For this reason, newly learned movement patterns and behavioral structures should be performed over a period of three months to allow the body's adaptation process to take place continuously. The human body is a genius in adapting to new structures and environments, which is evident in evolution. Therefore, everyone can decide to change something. So why not help your performance get optimized?

10.4 MOVEMENT SPECIFICS

Your training should always be movement specific, regardless of which exercise or which skill you wish to master. Each of the exercises introduced in section 10.1, "Overview of Basic Exercises," can be supplemented with other exercises that work the same muscle groups (assistance exercises). Many have a positive carryover to the final target movement and can reduce existing weaknesses. But it's always important to do the exercises yourself.

10.5 ASSISTANCE EXERCISES

Don't get too fixated on previously specified exercises, but instead, choose exercises that have the same objective just in a different way—exercises that carry over to the goal you're pursuing.

Here, we differentiate between two exercises that are very close to the motion sequence of the target exercise and exercises that strengthen individual areas (muscles). For instance, if you want to learn the pull-up, you can practice the *general motion sequence* of the pull-up with negative pull-ups, overhead band pulls, or ring rows. With exercises like a farmer's walk, hanging, face pulls, or a standing row with a barbell, you can specifically work the muscle structures that participate in the pull-up. The goal of all these exercises is to increase tractive power and strengthen the participating structures.

10.6 DIFFICULT EXERCISES MADE EASY

Movements can be seen as a building project that consists of individual elements and is assembled with the help of a tool kit. Even the seemingly simplest exercises are more complex than they appear. I'd like to explain this by using the example of the pull-up. The pull-up consists of three movement phases (**concentric, isometric, eccentric**) and, during its execution, is divided into three main movements. These take place in a fluid transition and primarily allow for the physiological gliding of the shoulder blades along the ribcage.

- **Concentric:** = the ascending phase
- **Eccentric:** = the descending phase
- **Isometric:** = the holding phase

- Phase one: the *initial movement*, from passive to active hanging, that results from the shoulder blades moving into retraction or depression (see section 10.9, "Shoulder-Blade Positions")

- Phase two: *activation of the latissimus dorsi* (large back muscle) via the externally rotated shoulder (break-the-bar principle; see section 10.9, "Shoulder-Blade Positions"), in which the m. infraspinatus participates

- Phase three: *elbows bending* close to the body at the pull-up's highest point, with the chin over the bar, whereby the shoulders stay back and down

But during this execution, we're looking at the way only the shoulder blades work, which, along with the latissimus dorsi, are significantly involved in the pull-up motion. There are, in fact, other factors that must be taken into consideration. The position of the hands, thumbs, and head and the involvement of the core (trunk) don't require additional explanations to help one ascertain how complex this simple exercise really is. A detailed description of this basic exercise can be found in section 11.3, "Pull-ups and Possible Progressions."

Not all the individual elements function equally well. Each has different strengths and weaknesses. We refer to **sticking points** or **weak links**. These must first be worked up separately with the use of certain tools from the tool kit (training methods, equipment, etc.) before they can be optimally inserted as a whole into the building project. In other words: beginners must first purposefully strengthen the individual movement phases of the pull-up before they can execute it as a complete pull-up.

10.7 STICKING POINTS

Sticking points or weak links means that certain radii of movement within a movement pattern to be executed are too weak—be it due to restricted range of motion, difficulty with control, or lack of strength—and must therefore be specifically worked on with special exercises. Sometimes this requires abstaining from calisthenics exercises and integrating other assisting-strength exercises, mobility training, or both.

Use a kettlebell to work on shoulder stability, hold dumbbells to isolate your rotator cuffs, or use assisting resistance bands for active mobility exercises. And don't underestimate the effect of **unilateral training** (one half of the body does most of the work) to correct imbalances between your right and left sides.

I've stopped doing only calisthenics exercises, because after my injury, I learned how important it is to remain versatile. It's the only way to give the body diverse input for processing, which will largely determine whether you'll stay in the middle or leave everyone else in the dust.

Sticking points must be eliminated as soon as you become aware of them, before imbalances occur and pain sets in. Since these problems are of a very individual nature and often stem from one-sided loading, we dedicate an entire section to this topic, section 2.7, "How Mobility Makes You Stronger." The relationship between strength and mobility is vital when it comes to training that keeps you healthy. If you either lack the necessary joint stability or have limited range of motion, that implies a lack of mobility or injuries.

10.8 FULL RANGE OF MOTION

The guiding principle for all calisthenics exercises is to perform them using full range of motion (FROM).

Stimulus to muscles, tendons, and ligaments is different than with FROM when the movement isn't completed. This is because of the participating structures. Due to the stretching in the end positions, more muscle fibers are recruited during FROM. Take the classic pull-up—you can achieve such an effect if you end the pull-up by completely hanging before initiating the next pull-up and moving your chest toward the bar until at least your head is above the bar. This way, the primary target muscle, the large back muscle (latissimus dorsi) can unfold all its strength.

Calisthenics Fundamentals: What You Need to Know

10.9 SHOULDER-BLADE POSITIONS

The shoulder girdle is a calisthenics athlete's key element. And because it plays such an important role, we've dedicated a section to its anatomy and biomechanics (see section 10.17, "Shoulder Joint").

The following photos show the shoulder-blade positions along with their descriptions::

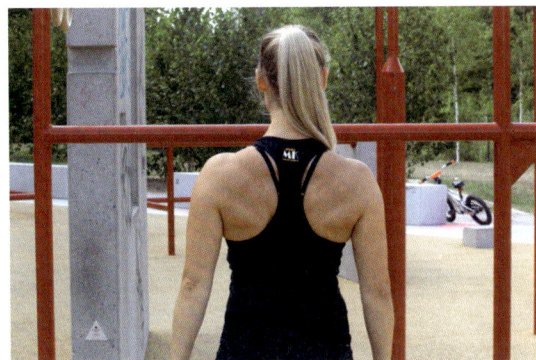 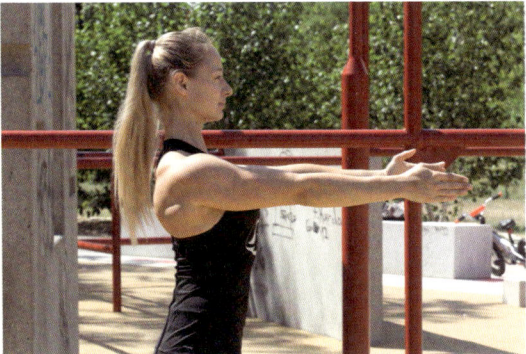

Depression: shoulders blades move away from the ears.

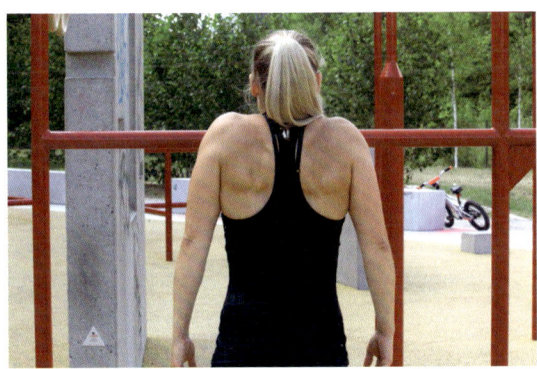 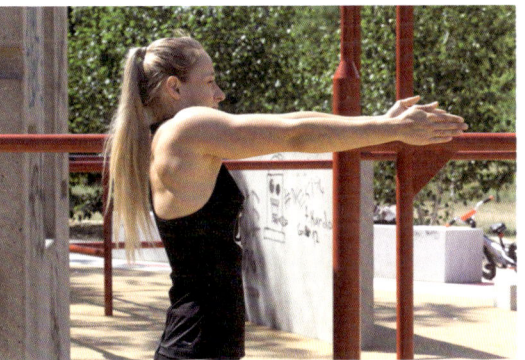

Elevation: shoulder blades move toward the ears.

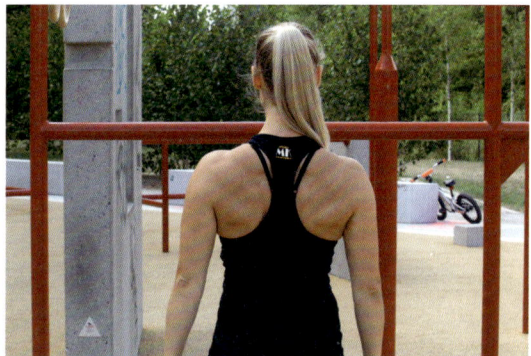
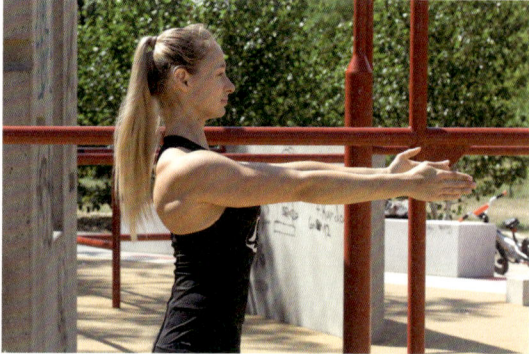

Retraction depression: shoulder blades push back and down (imagine holding a tennis ball between your shoulder blades)

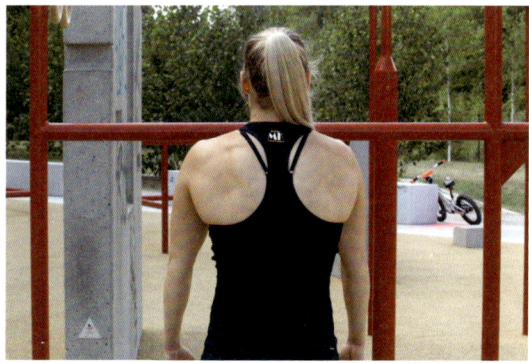
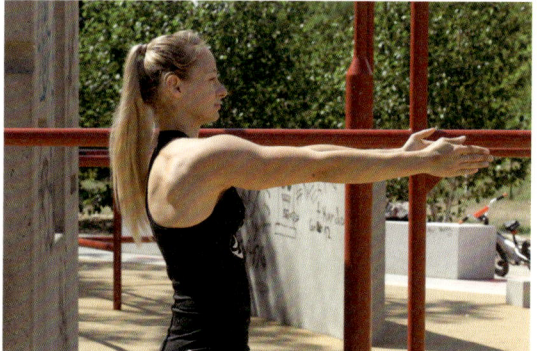

Protraction depression: shoulder blades move away from each other and are pulled apart (cat pose).

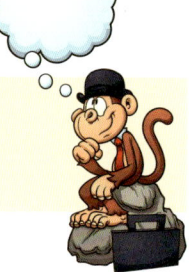

Here, you can memorize the following principle: **shoulders and ears don't get along**. (Thank you, Sebastian Müller, kettlebell trainer in Erfurt, Germany, for this.) You generally need elevation only for overhead movements, like a handstand.

Shoulder blades should move into position against gravity. Only then can you ensure that, along with an external rotation, which the m. infraspinatus supplies, the humeral head rests securely in the socket. This guarantees that the subacromial space, between the shoulder joint and acromion, is large enough to prevent rubbing and thus prevent pain and injuries.

Calisthenics Fundamentals: What You Need to Know

Since the shoulder joint is supported almost exclusively by the muscle-tendon-ligament apparatus but its shape is barely held by bony structures, it's particularly vulnerable to injury. This is one reason why a sport like CrossFit is suitable for an absolute beginner athlete only if she's first mastered the basics and her muscular and neuronal structures have been appropriately strengthened. Kipping pull-ups, for instance, follow a complex motion sequence that can't be safely executed if the basic strength and understanding of the motion sequence are lacking.

> As an example, when doing a push-up, gravity would pull the body (horizontal) downward in the area of the shoulder blades, which is why the shoulders must be protracted.

These shoulder positions should be specific to calisthenics. Ultimately, it's about already assuming during the basics fundamental positions that will later transmit force during advanced skills.

Many have difficulty controlling their shoulder blades independently of other joints and without compensating movements. This inability can become problematic. Exercises from the mobility part of the book as well as exercises listed as *regression* can help.

EXTERNAL SHOULDER ROTATION

External shoulder rotation means pointing your elbows forward.

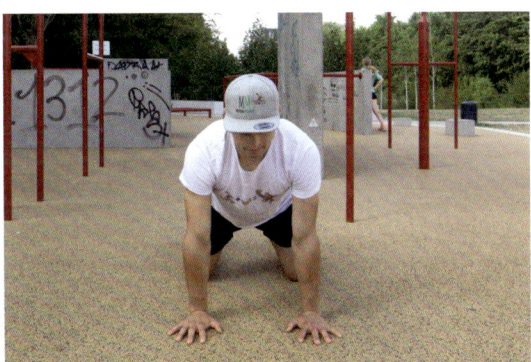

This external rotation should be maintained during both types of exercise—pulling and pushing. Regardless of the basic exercises, the external rotators should be worked with assistance exercises specifically. During support exercises, the inside of your forearms should face forward. Pulling exercises, like pull-ups and rowing with the bar, and bench presses require the *break-the-bar* strategy.

This is the break-the-bar strategy: imagine yourself breaking the bar from the inside.

When your external rotators are strong, you ensure healthy shoulders, more stability in the shoulder girdle, and thus a powerful performance.

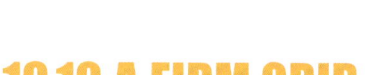

10.10 A FIRM GRIP

Regardless of whether you're on the bar, the rings, the parallel bars, the parallettes, or whatever you can get your hands on, if you increase your basic tension from the start, you give your nervous system a sense of control (safety), which allows you to greatly increase your force potential. For more background information, read (or reread) chapter 2, "Understanding the Mobility Myth," in which Leon explains how basic tension affects not only mobility but also strength.

10.11 HOLLOW-BODY POSITION

I look at calisthenics as a holistic sport primarily because of one important position: the hollow-body position (body swing or boat pose). As shown in the photos, it ensures that the core (the body's midsection) is activated during all exercises, be it basics or skills. It stabilizes the lower back in the area of the lumbar spine and protects you from the effects of carelessness. In addition, the core gets worked during practically all the exercises.

This makes it possible for advanced athletes to barely need any core and abdominal exercises to get that desirable six-pack unless their midsection is a sticking point that's resulted in injuries or threatens to do so. But beginners should first practice and solidify the hollow-body position and perform other core-stabilizing exercises to achieve a greater strength potential, because core tension is often a weakness. No, no sit-ups!

Generally speaking, more core stability results in a posture that prevents injury, which is also important in other strength sports. You can think of your spine as your body's support pillar. If it's unstable, it'll break away, and you'll collapse like a house of cards.

Calisthenics Fundamentals: What You Need to Know

Your spine houses the spinal cord, which sends all the information it receives from your surroundings and your body to the brain and back into the periphery. Since the brain is the control center of all your vital needs, including movement, this conduit must be protected. The core that surrounds it serves as a protective covering for your support pillar and absolutely must be cared for.

The practical implementation of the hollow-body position is that you tilt your pelvis back (**posterior pelvic tilt**), whereby you firmly squeeze your buttocks together. Your upper body doesn't move at all; only your pelvis is activated. Imagine your pelvis as a bowl that threatens to spill when it's tilted forward.

A good way to demonstrate this is the hollow-body position while lying on the ground. The idea is to close the gap between the lumbar spine and the ground, with the spine in its natural curve. Proceed as follows:

1. Lie on your back on the ground in a relaxed position with your legs extended. Now squeeze your buttocks together and actively push your pelvis toward the ceiling or sky.

2. Lift your legs and feet (**pointed toes**) off the ground while maintaining muscle tension in your legs.

3. Lift your shoulder blades off the ground.

4. Tighten your core like you're trying to perform a static crunch.

5. Extend your arms over your head.

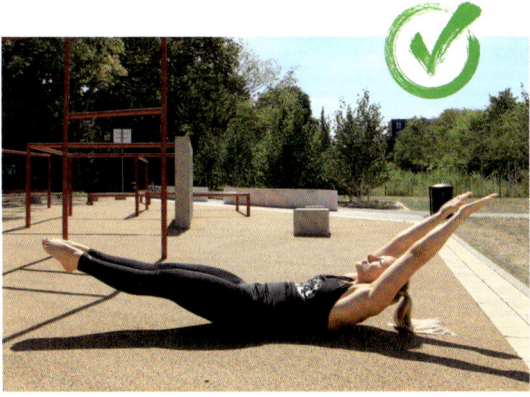
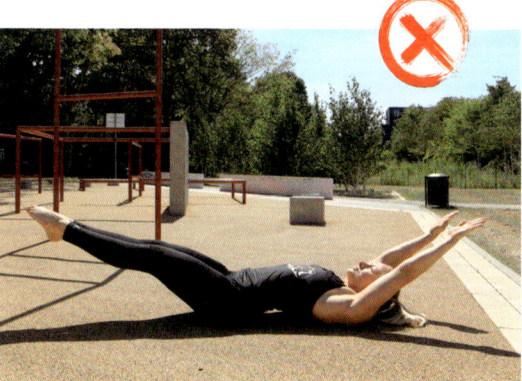

The goal is to find a position that allows you to keep your lower back on the ground. This is where the levers of your arms and legs come into play, which I describe in section 10.12, "All about Levers." Next play with the leg lever and angles in the hollow-body position. Then extend your arms over your head.

TIP

Imagine your pelvis as a bowl that's tilted forward and about to overflow.

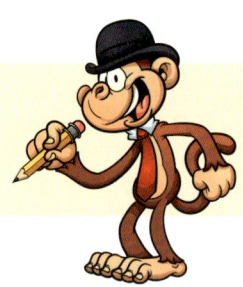

10.12 ALL ABOUT LEVERS

The body's *levers* determine the **degree of difficulty of the exercises**, particularly during static skills or the hollow-body position. Here, the arms and legs are the body's levers. The core is the stable part. The closer you bring the muscle insertion and muscle origin together by bending the elbow, hip, or knee joints, the shorter the lever gets, which makes the exercise easier.

The following photos show the different degrees of difficulty, starting with the easiest one:

TUCK

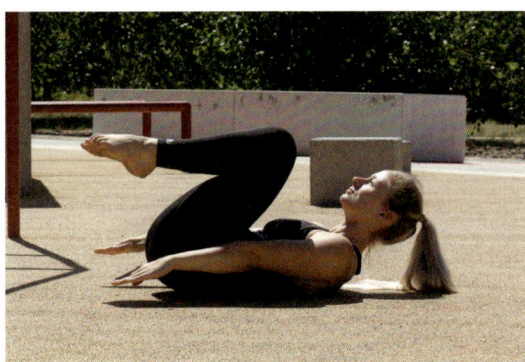

Knees are bent close to the chest.

ADVANCED TUCK

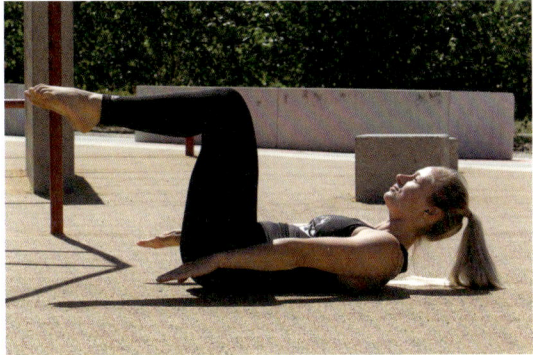

There's a 90-degree angle between the thighs and trunk.

ADVANCED TUCK STRADDLE

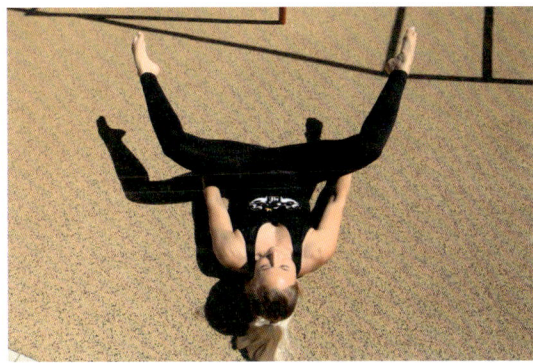

Legs are in a straddle with a 90-degree angle between the thighs and trunk.

STRADDLE

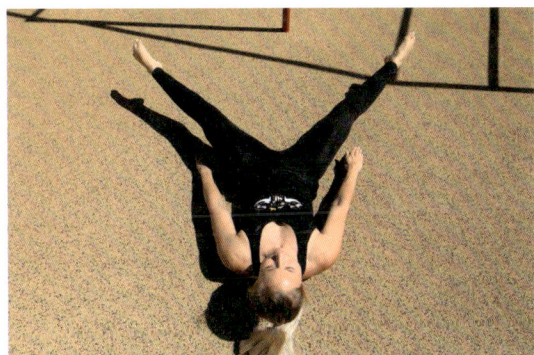

Legs are in a straddle position.

ONE-LEGGED POSITION

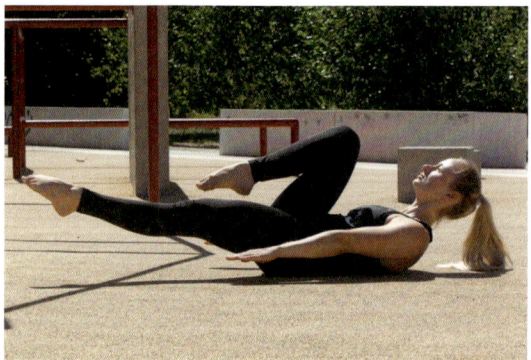

One leg is pulled in to the chest, and one leg is extended.

FULL

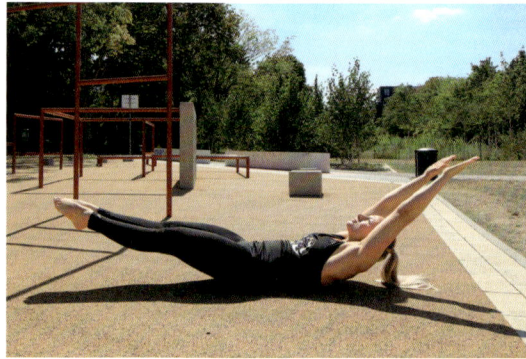

Body is in a full hollow-body position.

Empirically, though, the one-legged position has turned out to be difficult to implement. Many people are unable to maintain an active hip extension. Instead, they arch their back during the back lever or flex their hip during the front lever, because they're unable to overcome the forces of gravity.

But strength is most effective at approximately a 90-degree angle because that's where the muscle's ability to contract is greatest. That's why some people find the beginning and ending motions of certain exercises the most difficult.

10.13 REPETITION: THE MOTHER OF SKILL

The body must first create an image of the movement. This is done by **continuously repeating the movements to be learned**. The more often you perform these movements, the more *automated* they'll become in your brain so you can draw on these abilities at any time. Since the basics of calisthenics and the muscles that perform them are hardly used in this manner in our everyday life and are thus not a common function, they must be specifically trained.

10.14 STRAIGHT-ARM STRENGTH

Most exercises are performed with bent elbows. This is also true in our daily life. Our strength when our arms are extended, like during a full plank, and not on the forearms has deficiencies. The same is true for other exercises that require supporting strength: straddle sit, handstand, *L*-sit, press to handstand, and planche and its regressions, such as the lean. Exercises like the overhead walk with kettlebells are useful here. **RTO** (rings turned out), first in the push-up position and later in the support hold, is a great way to increase **straight-arm strength** (see sections 11.4 "Push-ups and Possible Progressions," and 11.5, "Dips and Possible Progressions").

10.15 TRAINING ON RINGS

I absolutely recommend training on rings. I'd almost say that anything you can do on the rings you can also do on the ground or the bar. But the muscle-up (combination of pull-up and dip) is easier to learn on the rings because you don't have to get past a bar in front of your chest. You have to move your arms past your sides to get into a support position. The muscle-up on the bar requires considerably more strength and explosiveness.

> The general rule for anything you do on the rings as a beginner is this:
> stay firm and compact

That means keeping your core absolutely stable and always keeping the rings close to your body so you don't start to wobble in the rings. The higher the rings are mounted, the more difficult it is to balance them.

10.16 CALISTHENICES AND LEG TRAINING

Do you want muscular legs? Then bend the legs and lift with heavy weights. Squats with just your bodyweight, as well as other free leg exercises, won't get you to your goal. Human beings are used to standing on their legs, be it by walking, standing, or running. Hence you're hardly providing any new stimulus to get your leg muscles to grow. But if it must come by free leg training, integrate plyometric (explosive jumps) and unilateral exercises as well as sprints.

Deadlifts and knee bends with weight (back and front squats) are lower-body exercises that are fundamental for building a strong foundation. Yes, really thick legs mean more weight and make static and dynamic exercises more difficult. But without any leg training, you risk muscle imbalances that can be accompanied by injuries to other structures, such as your shoulders.

Having heavy legs and still being able to perform spectacular skills is ultimately more impressive than being a flying lightweight on the bar. Adjust yourself and your performance to your physical characteristics, even if it means pulling some extra weight over the bar.

10.17 SHOULDER JOINT

The shoulder is the most mobile joint in the body.

In calisthenics, the shoulder is the primary movement joint. It's therefore particularly important that you take care of the health and functionality of the shoulder girdle.

The more you know about your shoulder, the safer you'll be when performing the various calisthenics movements.

The shoulder girdle consists of the shoulder joints (scapula and humeral head), which are connected, via the collarbone, to the ribcage and its first rib. The shoulder girdle is a functional unit that's secured primarily by the muscle-ligament apparatus. Since, unlike the hip, the shoulder lacks the stability provided by surrounding bony structures, it's very susceptible to injury.

Functionally, your shoulder joint is referred to as a ball joint. Stabilization and centralization of your humeral head take place on a reflexive basis. This means that your shoulder muscles, particularly the muscles of the shoulder girdle (rotator cuff: m. infraspinatus, m. supraspinatus, m. teres minor, m. subscapularis), must be strengthened.

But you must strengthen your shoulder muscles not only with isolated exercises for your external rotation, like banded press (see section 11.8, "Rehabilitation and Prehabilitation Exercises"), but also by training on rings and with kettlebells, because this is where the reflexive component comes to bear.

The m. trapezius, m. rhomboideus, m. serratus anterior, m. serratus posterior, and m. serratus posterior inferior as well as the latissimus dorsi are all important muscles that must be worked to maintain a healthy shoulder girdle.

Moreover, in a pull-up, it's not only the movement of the shoulder joint that's important. Moving the shoulder joint by moving the arms is always linked to movement of the scapula.

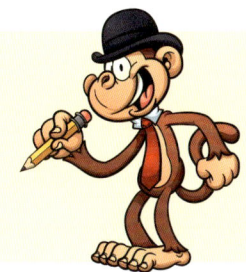

Try raising your arm while keeping your shoulder blade depressed (see section 10.9, "Shoulder-Blade Positions"). You'll quickly notice that you won't be able to raise your arm beyond a 140-degree elevation (a combination movement of bending the elbow and rotating the upper arm at the shoulder joint, which allows you to raise your arm).

To be able to raise your arm to the complete 180-degree elevation, as is needed for the starting position of a pull-up or handstand, the shoulder blade must move at an angle of 0–60 degrees, after which the rest of the motion takes place in the shoulder joint via the arm. This synergy between the **scapulothoracic groove** and the glenohumeral joint is called the *scapulohumeral rhythm*. That's why, in my chapter on the pull-up, I include exercises to strengthen the muscles around the scapula.

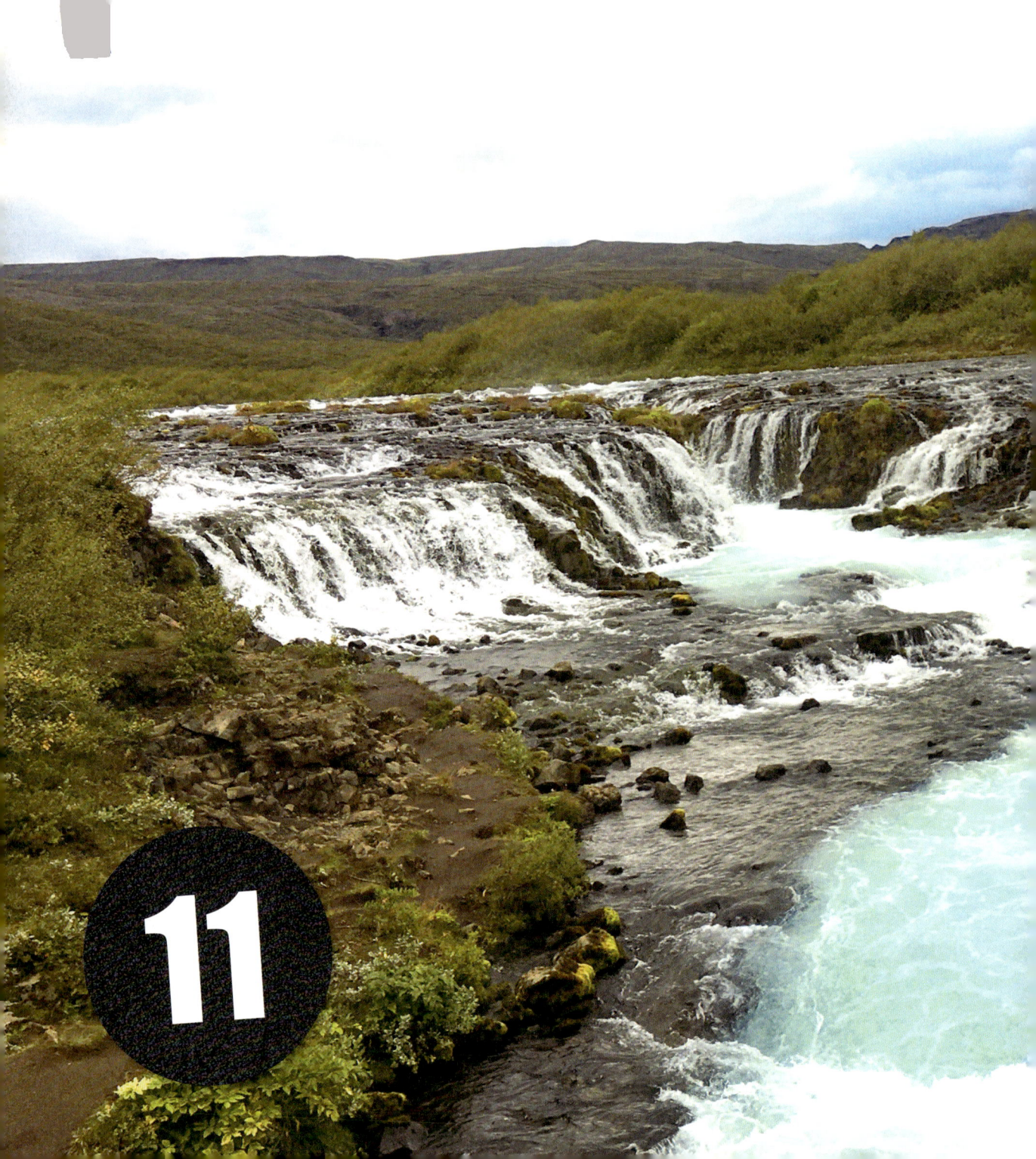

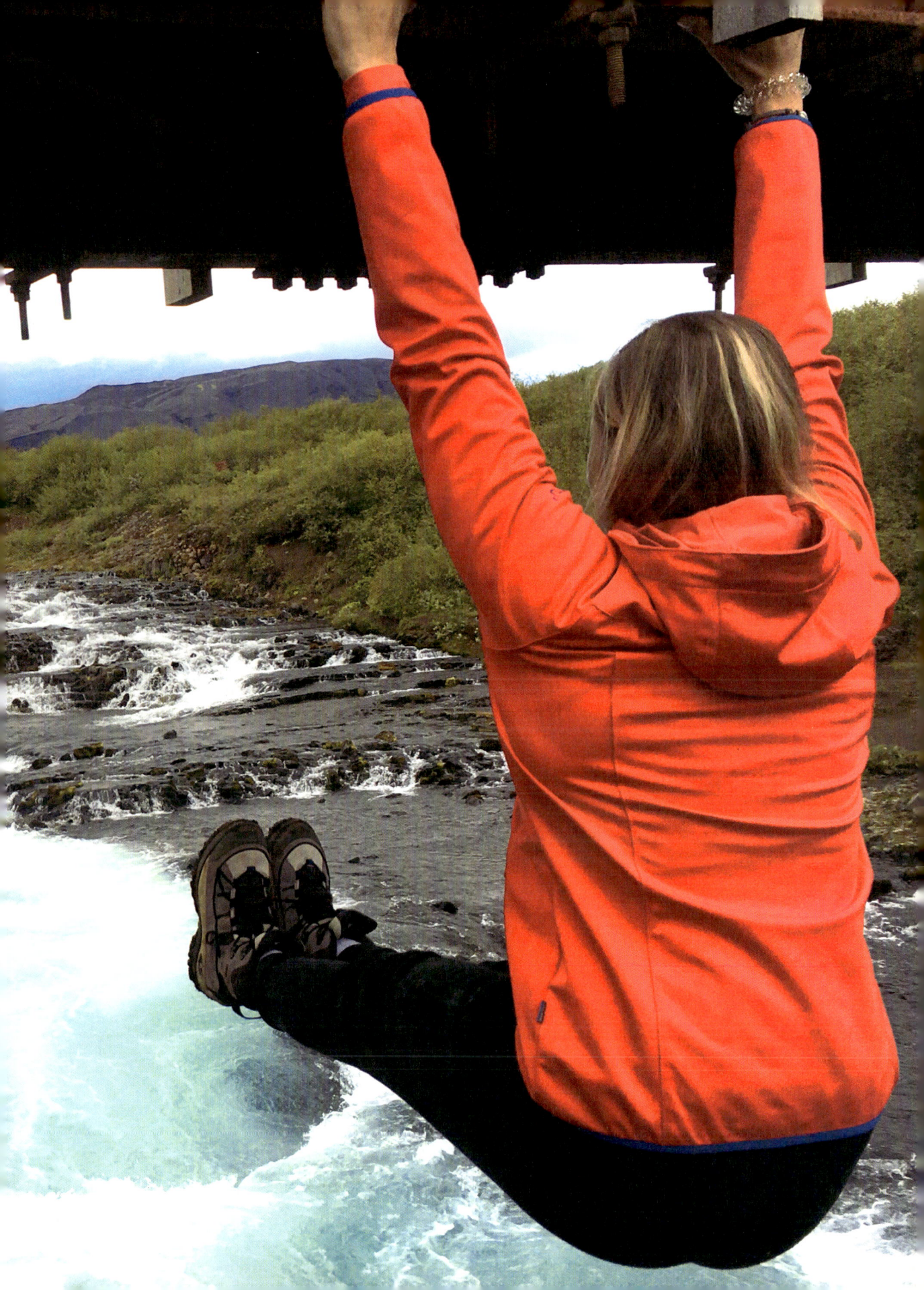

11 Beginner Basics and Their Possible Progressions

Following several chapters that provide a comprehensive overview, I lay out here the information most readers are, presumably, waiting for. I not only demonstrate the four *calisthenics basics*, but I also tell you what you need to pay attention to during the *execution*, which *basic prerequisite*s you must have, and which *feeder exercises (regressions)* are helpful, so you can master the basics and thereby build a strong foundation for advanced skills.

For my in-person newbies, the handstand is usually the first skill they'll learn. Of course, this requires overhead mobility and especially overhead strength. But most of all, the handstand requires room on either side, for sharing the knowledge with you in good conscience. Instead, over the course of this chapter, I introduce you to the skill of an *L*-sit.

Since calisthenics is referred to as progressive strength training with one's own bodyweight, I introduce the exercise regressions starting with the easiest exercise and progressively moving to more-difficult exercises. See chapter 12, "General Training Structure," to learn how to ultimately integrate them into your training.

An illustration shows the exercises divided into vertical and horizontal pulling and pushing exercises. When you look at the completed target shape of the basics, note that only the pull-up is a vertical pulling exercise, with horizontal pull variations as exercise regressions. By contrast, dips, push-ups, and squats are pushing exercises. Section 11.1 explains the importance of exercise variations on all planes.

Quality Beats Quantity

The technically clean and thus injury-free execution and the use of FROM in all exercises are top priorities. With all exercises, the main focus should be on performing the movements deliberately, slowly, and controlled instead of completing them as fast as possible. **Master the basics** before thinking about advanced skills. Your muscles need time to adjust to the loads. Don't rush something that you may come to regret later because an injury has sidelined you for an extended period of time, and trust your experience.

11.1 HEALTHY SHOULDER BALANCE WITH A COMBINATION OF PULLING AND PUSHING LOADS

Two mutually dependent guidelines fulfill an important function to ensure balanced loading of the shoulders. Training is based on these *pulling (tensile)* and *pushing (compressive)* exercises. They can be designated via two criteria, though there are also exercises that don't allow that particular allocation.

If the body's center of mass moves toward the hands, it's a pulling exercise. This includes not only the advanced back and front levers but also the basic pull-up. Here, all the upper-body muscles are activated. But when the body's center of mass moves away from the hands, it's a pushing exercise. Examples are the push-up, dip, and handstand.

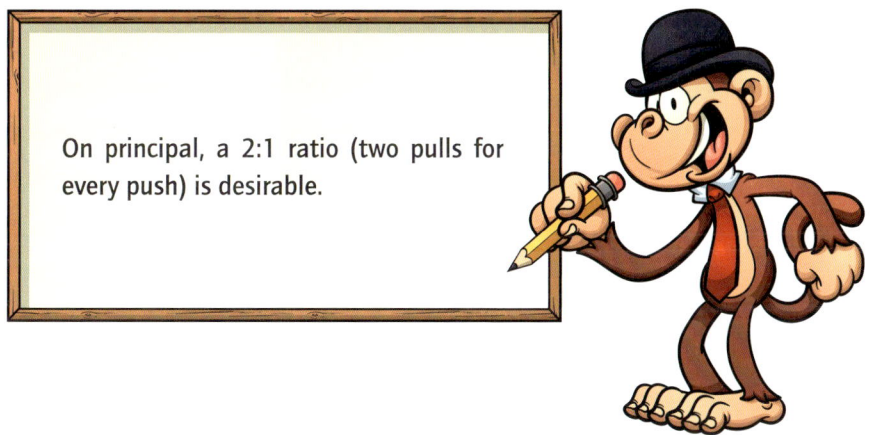

On principal, a 2:1 ratio (two pulls for every push) is desirable.

The reasons are simple. We do a lot of our work in front, especially in everyday life, which, to no surprise, is often spent sitting at a desk. The posterior chain and particularly the structures of the back are hardly utilized. Also, due to the anatomy of the shoulder girdle, pushing exercises present a greater strain, which is why they should be done less often than pulling exercises.

Ultimately, our body needs variety. To keep your body safe, work it on different planes and with different angles to set as many different impulses as possible, don't overwork certain muscle groups, and strengthen your body in every joint position.

11.2 ACTIVATION EXERCISES

As a total beginner athlete, regardless of your performance level, start by getting familiar with control exercises of the shoulder blades and the latissimus dorsi, which as stated in earlier chapters, are often weak links. Also, strengthen your rhomboids, trapezii, serrati, and the rotator cuffs (see section 10.17, "Shoulder Joint"). Consider the concept of **evaluation, isolation, integration, and improvisation** from Leon's chapter 3, "Mobility Fundamentals: What You Need to Know," which says you should first be able to activate joints separately from others before loading them (here with bodyweight). Slowly prepare your structures for the target movement by incrementally strengthening your shoulders with preparatory exercises.

Next, I introduce three exercises for shoulder-blade activation, which are also exercise regressions of the subsequently described basic exercises. The regressions are well suited as part of a warm-up but can also be part of a strength routine. I also describe resistance-band exercises that will prepare your shoulder blades for pulling exercises. You can review the information about shoulder CARs and wall slides in section 7.3, "Shoulders."

SCAPULA PULL-UPS

EXERCISE REGRESSIONS FOR PULL-UPS

1. Pull yourself from passive hanging to active hanging.

2. Keep your arms straight.

3. Briefly hold the position and then return to passive hanging in a controlled motion.

TIP

If you can't activate your shoulders during hollow-body position while hanging actively, release the hollow-body position and focus more on your shoulder blades.

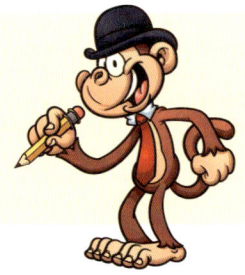

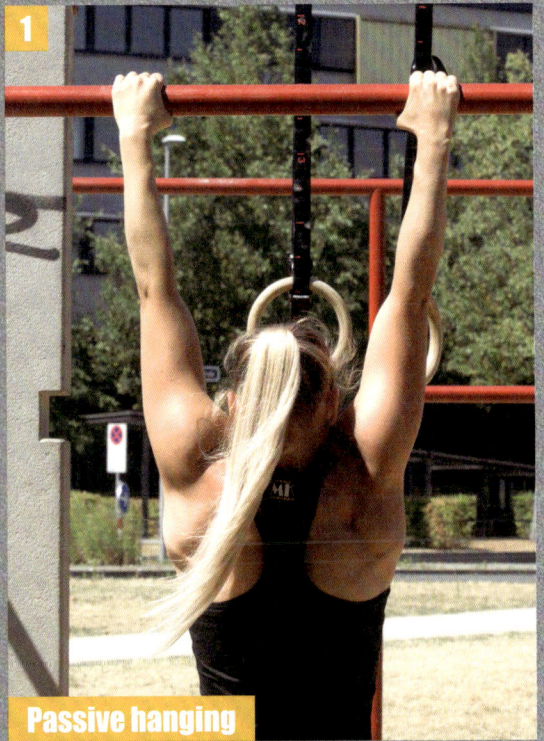

Passive hanging

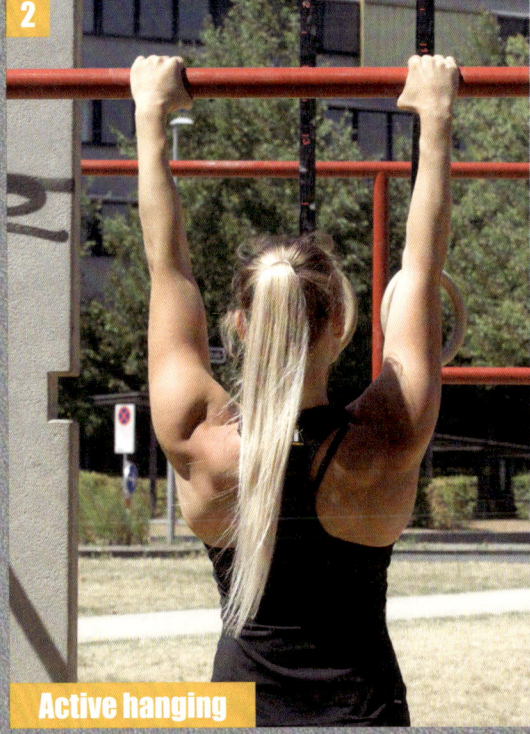

Active hanging

SCAPULA PUSH-UPS

EXERCISE REGRESSIONS FOR PUSH-UPS

1. Get in a push-up position.

2. Maintain the hollow-body position.

3. Alternate between protraction and retraction of the shoulder blades.

TIP

If you're unable to focus on your shoulder blades without also including your trunk, shorten the lever by resting your knees on the ground.

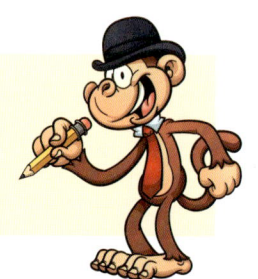

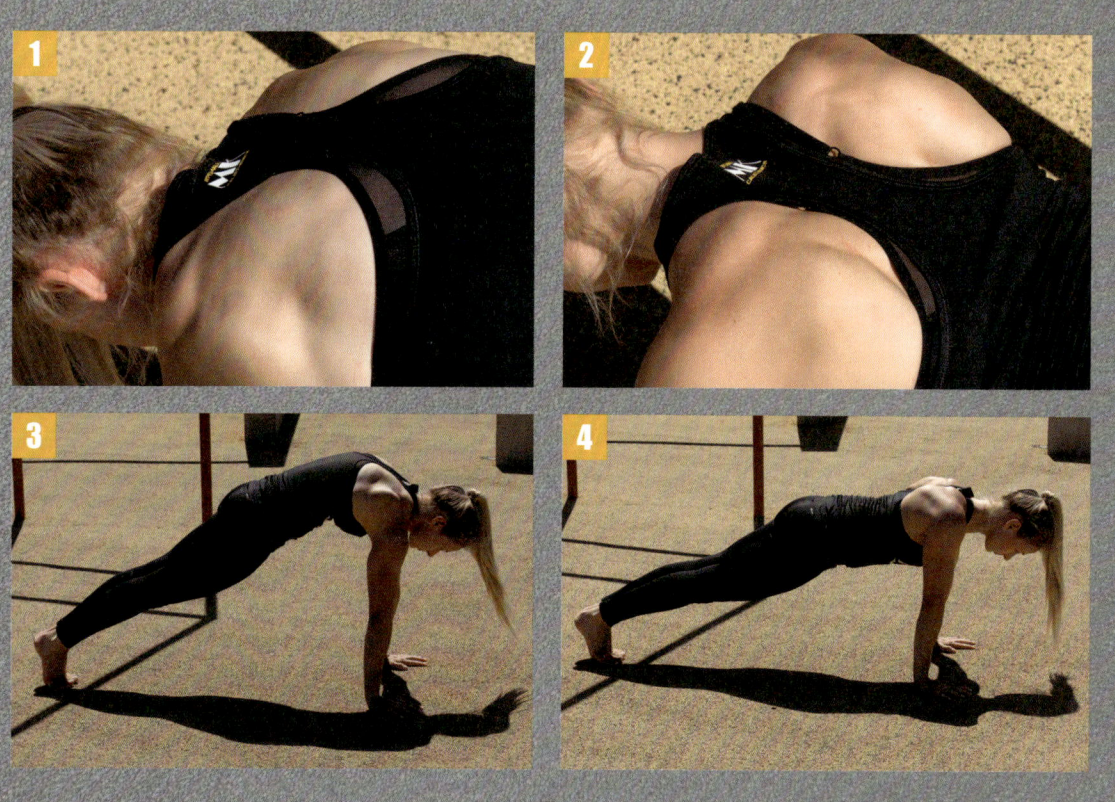

SCAPULA DIPS

EXERCISE REGRESSIONS FOR DIPS

1. Support yourself on the parallel bars.

2. Externally rotate your shoulders.

3. Alternate between shoulder retraction and protraction.

> **TIP**
>
> The more you can push into protraction, the farther forward you will automatically lean.

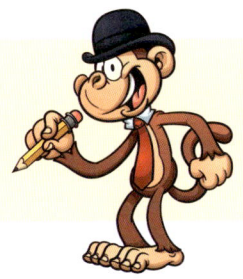

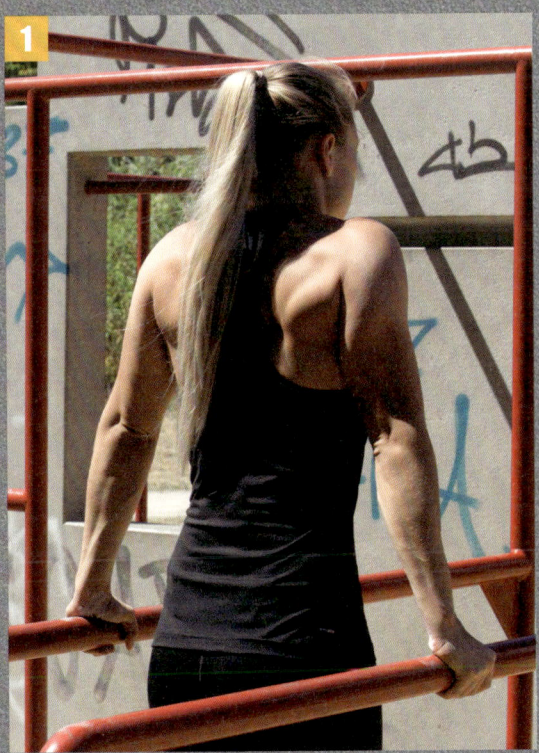

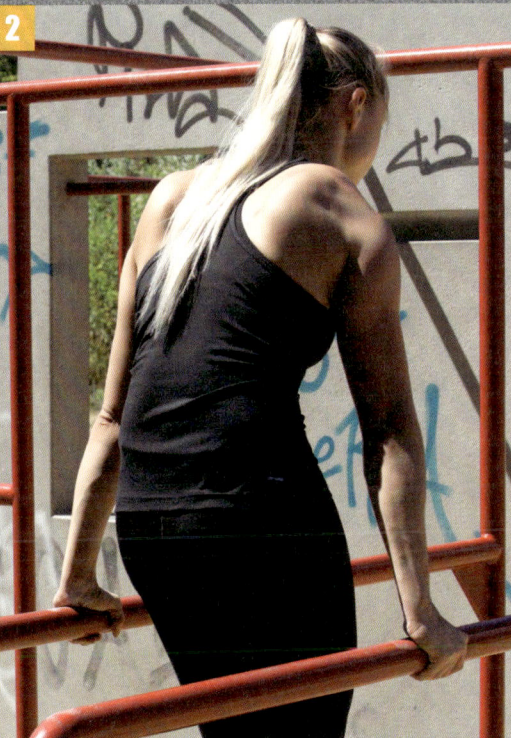

FRONT BAND ROW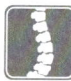

1. Sit with your legs extended in a straddle on the ground and hold the resistance band, attaching it with a neutral grip at chest level
2. Add pre-tension to the band.
3. Pull the band in to retraction and depression of your shoulder blades.
4. Keep your elbows close to your body.
5. Pull only as far as you can without your shoulders dropping forward.
6. Return your arms to a forward extension.
7. If retraction is your sticking point, hold that position on your way back.

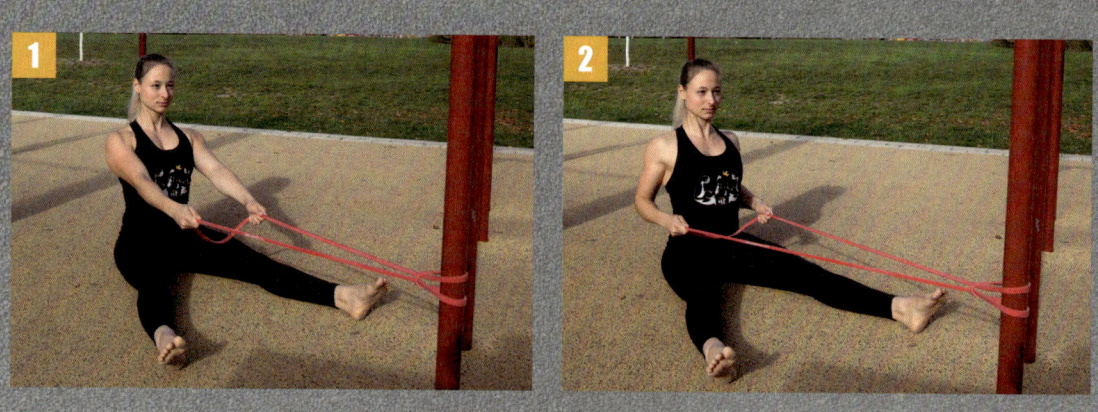

TIP

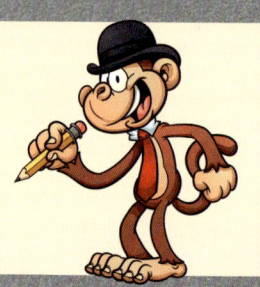

If you have no problem activating your shoulder blades in this position, you should view this exercise as merely part of your warm-up, and you can use your FROM by allowing a controlled protraction of the shoulder blades as you return to the starting position.

BAND PULL FROM ABOVE

  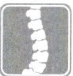

1. Attach a red or black resistance band to a high bar.

2. Get into a high kneeling position and, with a neutral grip, hold the band vertically below the bar.

3. Initiate the movement by depressing and retracting your shoulder blades.

4. Move your arms downward, keeping them close to your body, with your elbows pointing forward.

5. If retraction is your sticking point, maintain it on the way back to the end position with arms extended.

6. Use your FROM if you have no problem activating your shoulder blades.

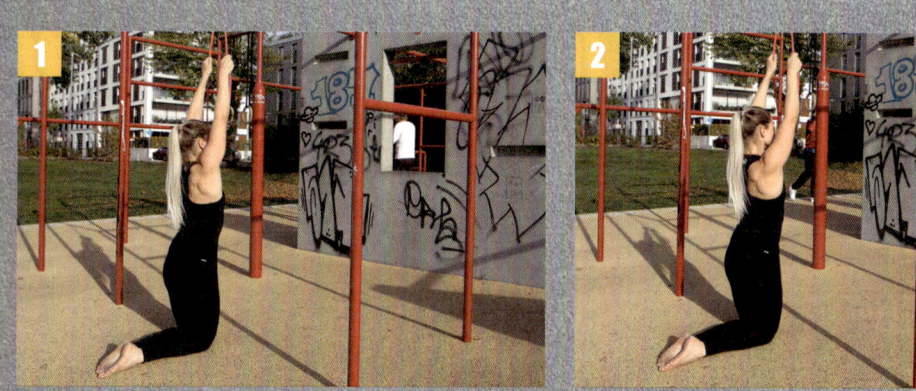
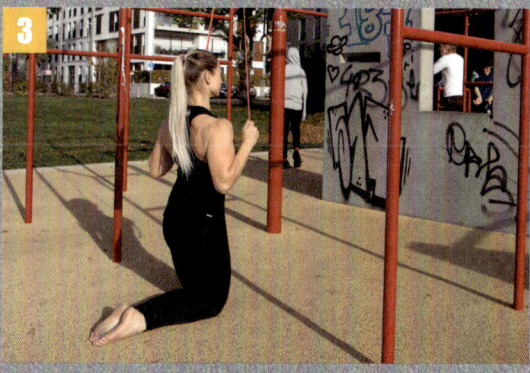

11.3 PULL-UPS AND POSSIBLE PROGRESSIONS

The pull-up seems to be particularly difficult for women. From an anatomical perspective, a woman's latissimus dorsi is, in fact, weaker, which is why targeted training is essential. If you don't practice it with focus and several times a week, you won't be able to master it.

In light of the rare activation of the large back muscle in our daily life, the pull-up requires more patience than the push-up or the dip until a decent, elegant pull-up has been mastered. But the result is worth it. Think about how it'll make your daily life easier and improve your posture when you strengthen the back with pull-ups. Instead of slumping shoulders and the associated rounded back, a strong back muscle helps to stabilize the spine and allows it to keep its natural shape.

That very first pull-up—it's an incredible feeling, especially when you want it as badly as I did back when I did it. I want you to experience that feeling, too, and in this section, I address frequent mistakes and sticking points and show you exercise regressions that will help you. Next to the classic pull-up, there are other progressions and thereby exercises that make the traditional pull-up more difficult. I mention some of these briefly at the end of the chapter.

11.3.1 WHAT YOUR PULL-UP SHOULD LOOK LIKE

A pull-up is best done on a bar or on rings. It's important that the bar or rings are high enough for you to hang freely, without your feet touching the ground.

The goal is to raise your chin above the bar and possibly bring your collarbones to the bar. The classic pull-up is done with an overhand grip, so the backs of your hands point toward your face..

1. The exercise begins with a firm, approximately shoulder-width grip while you hang passively. Grip the bar with both thumbs while using the break-the-bar principle to initiate an external shoulder rotation

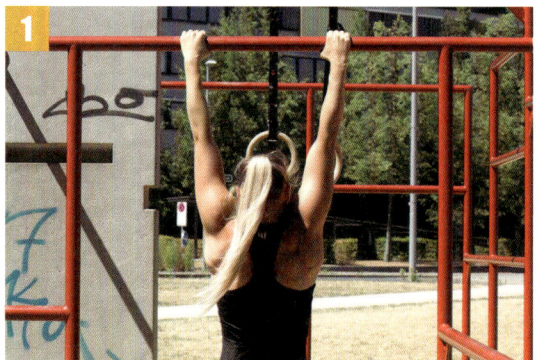

Beginner Basics and Their Possible Progressions

2. Activate your core. Assume the hollow-body position. Your feet should be slightly in front of the bar, not vertically below it.

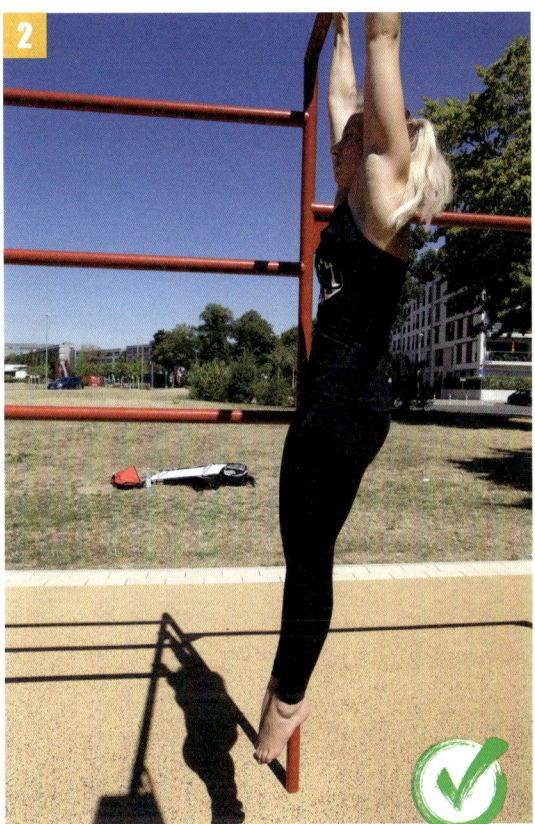 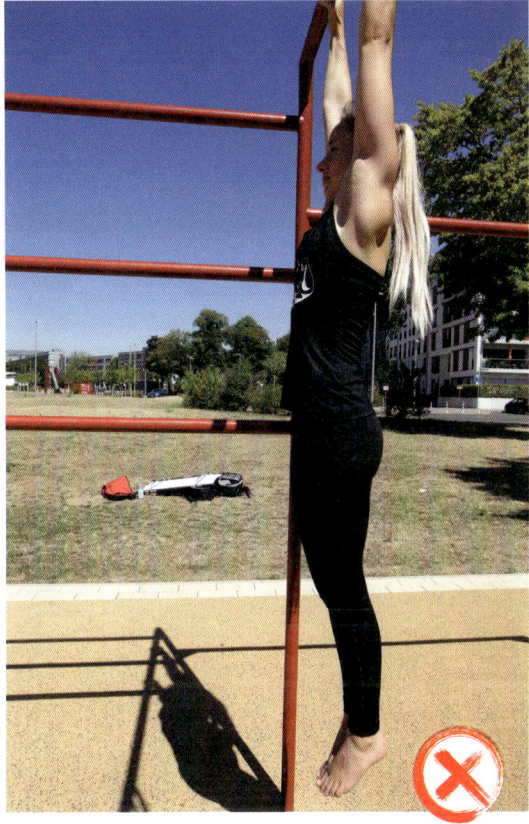

3. While maintaining the hollow-body position, pull yourself from a passive hanging position into an active one. At the same time, activate your shoulder blades (pulling them back and down) and thereby move them from elevation into depression and retraction.

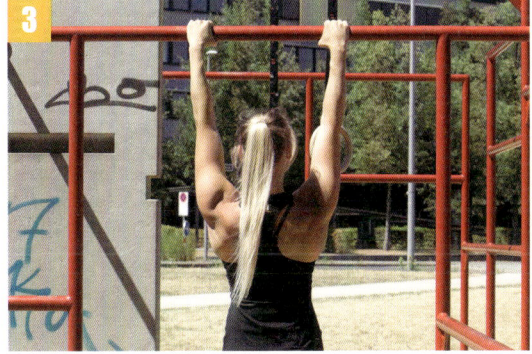

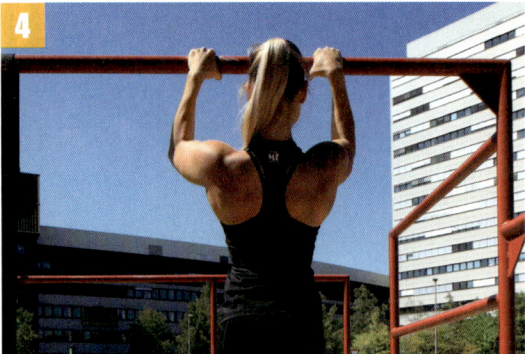
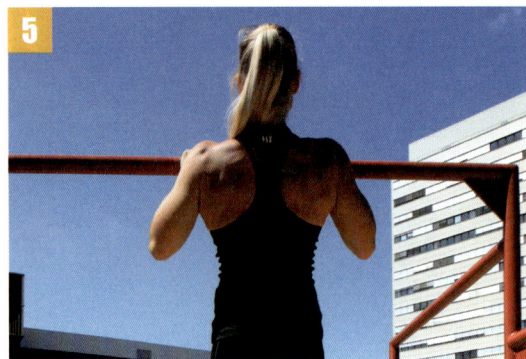
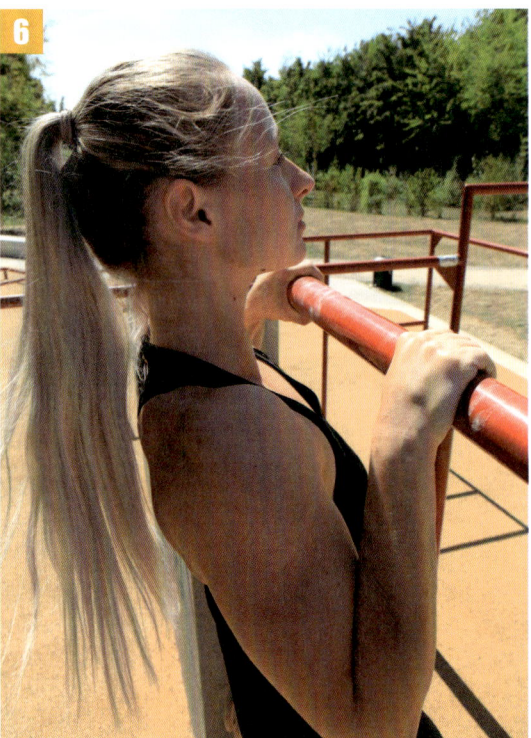

4. Bend your elbows by pulling yourself up so your chin passes above the bar. At the same time, let your elbows move back, close to the body, from about 90 degrees (shoulder retroversion) but only far enough to keep your shoulders from pitching forward. (Imagine describing a curved motion with your hands from your head to your chest.) Maintain depression and retraction at the highest point of the pull-up.

5. Keep your head in a forward-facing position to prevent hyperextension or bending of the cervical spine.

6. Activate muscle tension in your legs and keep them in an extended position. Due to the hollow-body position, which causes slight flexion of the trunk, they'll likely be in front of the bar. This means you're not hanging completely vertically below the bar while you're pulling yourself up.

7. After you've pulled yourself past the bar technically clean and using your FROM, reverse this movement on the way back down. It's important that you return to the passive hanging position slowly and in a controlled manner and don't let yourself drop into your shoulder joints, wrists, and elbows.

8. A complete pull-up has been achieved when the starting position of the dead hang has been assumed, meaning the elbows are straight and the shoulders are back to elevation in a passive hanging position. This is the only way to ensure that you'll use your FROM during subsequent pull-ups and that the participating muscles will be able to unfold their full strength potential to grow stronger.

The pull-up should be performed in a way that facilitates a fluid motion at the end. Make sure your shoulder blades glide dynamically along your ribcage.

11.3.2 TYPICAL MISTAKES

Based on these technically clean pull-ups, we often see mistakes that must be avoided to achieve the desired training effect and prevent possible injuires. Also, some people deliberately perform the movement incorrectly to, for instance, achieve record times in CrossFit or Freeletics. The following are some of the mistakes:

- Swinging the legs to be able to get the chin over the bar. As an initial impression of the movement pattern, this is more or less acceptable. But it shouldn't become a habit, as it's not in line with the form of a classic pull-up and strength isn't generated exclusively by the shoulders and back muscles. As a result, the back muscle, which is the focus of the exercise, isn't getting an optimal workout.

- Lowering too quickly from the bar back into the starting position should be avoided for the sake of the shoulder joint,

- Crossing the legs in back. (This is another pull-up variation. Read more in subsection 11.3.6, "Arched-Back Pull-ups.")

- Hyperextending the head at the highest point to get the chin barely over the bar (giraffe neck)

- Gripping the thumb at the top of bar (monkey grip) instead of around the bar (closed grip)

- Interrupting the movement amplitude prematurely, skipping the passive hanging position with extended arms at the lowest point

11.3.3 FREQUENT STICKING POINTS

LACK OF GRIP STRENGTH

The forearms are the weakest link during a pull-up. Although what's primarily working, the latissimus dorsi, still has strength, the forearms fail first.

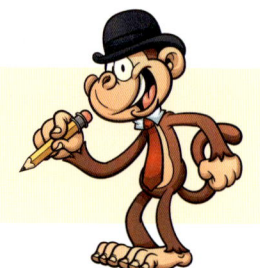

Grip strength has a proportionally positive effect on pull-up performance, which is why specific grip-strength training should be a regular part of your training schedule.

To do grip-strength training, hang from the bar or rings; find different ways to move hand over hand on the monkey bars; integrate loaded carries, like the farmer's walk (two heavy kettlebells carried like grocery bags); or use Captains of Crush grippers (grip-strength trainers) or dumbbells for targeted strengthening of the forearm muscles. You can also do rock climbing for a balancing workout.

At this point, I want to explain more about the correct thumb position while gripping the bar. The thumbs should reach around the bar and not be placed on top of the bar (monkey grip)—except if the bar is so thick that the thumb can't reach around the bar (closed grip). First of all, this position ensures a firm grip, and secondly, it has the advantage of the forearms being more involved while simultaneously working on the essential grip strength. Try it and feel the difference between the two thumb positions. Thumbs on top of the bar usually feels easier because the limiting factor of the forearms in the movement chain is minimized. But since we like to make things as difficult as possible in calisthenics so easier variations feel like child's play, we prefer *thumbs around the bar*.

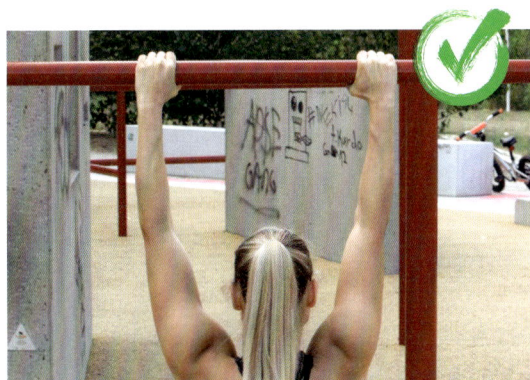 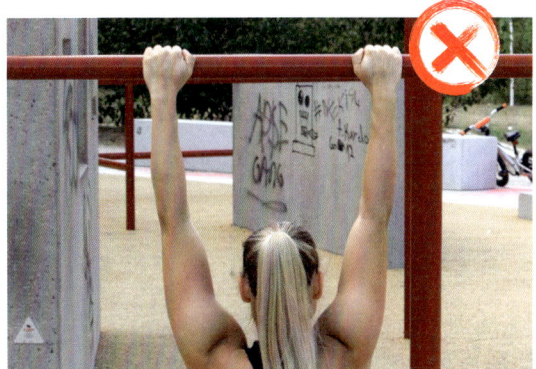

HUNCHBACK POSITION

Every day, I see people whose posture is reminiscent of a question mark: shoulders pitched forward and a *visible hunchback* in the area of the thoracic spine and *extreme lordosis* in the lumbar spine. The *muscle imbalances* that are the cause don't allow the thoracic spine to straighten. This means the prerequisite of using FROM while executing a pull-up doesn't exist.

The cause is *limited mobility* of the thoracic spine as well as *poor activation-ability* of the shoulder blades and the latissimus dorsi. In the pull-up, this is apparent in the frequently forward-pitching shoulders at the highest point of the pull-up, meaning the shoulders can't be sufficiently moved into depression and retraction. In this case, the strength of the actually participating muscles is inadequate, which is why there are compensating movements. Shoulders and the neck take on functions that result in incorrect weight bearing. This frequently results in pulled muscles in the neck or even shoulder pain.

It's therefore important to integrate correcting exercises into your training that primarily target the latissimus dorsi, rhomboids, trapezii, serrati, and rotator cuffs. These muscles make sure the shoulders are pulled back and down so you can assume an upright posture.

If you have trouble pulling your shoulders back and down, practice this position in particular by doing exercises like the band pull from above and the ring row, which are described in subsection 11.3.6, "Arched-Back Pull-Ups." Don't use your FROM, but leave your shoulder blades depressed and retracted with arms extended.

EXTERNAL ROTATION THAT'S TOO WEAK

While I address this in chapter 10, "Calisthenics Fundamentals: What You Need to Know," this item can't be left out here. Weak external rotators cause the shoulders to internally rotate, which results in a narrowing of the subacromial space and increases the risk of inflammation.

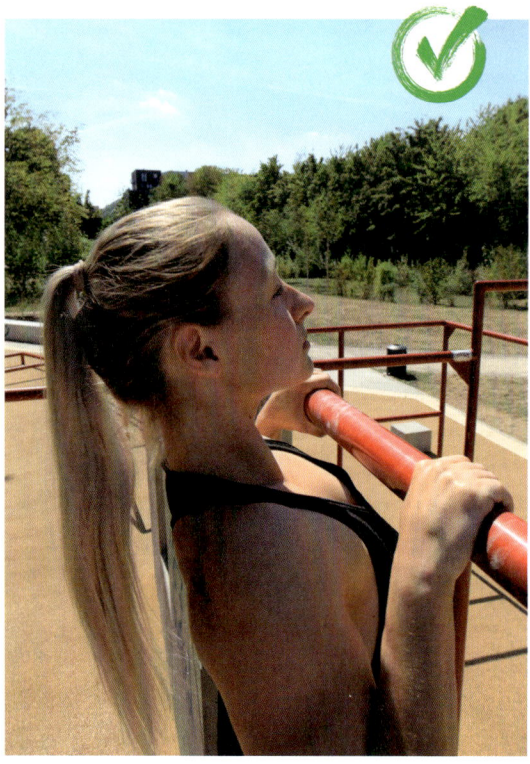 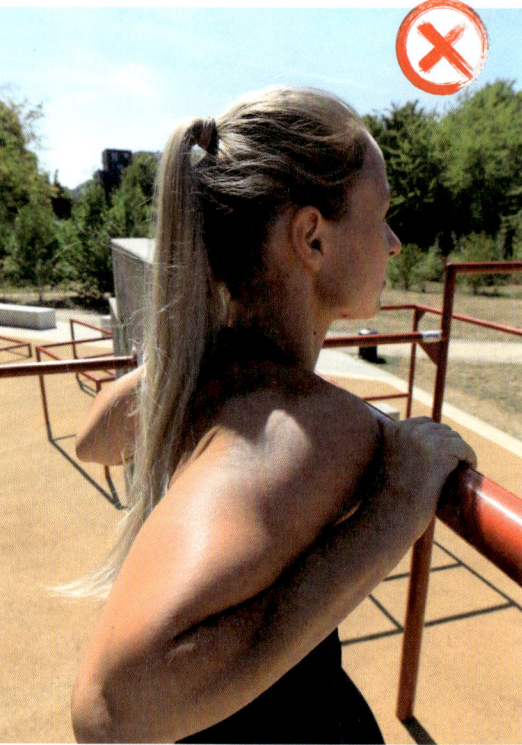

11.3.4 GRIP VARIATIONS

First, let's discuss the different grip techniques that can be used variably for all preparatory exercises, determine the degree of difficulty, and work other portions of the forearm muscles.

I introduce the grip variations from the easiest to increasingly more-difficult positions, starting with the *underhand pull-up*, also called a *chin-up*. Palms and fingers should point toward the face. In this supine-forearm position, the shoulders are already externally rotated, which is why no additional strength must be mustered for the break-the-bar principle.

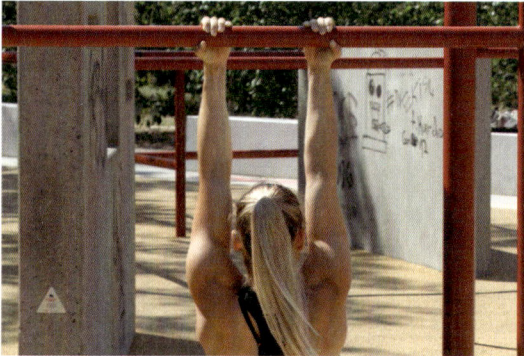

With the neutral grip (hammer grip), the backs of the hands point to the sides, and the palms face each other.

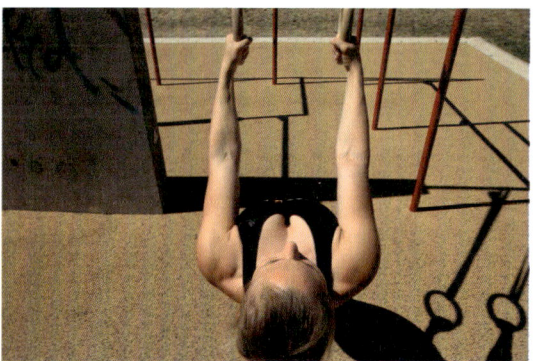

The *classic pull-up* is performed with the *overhand grip*, whereby the backs of the hands point toward the face. Due to the pronation of the forearms, the shoulders tend to rotate internally. Since this narrows the subacromial space between the humeral head and the socket, causing rubbing that can result in shoulder problems, it's necessary to externally rotate the shoulder joint via the break-the-bar principle.

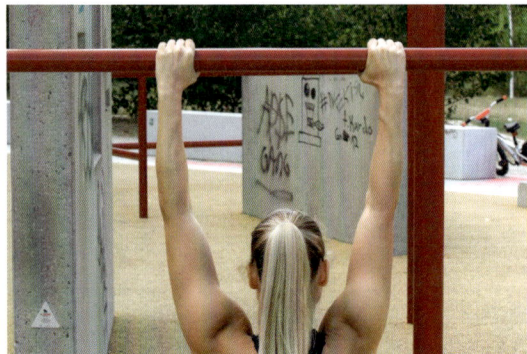

You can also vary the grip width from narrow to wide or use alternating grips (overhand and underhand). For a balanced workout, it's recommended to vary the grips. Ultimately, the different positions work other portions of the muscles, especially in the forearms.

TIP

Hold the rings with the neutral grip or underhand grip. The overhand grip on the rings makes it hard to achieve an active external shoulder rotation, which is why the shoulders are in a rather unfavorable internally rotated position.

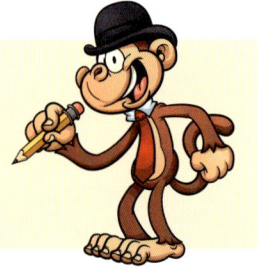

11.3.5 OVERHAND PULL-UPS VERSUS UNDERHAND PULL-UPS

Muscle activation is the same in both overhand and underhand pull-ups (chin-ups). Supine forearms merely involve the biceps more as an auxiliary muscle. The direction of movement during a chin-up is more specific, which is why compensating movements are less possible. In this case, the thoracic spine is straighter right from the start. But the pull-up with the overhand grip allows for more-compensating movements, with either the shoulders tilting forward or the elbows coming out to the sides.

Chin-ups use the lower, vertical fibers of the latissimus dorsi. Since most of the latissimus dorsi is made up of these fibers and diagonal fibers, this grip is easier to perform.

11.3.6 ARCHED-BACK PULL-UPS

ARCHED BACK PULL-UPS/
GIRONDA STERNUM PULL-UPS

This variation of the pull-up isn't appropriate for beginners, but I mention it here to answer this frequently asked question: Should pull-ups always be performed in the hollow-body position? No. Because variety is important. If you're able to perform technically correct classic pull-ups, integrate arched-back pull-ups into your training. Aside from variation, the reason can depend on your goals. But, first, let's talk about the execution of an arched-back pull-up.

The difference from the pull-up in the hollow-body position is that, in the arched-back pull-up (also called the *Gironda sternum pull-up*), you don't assume the hollow-body position, and thus your lower body, from the trunk down, doesn't participate in the movement chain, which places the focus on the retracted shoulder blades and an ideally goal-oriented activation of the latissimus dorsi. With your chest, you pull toward the bar with your upper body parallel to the bar and your legs hanging in a relaxed position until your chest touches the bar. So if you want to have a pretty wide latissimus dorsi, you should give preference to this variation. The arched-back pull-up is seen primarily in bodybuilding circles. Considering the description, this isn't surprising, since that sport is primarily about the best-possible hypertrophy of individual muscles.

TIP

The execution is quite a bit easier with a neutral grip.

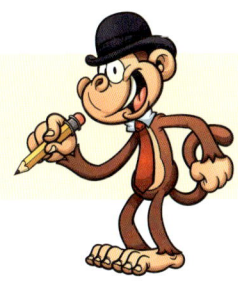

11.3.7 PULL-UP EXERCISE REGRESSIONS

AUSTRALIAN PULL-UPS/ RING ROWS/INCLINE ROWING

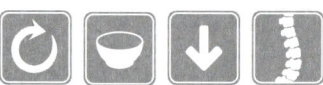

The Australian pull-up (also called the ring row or incline rowing), commends itself for beginning pull-up training. Rings are best suited because their height can be adjusted, making it possible to change the degree of difficulty. A bar at chest or stomach level would also work.

1. Position yourself at an angle to the rings and hold them with a neutral grip. The more parallel you hang to the ground, the more difficult the exercise.

2. Remember the levers. Knees slightly bent make the exercise easier than straight legs.

3. Lengthen the spine, keep your head in a neutral position, and maintain core tension.

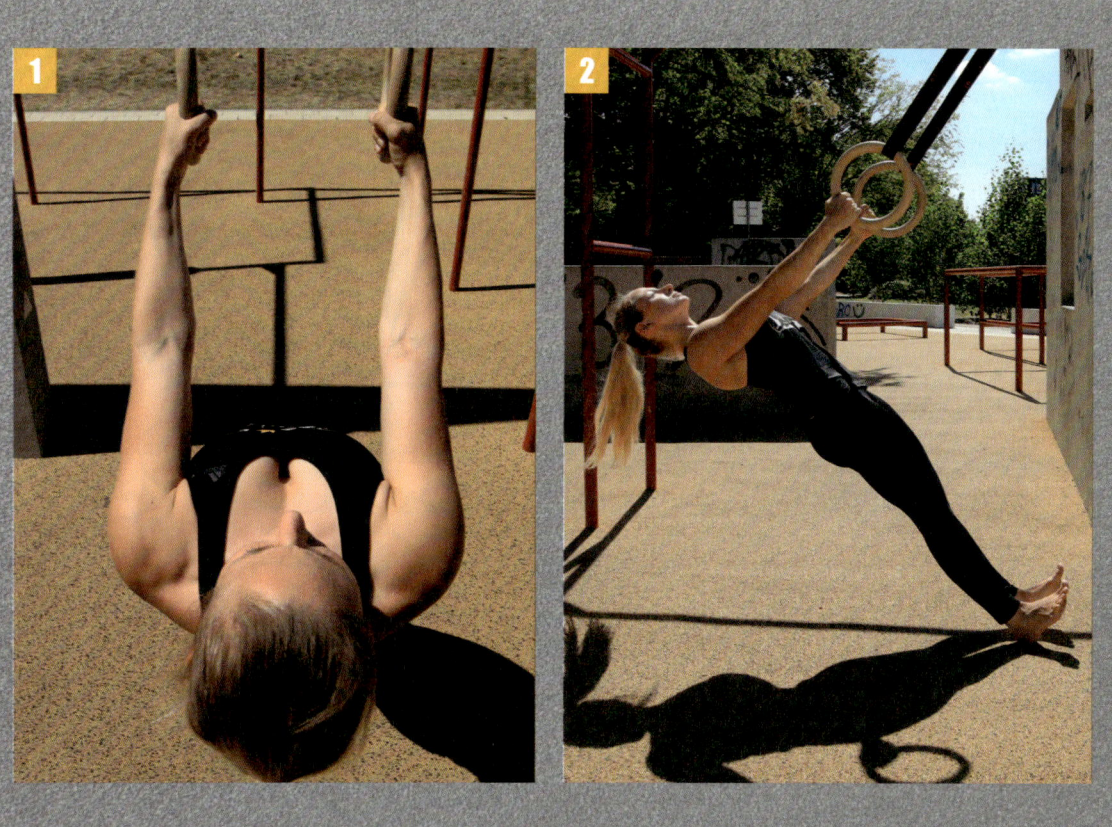

Beginner Basics and Their Possible Progressions   **213**

4. With your chest, pull yourself up to ring level, while keeping your elbows close to your body as they move past your ribcage.

5. Pull with your shoulder blades in a depressed and retracted position.

6. In a controlled motion, lower yourself back down to the extended-arm position.

7. If the lowest position is your sticking point, maintain depression and retraction of the shoulder blades at that lowest point.

8. Execute the movement with FROM by lowering your shoulders into protraction.

9. On a bar, you can vary the grip, either underhand or overhand, wide, or narrow.

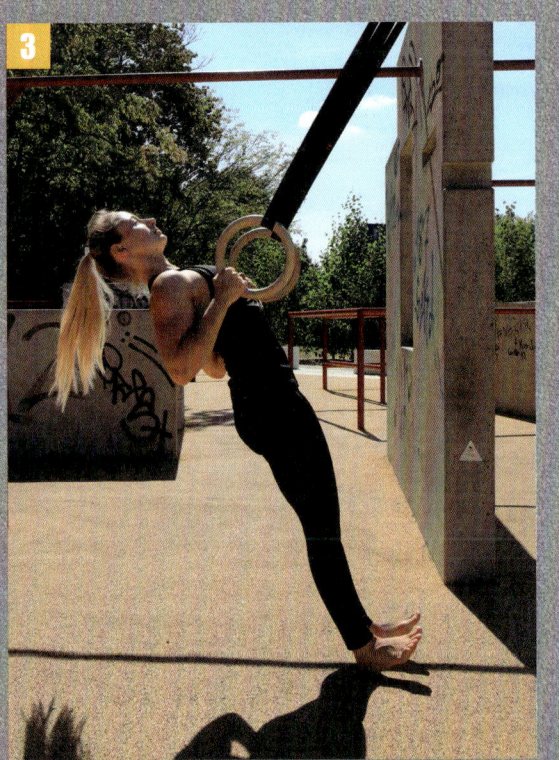

TIP

The more vertical your body is to the rings or bar, the easier the exercise.

While pulling, imagine you're squeezing a ping-pong ball between your shoulder blades.

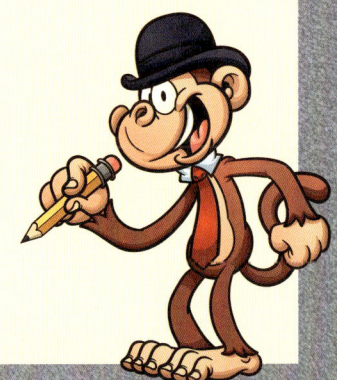

NEGATIVE (ECCENTRIC) PULL-UPS

1. Behind the bar or rings, set up a vaulting box for mounting.

2. Slowly lower yourself incrementally forward into the starting position of the negative pull-up.

3. Start with your chin over the bar and pull your shoulders back and down.

4. Lower yourself as slowly as possible into the passive hanging position.

> **TIP**
>
> Press your upper arms against your sides while maintaining the depressed and retracted shoulder-blade position. This creates more tension and allows you to lower yourself more slowly and in a more controlled motion.

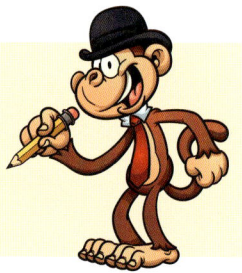

Now, you might be wondering how to do this exercise using a resistance band. The idea behind using bands is to reduce the bodyweight. For this purpose, bands come in different strengths. I'm not a fan of resistance bands. Especially not for the pull-up. Bands expose two obvious weak spots.

1. Beyond a 90-degree angle, you're on your own. The band supports you in only the initial third of the movement.

2. With insufficient core stability, the band pulls you diagonally forward into an unfavorable position. A beginner, in particular, relies too much on the band for support, losing core tension and giving the body and the brain an inaccurate image of the movement.

Overall, bands are great for creating positive experiences, and when used correctly with core stability, they help to internalize the motion sequence. But ultimately, you should focus on doing these exercises without bands. Negative pull-ups, in particular, generate the strength you need for the eccentric nature of the pull-up. Here, too, positive benefits are individual. The band works great for some people and not so much for others. Try it for yourself.

Beginner Basics and Their Possible Progressions

Awesome! You did your first clean pull-up. Now you need to work on increasing your repetitions. The pull-up, with its versatility, extends to other progressive exercises.

JUMPING PULL-UPS

These are done on a bar (or rings) that's high enough for your arms, extended, to reach them while your knees are slightly bent. Actively use your legs to push off the ground. Use this momentum to pull yourself up.

1. Choose a certain height for the bar or rings so you can still reach them with extended arms.

2. Actively use your legs, push off the ground, and use the momentum to pull yourself up.

3. In addition to the momentum created by your legs, pull with your arms.

TIP

During a jumping pull-up, you skip activation of the shoulder blades, which is why you also need to practice the other exercises, especially the scapula pull-ups.

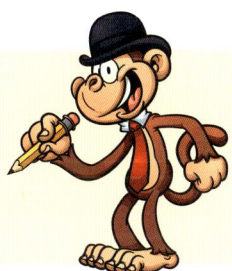

11.4 PUSH-UPS AND POSSIBLE PROGRESSIONS

I'd like to begin the pushing exercises with the classic push-up in its correct form as well as frequent mistakes and sticking points. These are followed by explanations of progressive intensification. Building on that are push-up variations, to highlight the versatility of the push-up.

11.4.1 WHAT YOUR PUSH-UP SHOULD LOOK LIKE

1. Place your hands shoulder-width apart in a force line vertically below your shoulders. Spread your fingers to enlarge the support surface. This will allow you to bring more strength to bear. Point your index fingers to twelve o'clock.

2. In the starting position, your arms should be straight. The crooks of the elbows point forward (external shoulder rotation). Imagine trying to screw your hands into the ground and toward the outside.

3. Move into push-up position.

4. Push your shoulder blades against gravity into protraction. Engage your core in the hollow-body position.

5. Your body should form a stable, straight line from head to toe. Your eyes should be looking at the ground. By doing so, your head forms a natural extension of your spine. Your feet should be very close together with your heels touching.

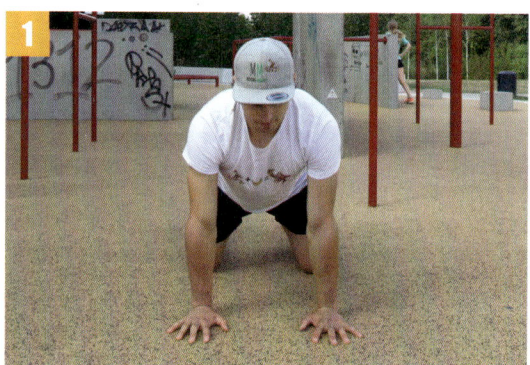
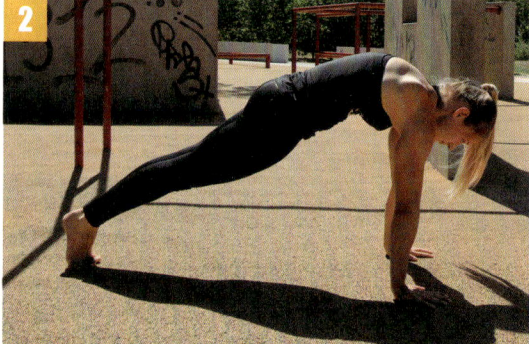

Beginner Basics and Their Possible Progressions   217

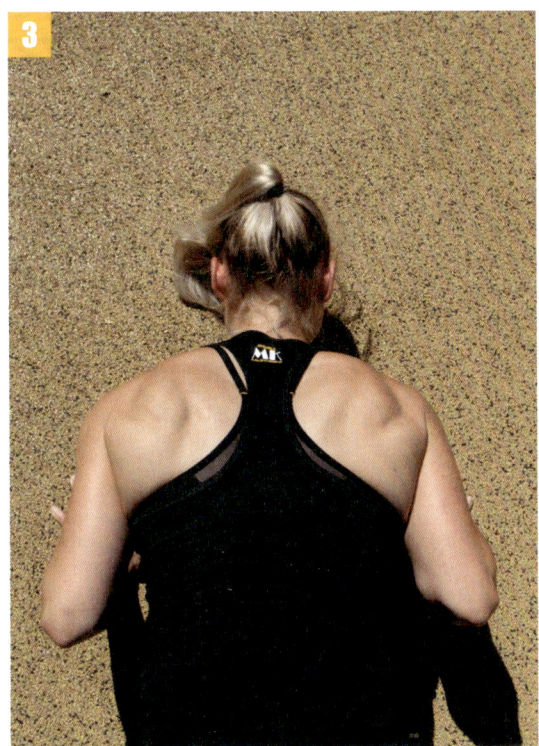
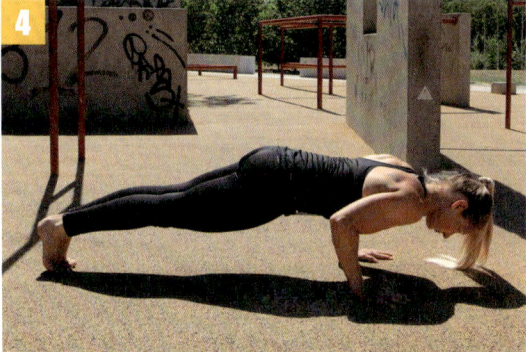
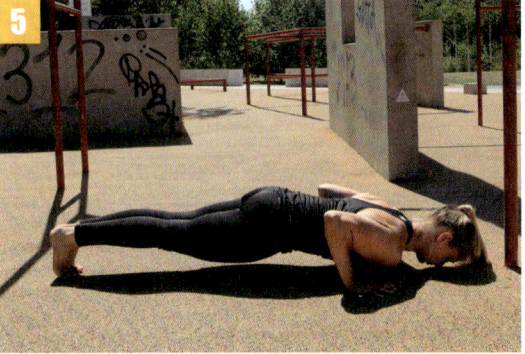

6. Now bend your elbows so they stay very close to your upper body (45 degrees max) and point back rather than to the sides. Lower your chest until your upper arms are parallel to the ground. Ideally, your chest should touch the ground for FROM. Don't lie on your stomach. Use parallettes for more FROM.

7. Make sure your shoulder blades glide smoothly along your ribcage.

8. From the end position, at the lowest point, you now need to push back up into a support position while maintaining body tension. In the starting position, your arms should be completely extended, and your shoulder blades should be in protraction before starting the next repetition.

11.4.2 TYPICAL MISTAKES

- Hands are internally rotated, which is why the elbows stick out to the sides and are at a nearly 90-degree angle to the body, so when looking down at the elbows from above, they form a line with the shoulder blades. In this case, people often compensate with the strength of their chest muscles because their triceps are too weak. In the long run, this lack of external shoulder rotation leads to shoulder problems.

- The chest lifts off the ground before the hips do.

- The exercise is performed with extreme tucking of the head toward the chest. This causes the cervical spine to abandon its position as a natural extension of the rest of the spine and can cause neck pain, which in turn can cause back problems.

- The movement amplitude isn't complete.

11.4.3 FREQUENT STICKING POINTS

LACK OF CORE TENSION

Insufficiently strong abdominal and back muscles prevent buildup of core tension, resulting in either hips sagging or the backside sticking up to compensate. Pushing your backside up activates the long psoas muscle (m. psoas major), which holds the hip in a neutral position more than the abdominal muscles. This can cause back pain, particularly in the area of the lumbar spine.

WEAK TRICEPS

Remember, a weak triceps can result in the primary power being shifted to the chest. Theoretically, this isn't a problem. After all, the chest and triceps participate in the push-up. During the upward movement, though, this is compensated for by the elbows sticking out to the side, resulting in the shoulders rotating inward.

11.4.4 GRIP VARIATIONS

Here, too, you can use all grip variations but only after you've cleanly executed the classic push-up several times in a row. Your hands can form a triangle (diamond [narrow] push-ups), whereby more effort is placed on the triceps. Or you can place your hands farther apart to activate the chest muscles.

11.4.5 PUSH-UP EXERCISE REGRESSIONS

The same criteria regarding proper execution also apply to the exercise regressions.

NEGATIVE (ECCENTRIC) PUSH-UPS

1. Get in the push-up position.

2. By bending your elbows, lower yourself to the ground as slowly and as controlled as possible.

3. Drop your knees to the ground to help push yourself back up to the starting position to perform more repetitions.

INCLINE PUSH-UPS

1. Choose a raised surface. You can also start with a wall.

2. The lower the surface, the more difficult the exercise.

3. Let your chest touch the surface.

4. Progressively lower the surface to pursue your goal of doing a push-up, one that's parallel to the ground.

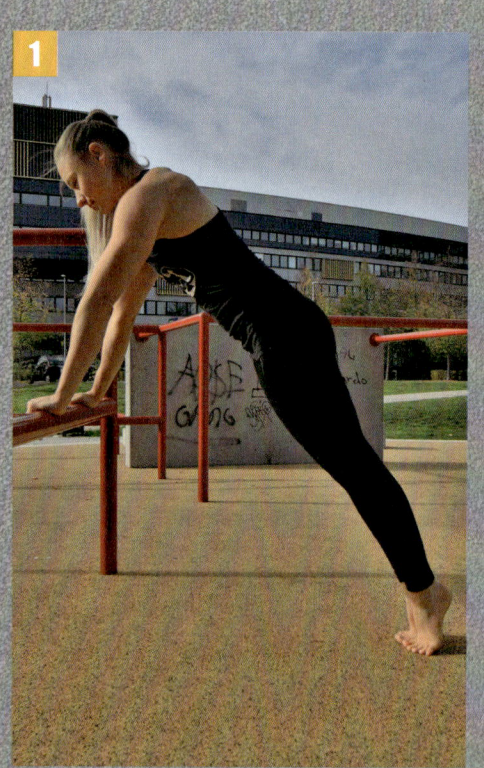

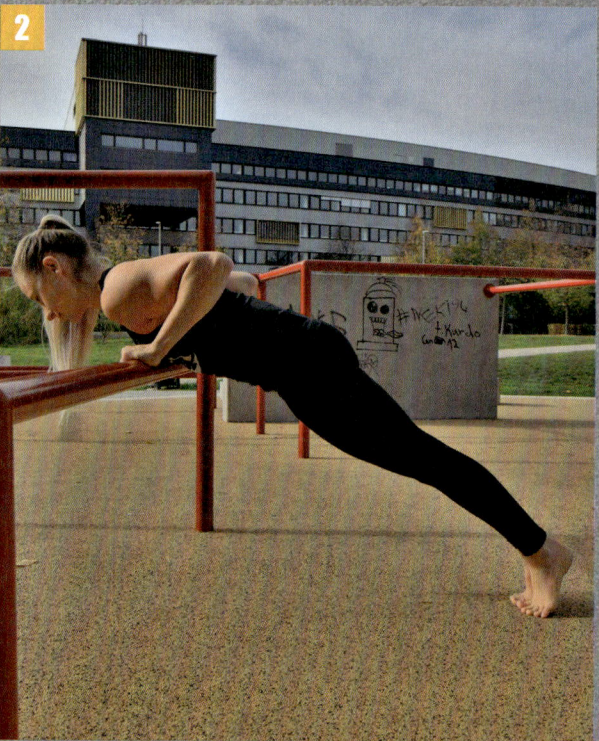

BAND-ASSISTED PUSH-UPS 💪(💪)

1. Attach a red or black resistance band to an overhead bar.

2. Reach with your arms through the loop and position it below your chest (underarms).

3. Move vertically into a push-up position below the bar.

4. The supporting tension of the band from above makes the concentric phase of the push-up easier.

DEAD-POINT PUSH-UPS 💪💪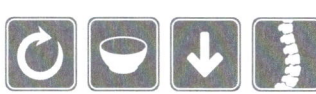

1. Lie on your stomach on the ground.

2. Place your hands next to your chest, close to your body.

3. Build up body tension (like a plank) and push yourself into the push-up, with your elbows pointing back.

RTO IN A PUSH-UP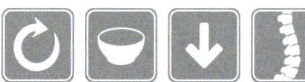

1. Hang the rings just above the ground.

2. Get in the starting position for a push-up in the rings. Use the neutral grip.

3. Now move the rings into RTO. Your elbows and palms should face forward.

4. Actively push out of your shoulders into protraction. In addition to turning the rings out, you must also push them in, toward each other, so you can stabilize the wobbly rings.

5. Hold this position briefly and then return to the neutral starting position. This exercise is also a preparatory exercise for RTO in free ring dips (see subsection 11.5.4, "Dip Exercise Regressions").

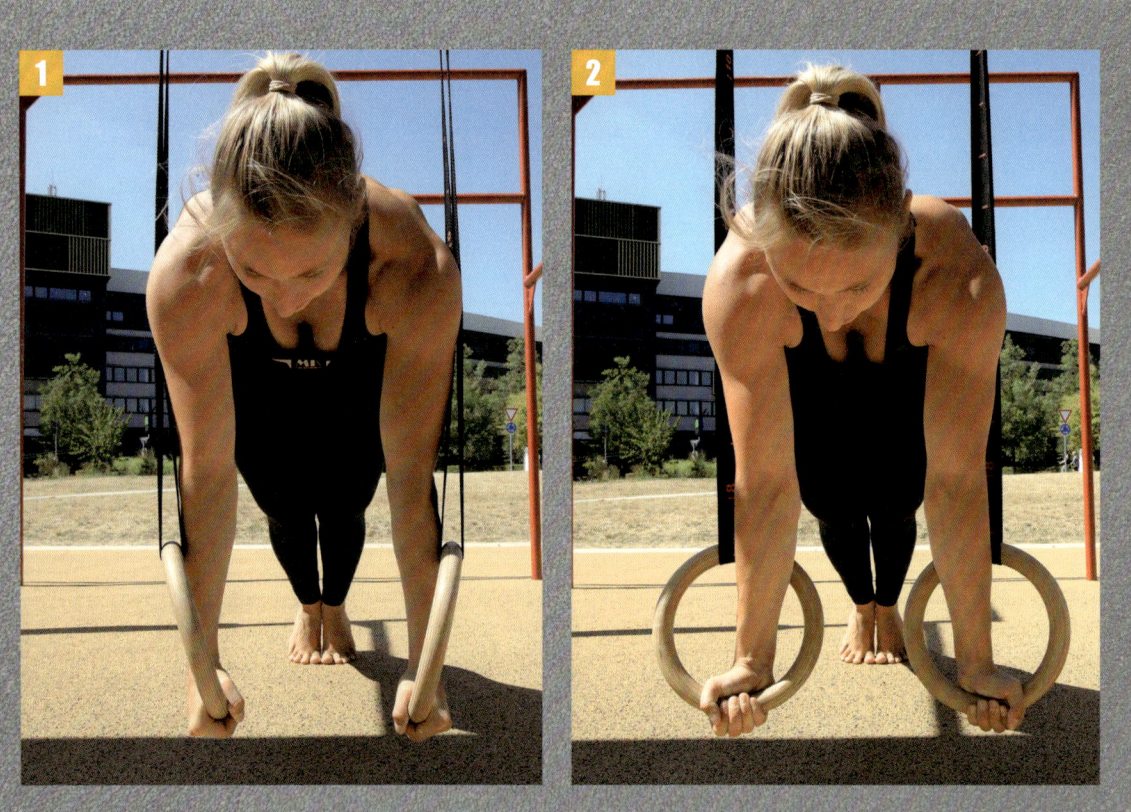

Another regression is an exercise that's often recommended but one I personally can't recommend as the previous exercises are better alternatives for learning the push-up. I'm talking about what are sometimes called *women's push-ups*, push-ups that are performed on the knees for support. The idea of shortening the lever by drawing in the legs in is a good one, but there are two problems with this type of push-up.

1. It's awkward and hurts the knees in the long term.

2. Beginners usually aren't able to focus simultaneously on all the technical aspects, which is why the all-important core tension is often not maintained in this position.

By the way, this is also true for doing push-ups with your legs in a straddle. Yes, it does provide a wider support surface and makes the push-up easier, but aside from the lack of health-promoting stabilization of the lumbar spine, the aforementioned lack of core tension makes the push-up look saggy.

Once you can perform these preparatory exercises correctly, you can try the classic push-up.

Here are options for increasing the difficulty: ring push-ups; decline push-ups (feet on a raised surface); deficit push-ups, for which the hands rest on parallettes to allow for more range of motion, placing the chest muscles in a stretch position and recruiting more muscle fibers; typewriter or archer push-ups, which are preparatory exercises for the one-armed push-up; pseudo planche push-ups; and pike push-ups, which can be considered exercise regressions for handstand push-ups against a wall and subsequently build up strength for free-standing handstand push-ups.

11.5 DIPS AND POSSIBLE PROGRESSIONS

We now get to the dip as a vertical and thus more-difficult pushing exercise. But first, for your sake and the sake of your shoulder health, it's important to make sure that the width of the parallel bars matches your individual dip width. You can measure the width by holding one forearm plus two fingers arm horizontally in front of your chest and touching it to the opposite hand.

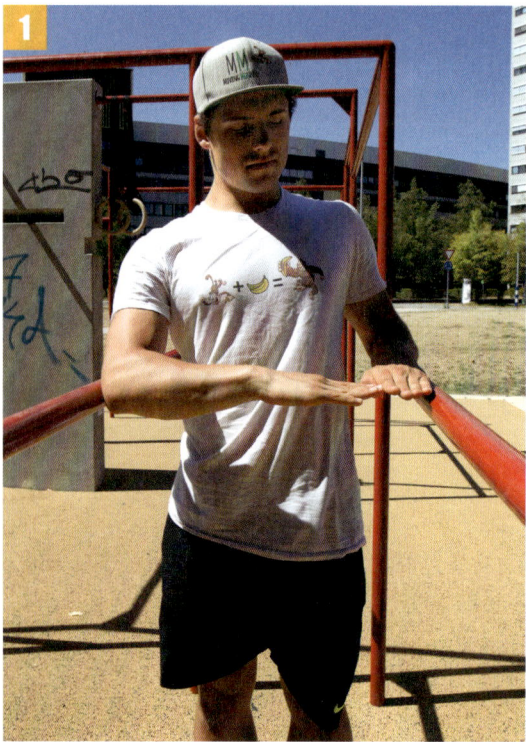
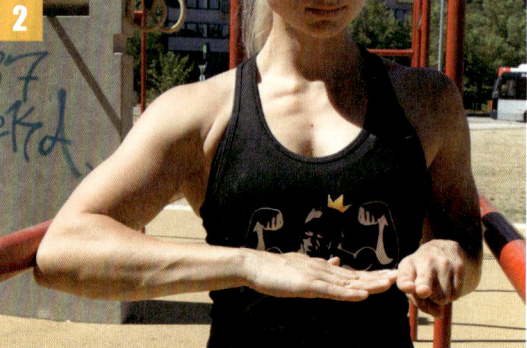
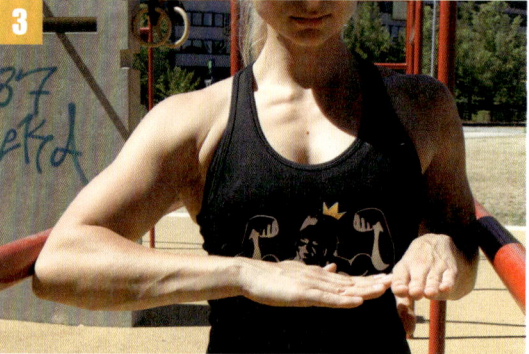

In terms of guidelines, follow the directions for the push-up (only now you're vertical instead of horizontal).

11.5.1 WHAT YOUR DIP SHOULD LOOK LIKE

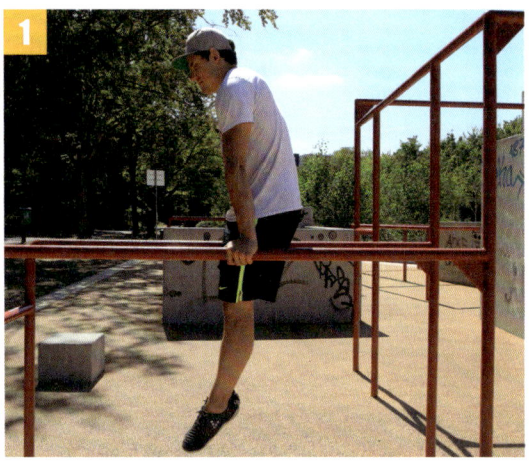
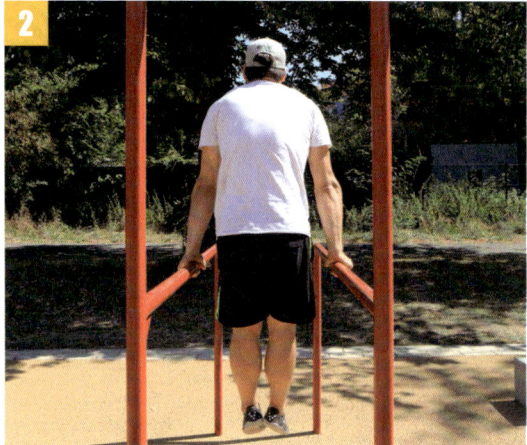

1. Use straight arms to support yourself on the parallel bars. If the bars are too high for you, stand on a box to get in the starting position more easily.

2. Don't bend your wrists. Keep them as neutral as possible to protect them.

3. Rotate the inside of your elbows forward again to externally rotate the shoulders. Push out of the shoulders into shoulder protraction.

4. Assume the hollow-body position. Your feet will likely be slightly more forward.

5. Lean forward with your chest.

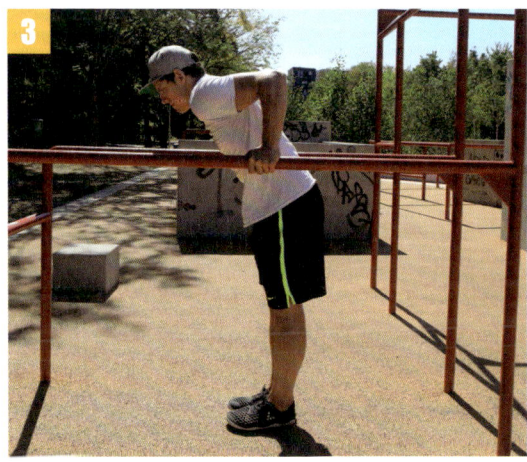
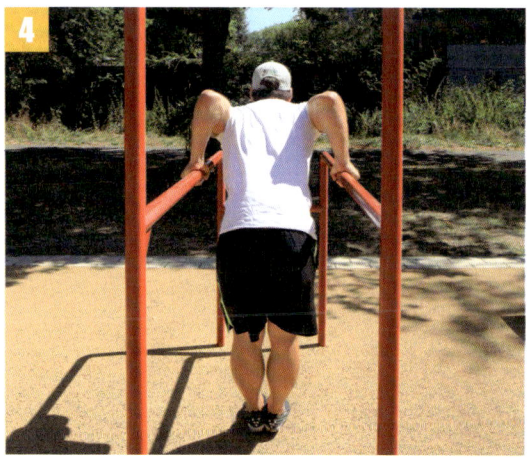

6. Now bend your elbows to 90 degrees or more for ROM, but only if your shoulders don't bother you in this position. Your elbows should stay very close to your body as they move back. Forearms should remain vertical to the bars.

7. Without letting your elbows move to the outside, push yourself up into the starting position with shoulders protracted. Then—and only then—start to initiate repetitions.

11.5.2 TYPICAL MISTAKES

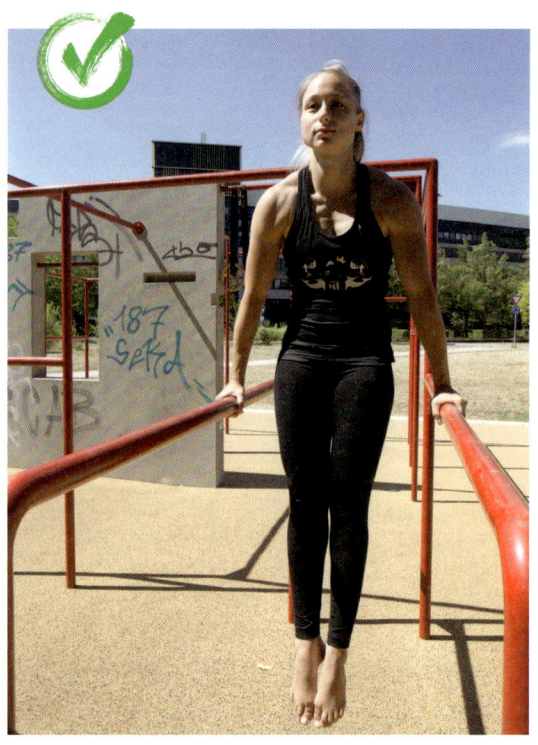
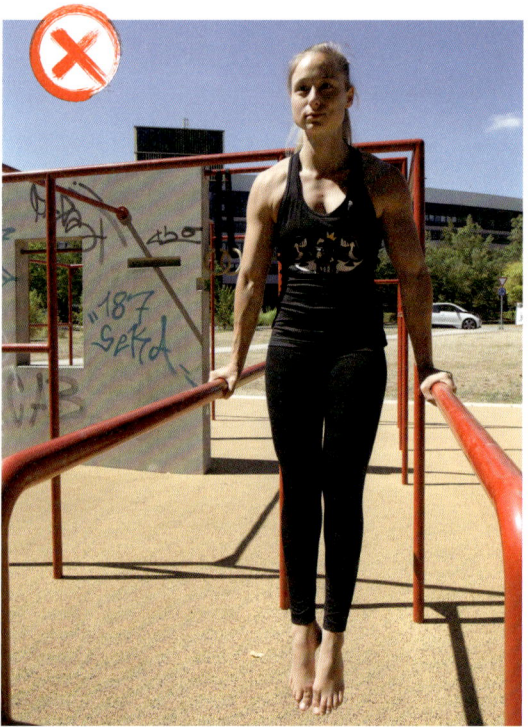

- bent wrists
- elbows moving to the outside when pushing up
- movement coming almost entirely from bending at the hips—something that's evident in the feet, which aren't moving up and down
- not being able to maintain hollow-body position
- legs are angled backward
- movement not being executed to completion

11.5.3 FREQUENT STICKING POINTS

TRICEPS TOO WEAK

Due to the lack of strength in the triceps, the chest muscles compensate, whereby the elbows stick out to the sides, forcing the shoulder into internal rotation.

CORE TOO WEAK

The lack of core tension causes upward lordosis, and the legs compensate by moving behind.

LACK OF SHOULDER-BLADE ACTIVATION

If the shoulders can't be fully moved into depression or protraction, we recommend shoulder-blade activation exercises in a support position.

LACK OF ARM STRENGTH

Movements on fully extended arms are rather rare in general training and show deficiencies. When we think of advanced exercises like the handstand or planche, it quickly becomes apparent that these exercises require a good amount of strength on extended arms. It's generally good advice to do support exercises on extended arms and in different planes, like doing overhead carries with kettlebells.

11.5.4 DIP EXERCISE REGRESSIONS

BENCH DIPS

 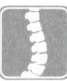

1. Place your hands behind you on a raised surface.

2. Support yourself on fully extended arms so your back remains vertical to the surface while you perform the exercise.

3. Extend your spine and bend your elbows to 90 degrees or more.

4. Keep your legs together and extended.

5. You can make the exercise easier by bending your knees to shorten the lever.

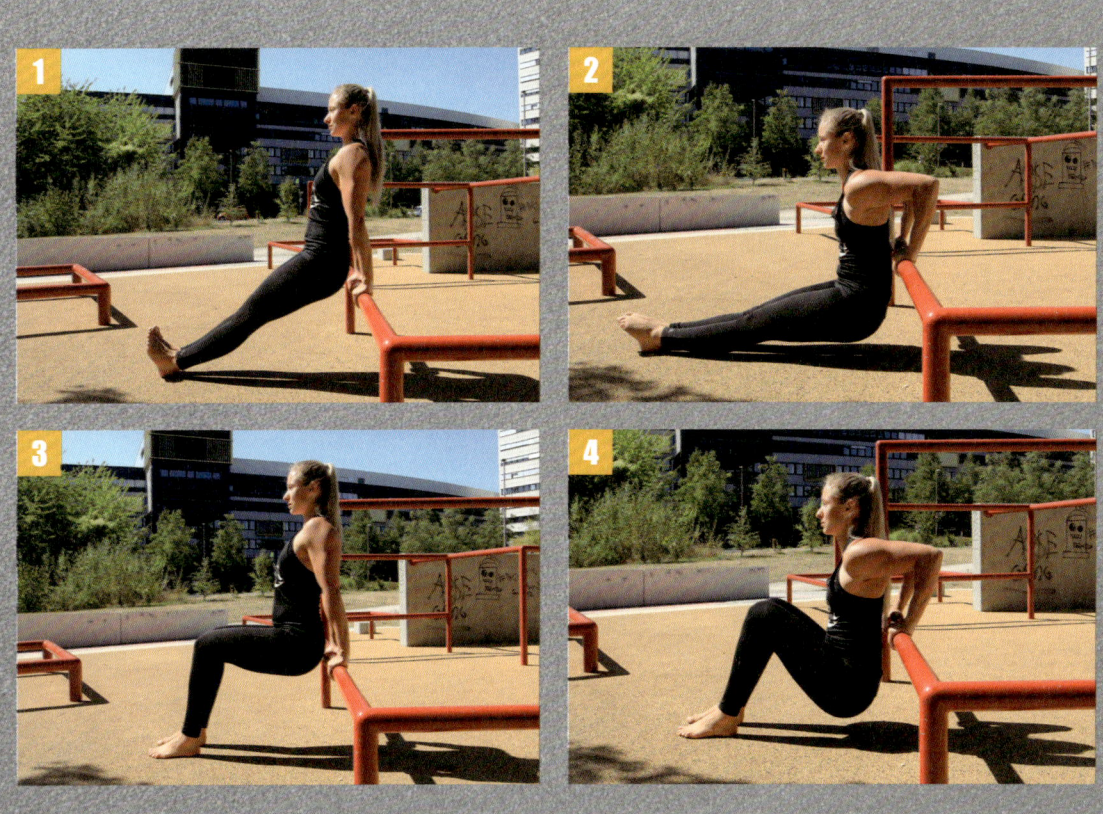

NEGATIVE DIPS

1. Set up a box behind you to ensure a safe mount and dismount on and from the parallel bars.

2. From the support starting position, lower yourself to a 90-degree arm position.

3. At the lowest point, rest your feet on the box to be able to then perform additional repetitions.

TIP

Resting your feet on the box keeps you from falling into the potentially too-high parallel bars should you lose your strength and lose control.

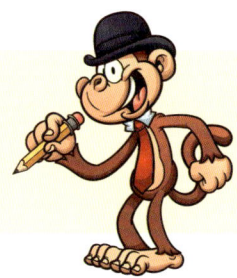

RTO IN HANGING DIP PUSH-UP

As a progressive exercise for the RTO push-up, this one is considerably more difficult. Here, too, there are possible differentiations. Support yourself on rings hung high enough so your feet don't touch the ground when your arms are fully extended. Now turn the inside of your elbows forward into the RTO position. At the same time, push the rings toward each other.

1. Support yourself with neutral wrists on rings hung high enough so your feet don't touch the ground when your arms are fully extended.

2. Turn the inside of your elbows forward into the RTO position and push the rings toward each other.

3. Briefly hold this position and return to the starting position.

Important: Stay compact and maintain core tension to avoid wobbling. If you still find this exercise too difficult, support yourself with your feet or toes on the ground. To do so, you'll have to lower the rings slightly.

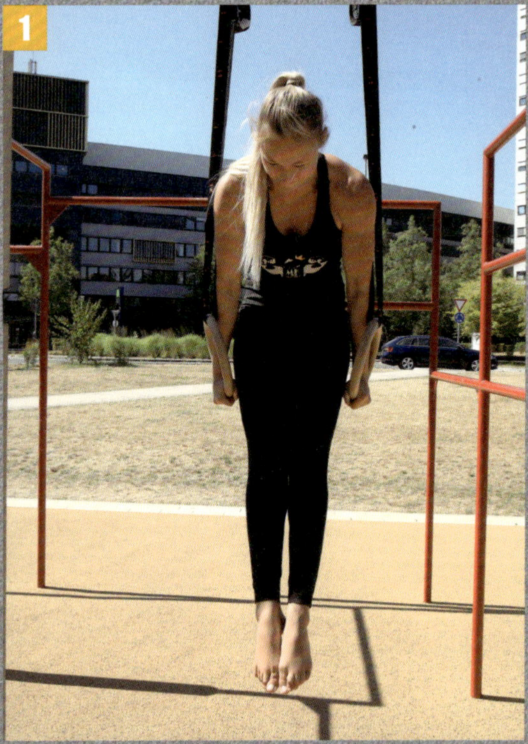

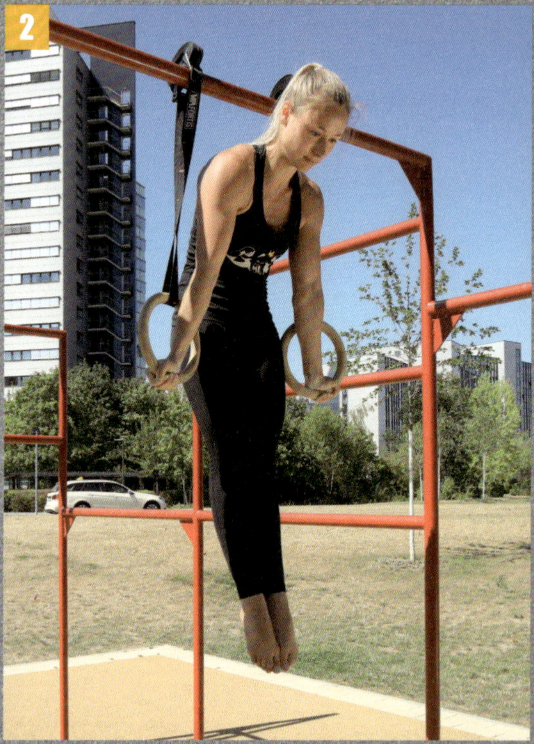

Once you've mastered your first dips and several consecutive repetitions are getting too easy, try doing dips on the rings. Here, the *end range of motion* is achieved via RTO. Try doing straight-bar (single-bar) dips as part of your exercise regressions for the bar muscle-up. Russian dips, Bulgarian dips, and Korean dips are other advanced exercises that build on the classic dip.

11.6 SQUATS AND POSSIBLE PROGRESSIONS

The squat is a hip-dominant exercise for strengthening the legs. But before we get into the specifics, I want to briefly dispel a few myths:

- Myth 1: It's dangerous for your knees to cross the toe line.
- Myth 2: It's dangerous to go lower than your knees being bent 90 degrees.
- Myth 3: You should always squat with your legs hip-width apart and toes pointing forward.

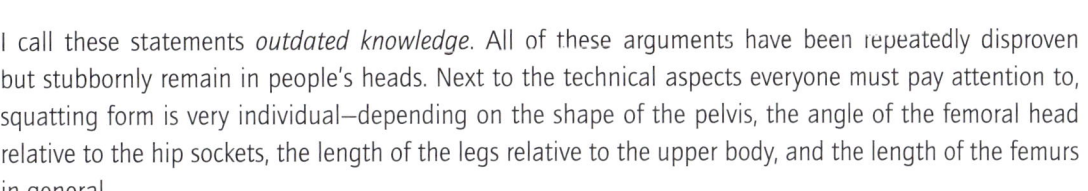

I call these statements *outdated knowledge*. All of these arguments have been repeatedly disproven but stubbornly remain in people's heads. Next to the technical aspects everyone must pay attention to, squatting form is very individual—depending on the shape of the pelvis, the angle of the femoral head relative to the hip sockets, the length of the legs relative to the upper body, and the length of the femurs in general.

The different leg and hip shapes and angles vary the width of the stance, the angle of the toes, and the depth of the squat, among other things.

But first, one must have some basic hip mobility to be able to perform a squat with FROM, because a lack of mobility is no excuse for a technically poor execution.

11.6.1 WHAT YOUR SQUAT SHOULD LOOK LIKE

SQUAT 💪💪

 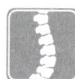

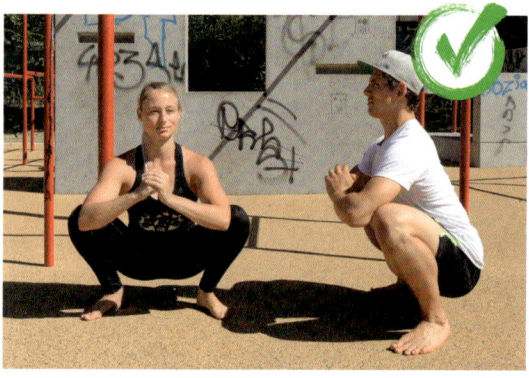 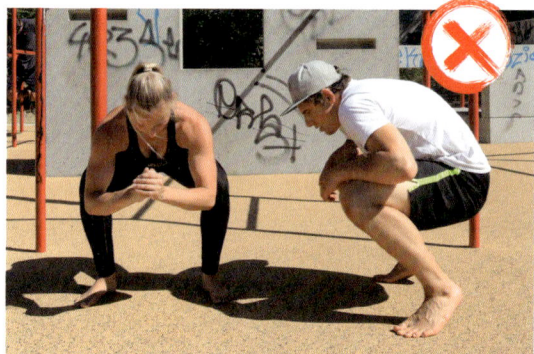

1. Take an approximately hip-width stance.

2. Try to see if pointing your toes forward or slightly to the side works better for you.

3. Extend your spine as though someone were pulling you, by your hair, out of the water (always keep your spine extended).

4. Imagine screwing your feet into the ground. (Your feet don't actually move; your knees are turned out slightly.)

5. Tighten your backside by externally rotating your hips.

6. Take deep belly breaths and maintain the resulting core tension throughout the exercise.

7. Next, push your hips back just a little (imagine sitting in a chair).

8. Push your hips back only enough to keep your head at the same level. (When you push them too far back, you have to lean your upper body too far forward to create a counterbalance.)

9. Bend your knees.

10. Throughout the exercise, make sure your heels remain on the ground.

11. Your knees should come out over your toes in the direction your feet are pointed.

12. Bend as low as you can under the specified technical requirements.

13. When you rise back up, make sure you push up over the midfoot. (Your weight should be centered over the center of your feet.)

14. Continue to make sure your spine is extended and simultaneously open your knee and hip angle (meaning avoid lifting your pelvis too soon).

As you perform the exercise and take into account the listed aspects, it's important to make individual adjustments as described.

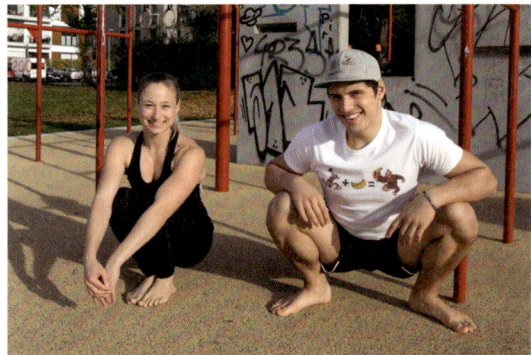

Maybe try using a wider stance, turning your feet out a little more, or something else.

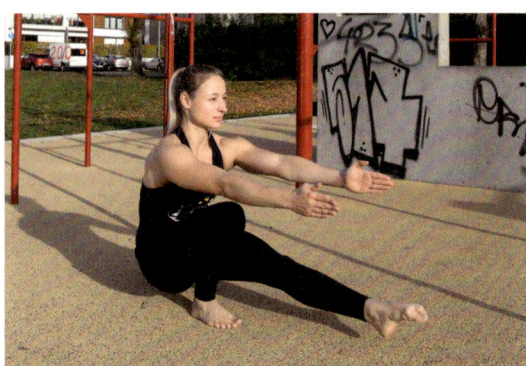

You can try the pistol squat (one-legged squat) to make this exercise more difficult.

11.7 REGRESSION—THE *L*-SIT

Since the *L*-sit builds on basics taught elsewhere in the book, I won't break it down and offer step-by-step directions as I do with the other exercises.

As a static skill, the *L*-sit hanging or in a support position is good for linking several elements or for creating a nice starting position for a handstand ascent. In terms of participating muscles, the L-sit is a great core and hip-flexor exercise. Since we know from experience that the core is a weak spot but has a key function in stabilizing the spine, it must be worked accordingly, particularly in the beginning stages.

Beginner Basics and Their Possible Progressions   **235**

But instead of choosing sit-ups or crunches as the exercise of choice, you should choose more-natural forms of movement for strengthening. Isometric holds or slow, controlled movements with maximum contraction are more effective than dull repetitions of thousands of six-pack abdominal exercises.

If you've read everything up to this point, the lever principle is probably clear. If it's not, review 10.12, "All about Levers" This principle can, of course, also be applied to exercise regressions of the *L*-sit. As a simple progression, in a static support or hanging position, you can also pull your legs, bent at 90 degrees, in to your body. If that's too difficult, pull your knees closer to your chest. Learn to master this position so you're able to take relaxed breaths while holding it. If that's too easy, slowly open your upper- and lower-leg angle until you're able to extend your legs.

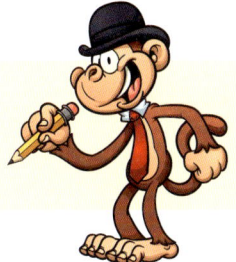

TIP

Pointed toes create even more tension.

11.7.1 HANGING *L*-SIT

HANGING *L*-SIT

1. Get into an active hanging position. Avoid the mistake of leaning back.

2. Fix your eyes on a point in front of you. Hold your head straight.

3. Raise your legs, extended, only as far as you can while keeping your back straight.

11.7.2 *L*-SIT IN A SUPPORT POSITION

L-SIT IN A SUPPORT POSITION

  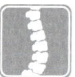

To make your form during the *L*-sit look really good, your arms, when seen from the side, should support your trunk in a vertical line, as shown in this photo. Your arms cover up your trunk. You should get in this position only if you have enough strength in your shoulder girdle to push your backside forward in this position. Actively push from your shoulders into depression.

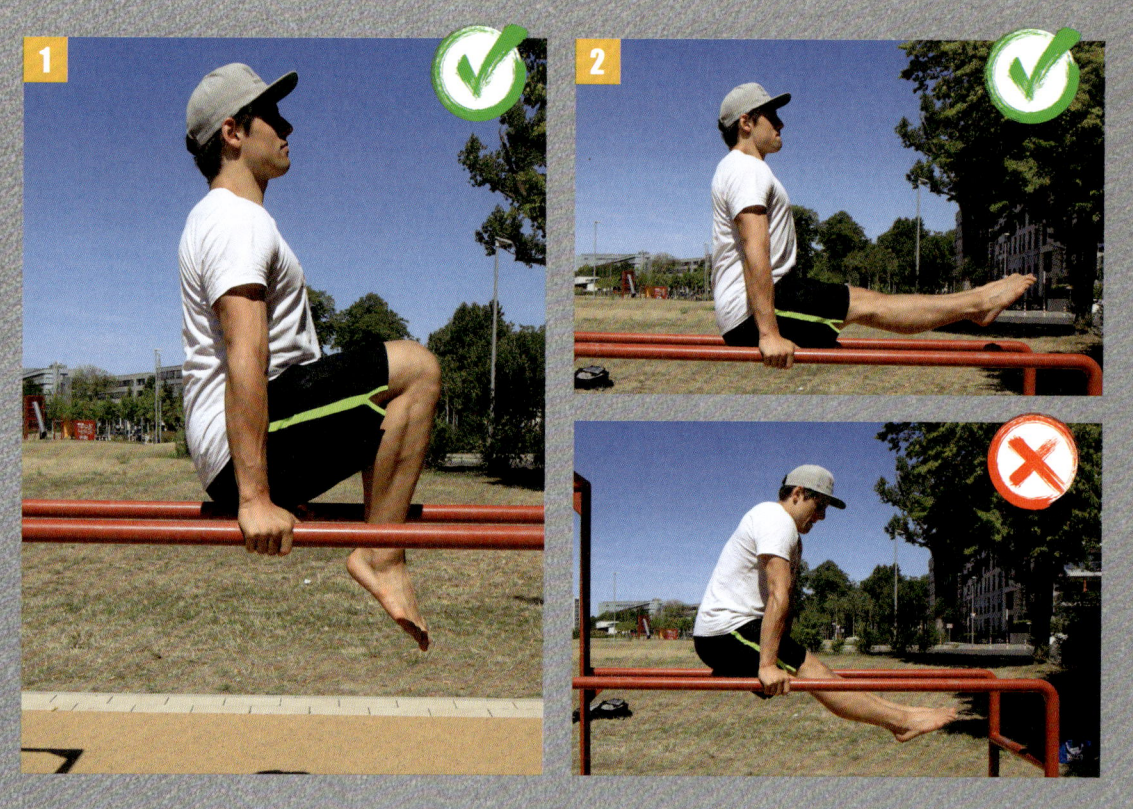

11.7.3 ASSISTING EXERCISES

Do the following exercises to strengthen your hip flexors.

PIKE COMPRESSIONS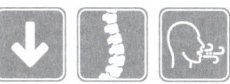

1. Sit on the ground, with your back straight and legs extended forward.

2. Support yourself with your hands on the ground next to your knees (farther forward, toward your feet, is more difficult).

3. Build up muscle tension in your entire body by taking deep belly breaths. Unlike the squat, allow your breath to flow.

4. Now lift your legs, together and extended (toes pointed), off the ground.

5. Lower your legs in a controlled motion until they almost touch the ground, then lift them again.

LEG RAISES

1. Hang from a bar or rings or support yourself on the parallel bars.
2. Build up body tension (breath).
3. Lift your legs.

Variation 1 : *Toes to the bar:* Touch your feet touch the bar, keeping your back vertical and your legs completely extended. Fix your eyes on a point in front of you.

Variation 2 : *Leg lifts:* Lift your legs, extended, only 90 degrees.

Variation 3 : *Knee raises:* pull your knees in to your chest (tucked).

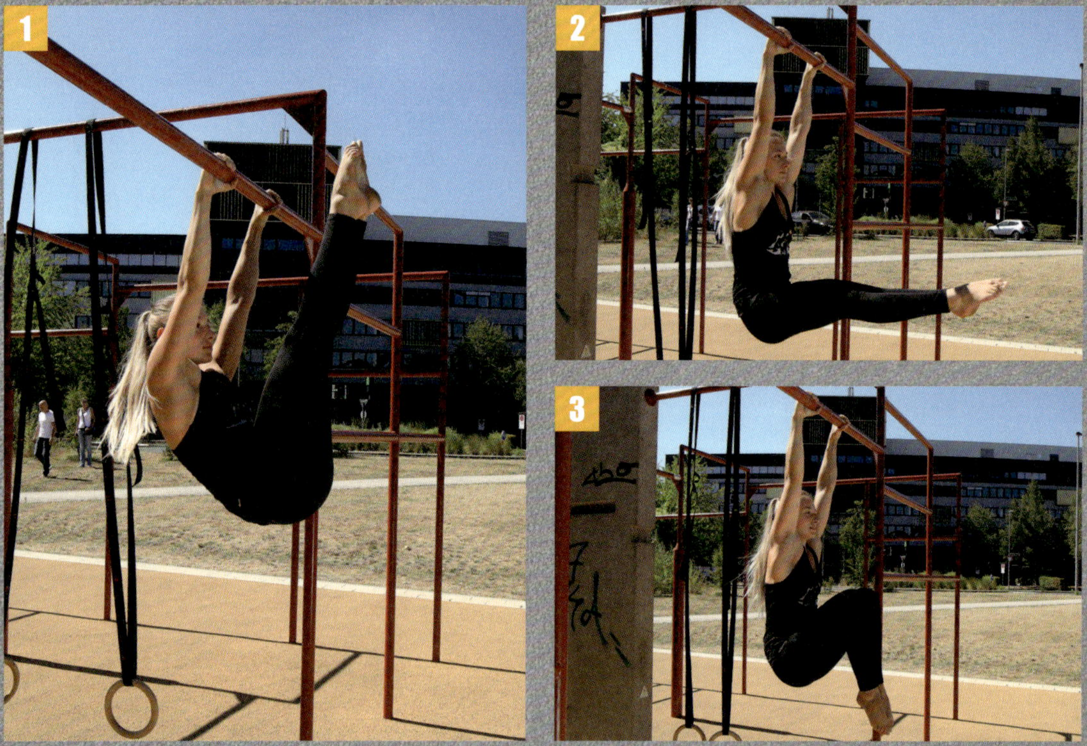

11.8 REHABILITATION AND PREHABILITATION EXERCISES

FACE PULLS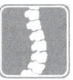

This exercise strengthens the rhomboids and trapezii and can be performed during rehabilitation as well as preventatively.

1. Grip the rings so the backs of your hands face each other.
2. From the rings, hang on a diagonal.
3. Pull the rings in close toward your ears while maintaining this hand position.
4. Leave your shoulder blades in depression and retraction.
5. Return to the starting position in the same way.

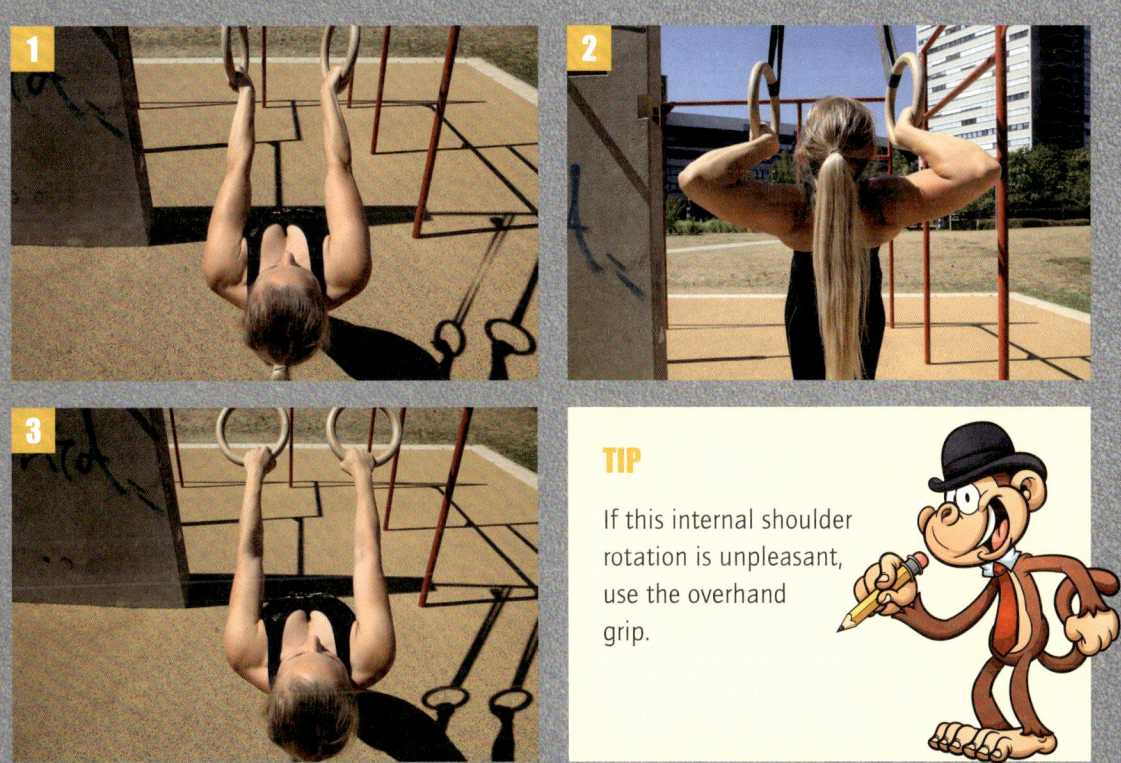

TIP

If this internal shoulder rotation is unpleasant, use the overhand grip.

EXTERNAL ROTATION: BANDED PRESS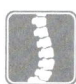

1. Attach a lightweight band at waist-level and stand next to it with your side to the band.

2. When you grip the band with your right hand, stand so the band's point of attachment is to your left.

3. Hold your forearm at a 90-degree angle to your upper arm.

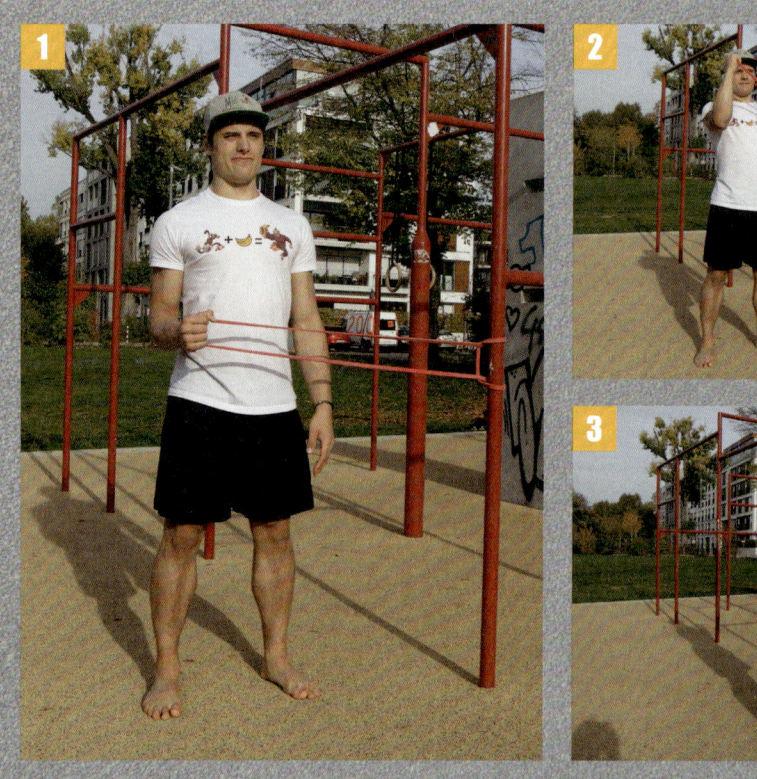

4. Raise your arm until your upper arm is at a 90-degree angle to your trunk.

5. Extend your arm overhead and to the side.

6. On the way back down, first return to the 90-degree angle of upper arm to trunk before lowering the arm.

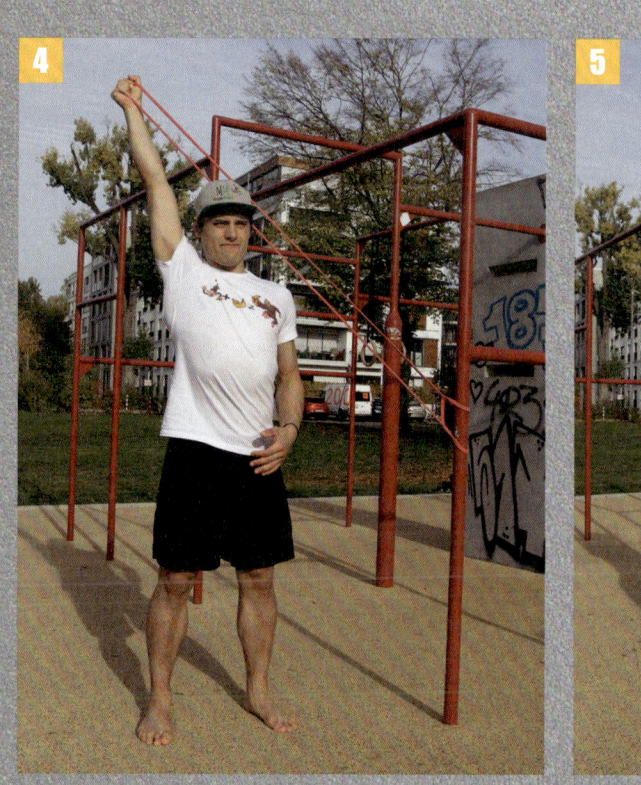 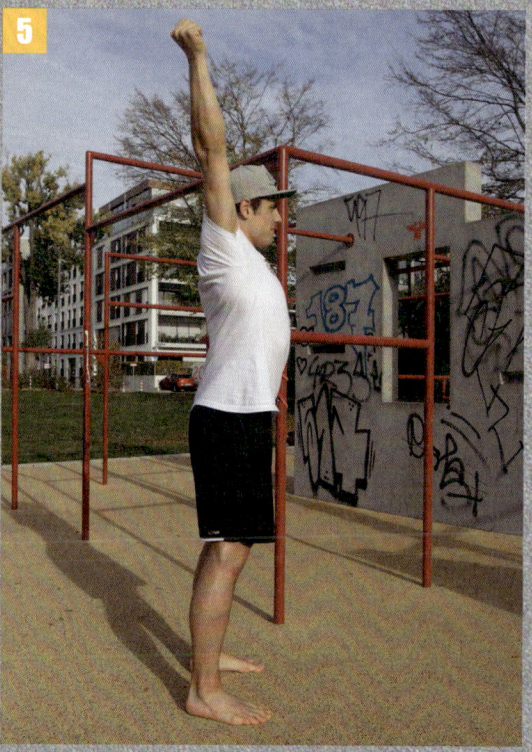

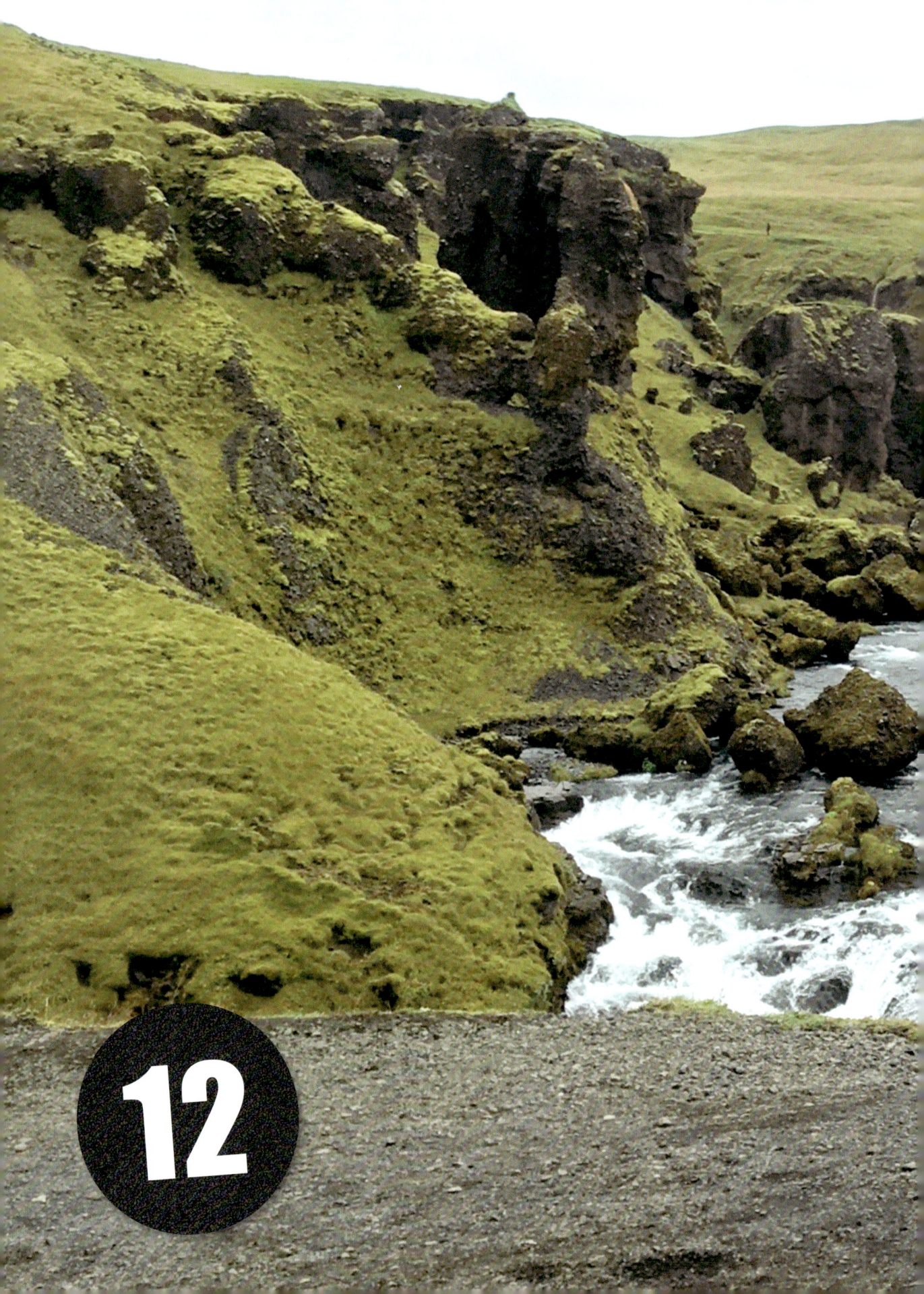

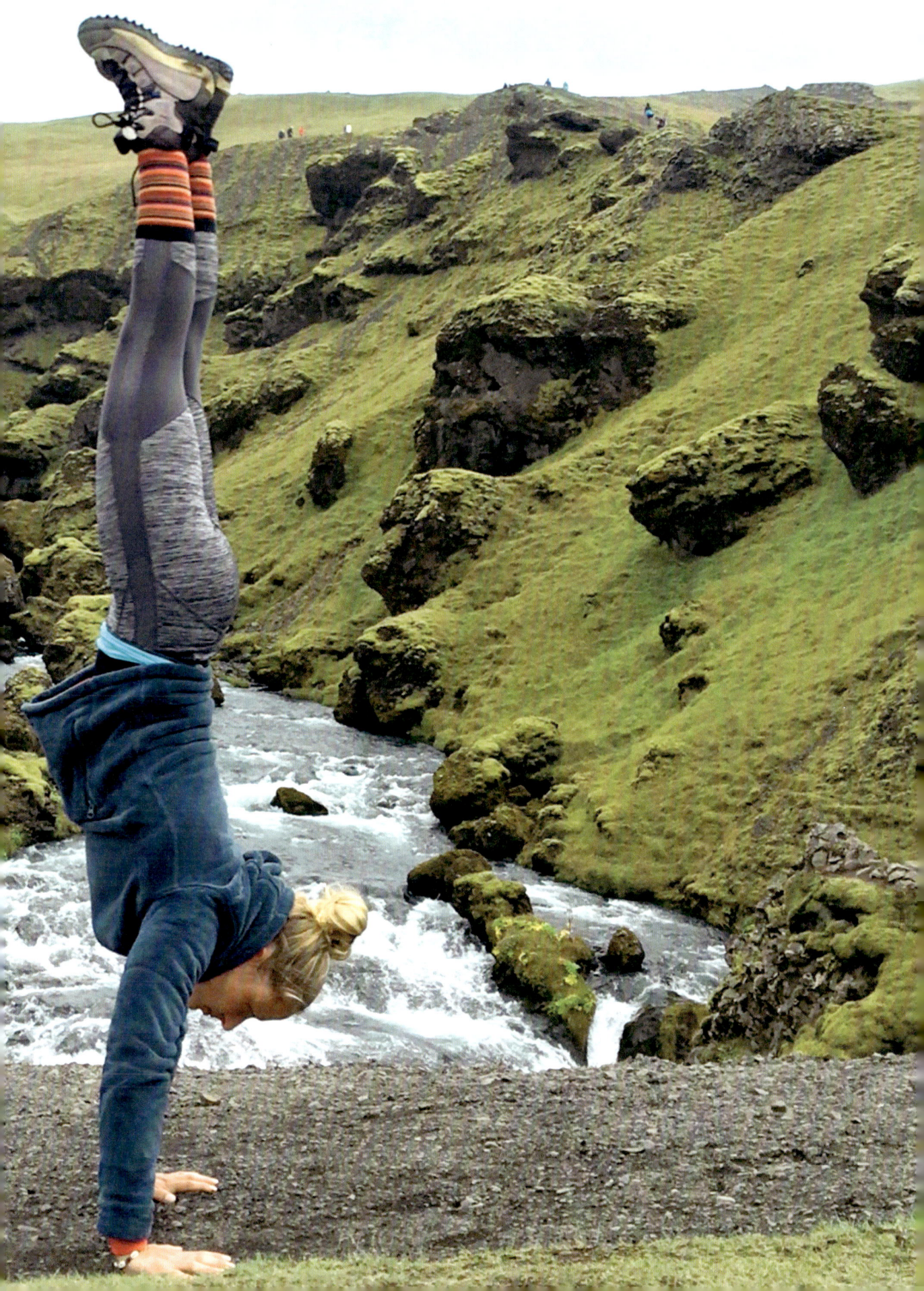

12 General Training Structure

This chapter focuses strictly on the general training structure and doesn't consider any special approaches to training plans. Chapter 14 includes a sample plan for a single day without a prespecified cycle, which you, as a beginner, can practice. It's important, though, that you understand the theoretical approach to training.

Many beginners get caught up in finding the perfect training plan or planning it themselves without really training. In the beginning, any simple plan will work to build basic strength. So make sure you start training first.

If you already have basic strength and have specific goals, then it should follow that you also have a well-thought-out plan. To build effective training that helps you achieve your goals and gradually improves your abilities, you need a training program *you* can train with. Once your goals are set, you need to find exercises to practice that will bring you closer to your goals. But these exercises shouldn't be randomly strung together; they must follow a specific structure that builds on itself, also called a *routine*.

On principal, every training session begins with a *warm-up*, which in turn consists of different components. You first choose exercises that kick-start your cardiovascular system and raise your body temperature so the chemical reactions in your muscles can take place more quickly. This optimizes the muscles' ability to contract and activates the nervous system. Heart rate as well as blood flow should be increased to supply the muscles with adequate oxygen and nutrients.

The warm-up is ideally geared toward training with bodyweight, meaning you should be doing exercises that prepare the muscles you'll be working. To be honest, I'm often tempted to neglect the cardio portion of the warm-up, even though I know it's useful. Don't fall into that trap like I sometimes do.

Mobility should be integrated into the warm-up as the second component. Mobility can be considered prophylactic and is important for preparing the muscles, joints, tendons, and ligaments so they can perform the training exercises with a FROM. Mobility training is an important part of functional strength training. Review section 2.7, "How Mobility Makes You Stronger."

There, you can also find an explanation of the difference between mobility training and mobilization. Static twisting should be avoided as it requires that a certain amount of muscle tension (muscle tone) be maintained to facilitate a strong muscle contraction. After this part, you can use *muscle-tension exercise*s for your core muscles, like the hollow-body position. These exercises should be performed only briefly and are merely intended to generate basic body tension, especially when they're followed by static skill training, like a handstand, back lever, or front lever.

The second focal point of training design is *skill training*. During this part of the routine, you refine existing skills and techniques well suited for beginners.

The actual strength training takes place during the third step of the routine, the *main portion*. To be effective, it requires the central nervous system to be highly stimulated. After the still low intensity of the first and second phases, here, the ideally maximum number of muscle fibers get their best workout. A good way to effectively work your shoulders and avoid imbalances is alternating between pushing and pulling exercises, which should be part of every training plan (see "Antagonist Training" within subsection 12.1.2, "Types of Training"). Leg exercises, like squats, pistols, and more should, of course, be included.

You can specifically work your core, meaning your stomach, pelvic, hip, and back muscles. For an advanced calisthenics athlete with good core stability, this usually isn't necessary, since the calisthenics exercises, if performed correctly, require extreme muscle tension in the midsection, thereby already working the core.

Based on the performance level, the exercises are set up in sets and repetitions, either as a whole-body routine in a circuit, which is particularly well suited for beginners as it builds overall basic strength, or as specific preparatory exercises (progressions) that work on a specific strength (push or pull strength) to learn certain skills, like the back lever or handstand. Of course, there's a wide range of training methods that vary the training volume, intensity, and duration as well as other factors. You can find some concepts in "Antagonist Training" within subsection 12.1.2, "Types of Training."

The fifth and final phase is the cool-down, which should be very diverse. It includes preventative, rehabilitative, and mobility work. Its purpose isn't only to relax the body after a workout, but it's also meant for focusing on improving physical abilities and preventing injuries. The elevated blood pressure that's still present after training makes the muscles more flexible, which is why mobility exercises are highly recommended in the cool-down.

Rehabilitation refers to working on weak spots in cases of injuries. Assuming there isn't an injury, it's always advisable to mobilize the shoulders as a preventative, since they're so important. You can find some good rehabilitation and prehabilitation exercises in section 11.8.

12.1 TRAINING METHODS

When you choose a training method, the focus here, too, is based on your goal.

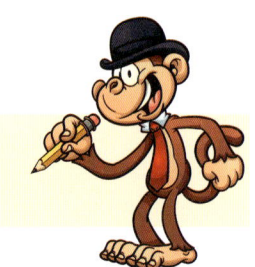

Regardless of how advanced you are or will be, the general rule is this: basics should still be a part of your training plan.

Set the stimuli based on your performance level. There are no blanket statements about prespecified set-and-repetition numbers. Every athlete should be seen as an individual. Some find that the method with lots of repetitions works for them, while others do better with repetitions in the maximum-strength range and get stronger that way. Especially in the beginning, it's important to get to know and understand your body so you'll know down the road how performance adjustments will work for you and where you can tweak them. If it's too easy and doesn't challenge you, adjust your plan accordingly. As you do so, remember the 80-percent rule (see section 9.12, "Calisthenics: Street Gymnastics").

As a beginner, the training plan is about being able to perform the learned basics at higher repetitions to be able to process the new stimuli for your body and your brain. Structural and neuronal connections must be reinforced.

12.1.1 FREQUENCY OF TRAINING, NUMBER OF SETS, NUMBER OF REPETITIONS, AND BREAKS

The question I most often get asked is probably this: "Should my training method work my entire body, or should it always focus on specific muscle groups [i.e., working on biceps (or back) and triceps (or chest) on one day and legs the next]?"

Full-body training has some advantages. You perform several related movement patterns in one workout that targets all muscle groups, which can be performed several times a week, taking into account recovery days. If you split up your training and, for instance, do pulling exercises on Monday, pushing exercises on Tuesday, and leg work on Wednesday, each workout can be done only twice a week, with Thursday as the recovery day. Full-body training is recommended, particularly for beginners, since it works simultaneously on strengths and weaknesses and the **frequency** of completed weekly units is greater. But if an advanced athlete's specific goal is working on skills, the broken split version can be advantageous.

There are many ways to design your training. You can make changes to each of the existing parameters, be it training frequency per week or training intensity. If you train hard based on the degree of difficulty of bodyweight exercises or external weight, you need only a few repetitions (three to five). If you choose exercises that feel easier, you can do more repetitions, but you'll be working at a lower intensity level.

Train at least twice—or, better yet, three times—a week to adequately challenge your muscles, to give them the opportunity to gradually adapt, and to allow the movements to be automated safely.

Ultimately, the *training volume* (number of sets multiplied by number of repetitions) determines whether you've set an adequate stimulus for the adaptation. The general consensus is that approximately thirty to sixty repetitions per muscle group should be completed across different exercises. Why is there such a wide range, between thirty and sixty repetitions? If you work at a lower intensity, you do more repetitions (sixty). If you work at a higher intensity (heavy), you should aim for thirty repetitions. That means you should already know what muscle groups you'll work with which exercise, to avoid overlap that could possibly overload you. Differentiating between pushing and pulling exercises is sufficient. You can also review chapter 11, "Beginner Basics and Their Possible Progressions."

One possibility is *ladder workouts*, in which sets consist of an ascending or descending number of repetitions. It could look like this:

A1: pull-ups with 2/4/6/8/10 repetitions (ascending ladder)

A2: dips with 10/8/6/4/2 repetitions (descending ladder)

Do A1 and A2, taking a thirty-second break in between and a one-minute set-break after both exercises.

Exercises A1 and A2 should be performed alternately, as a block. The numbers *1* and *2* following an identical letter mean that the exercises belong together. The ∕ symbol separates the sets, and the numbers indicate the number of repetitions for each set.

You can also complete this antagonist-training method separately, as individual exercises. Pull-ups would then be completed as part A before doing the dips as part B. Correspondingly, during the first set of a total of five sets, you'd do two pull-ups, take a thirty-second break, do ten dips, then take a one-and-a-half-minute set-break. In the second set, you'd do four pull-ups and eight dips and continue on in this way. You'd end up with a volume of thirty repetitions per exercise. Here, you can't simply multiply the number of sets by the number of repetitions, because each set has a different number of repetitions.

When doing a *pyramid*, you increase your repetitions and then decrease them again (e.g., 2/4/6/8/6/4/2 repetitions).

It also doesn't matter if you do 8 × 3 (eight sets with three repetitions each) or 3 × 8 (three sets with eight repetitions each). Ultimately, the volume is the same with twenty-four repetitions. Transferred to weights, it does make a difference whether you work out in the maximum-strength range (8 × 3) or the hypertrophy range (3 × 8).

It's important to adhere to the *break times*.

- *For maximum-strength training* (strength buildup: one to five repetitions), calculate two-and-a-half- to three-minute breaks. Your body and especially your nervous system will require this amount of time to be fully functional for the next set.

- In the *hypertrophy area* (muscle buildup: six to twelve repetitions), one and a half to two minutes is sufficient.

- Training beyond that is considered s*trength-endurance training* (twelve or more repetitions) and requires thirty seconds to one minute of break time. Ultimately, you'll decide when you're ready for the next set, but give yourself time and don't rush.

The listed ranges for the strength types vary, which is why you should also utilize *time under tension (TUT)*.

TUT is a way to assign time values (*tempo and cadence training*) to the strength phases (eccentric, concentric, isometric).

General Training Structure

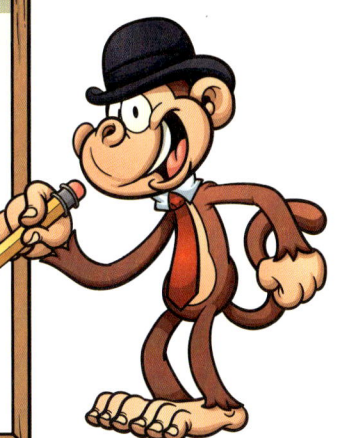

TUT defines the strength areas based on the required amount of time for the muscle to be activated while performing an exercise. All times are approximate.

- **Maximum-strength area:** four to twenty seconds
- **Hypertrophy area:** twenty-four to forty-eight seconds
- **Strength-endurance area:** more than fifty seconds

These values are based on an average of four seconds per repetition.

Muscle-fiber types 1 and 2 and their hybrids can't be worked independent of each other. You can only change the focus. The muscle stimulus (muscle-fiber recruitment) is generally greater in exercises that use FROM than those that are exclusively eccentric or isometric. But for beginners, eccentric training works to set a stimulus that helps overcome the concentric phases by reaching a TUT via the slow exercise execution that's equal to a normal FROM repetition so as many muscle fibers as possible are recruited. Tears in the muscle fibers occur, which stimulate protein biosynthesis to repair damaged tissue.

This metabolic stress makes itself felt in sore muscles. Do an internet search for **"cadences"** and "isometrics" to learn more about training them. If you want to set new stimuli, have trouble with certain movement phases, or are at a standstill, try these forms of training.

If you're asking yourself how to exchange or supplement a completed, random dynamic movement with isometric or eccentric exercises, the answer is in these examples:

- A *concentric* movement in approximately two seconds corresponds to an *isometric* movement execution.
- A *concentric* movement in approximately three seconds corresponds to an *eccentric* movement execution.

When using such methods, don't work at your limit but choose an intensity of approximately 60–75 percent. **The final repetition should be as clean as the first one.** When you notice your form slipping and your movement execution getting sloppy, end the set. You want to send positive signals to your brain to improve your movement quality. You don't want to internalize bad movement patterns.

Begin the main portion of strength training with the exercises you find most difficult and thereby work in the maximum-strength range. Then do the less-difficult exercises that allow you to train with more repetitions. You'll have then combined several types of strength in your workout. Of course, it's also possible to do them separately on different days. Try it to see what works best for you.

12.1.2 TYPES OF TRAINING

ANTAGONIST TRAINING

Choose antagonist training to implement the alternating push-pull exercises. When choosing the appropriate exercises, we generally differentiate between the muscle groups we plan to work. Since calisthenics exercises tend to be more holistic in nature, here, we differentiate between direction of movement and plane of movement. We ultimately combine pulling and pushing exercises. For instance, dips and pull-ups are performed one after another. Instead of combining only two exercises, you can also link multiple exercises in this way.

CIRCUIT TRAINING

A simple circuit of the basics with the corresponding exercise regressions is ideal for a beginner. String together basics exercises (dips, pull-ups, push-ups, and squat variations) so pulling and pushing exercises alternate and do a few rounds of these. You can also divide your circuit into multiple blocks. For instance, let's say you plan on doing nine rounds and choose different exercises for rounds one through three, four through six, and seven through nine. Put at the beginning exercises that are difficult for you and then choose easier exercises for the subsequent two blocks.

HIGH-VOLUME TRAINING

It helps to work with lots of repetitions to increase the repetitions you initially mastered. Knowing your maximum-strength values for the exercises is helpful for planning your training.

Example: You're able to maximally perform four clean pull-ups. Now multiply this number by three (4 × 3 = 12 repetitions total). Now divide in half (50 percent of your maximum-strength values) for the four clean pull-ups. That's two repetitions per set. So you must do six sets of two repetitions each to reach a total of twelve repetitions. Take a two- to three-minute break to keep the repetitions in each set consistent.

Since, when you first begin, you start out with one pull-up, work your way up with single reps. For example, do eight to twelve sets of one clean pull-up each.

A high training volume can also look different. For instance, the repetition numbers per set can go down. This works particularly well when the existing number of repetitions is already high. In general, the idea is to complete lots of repetitions with one method.

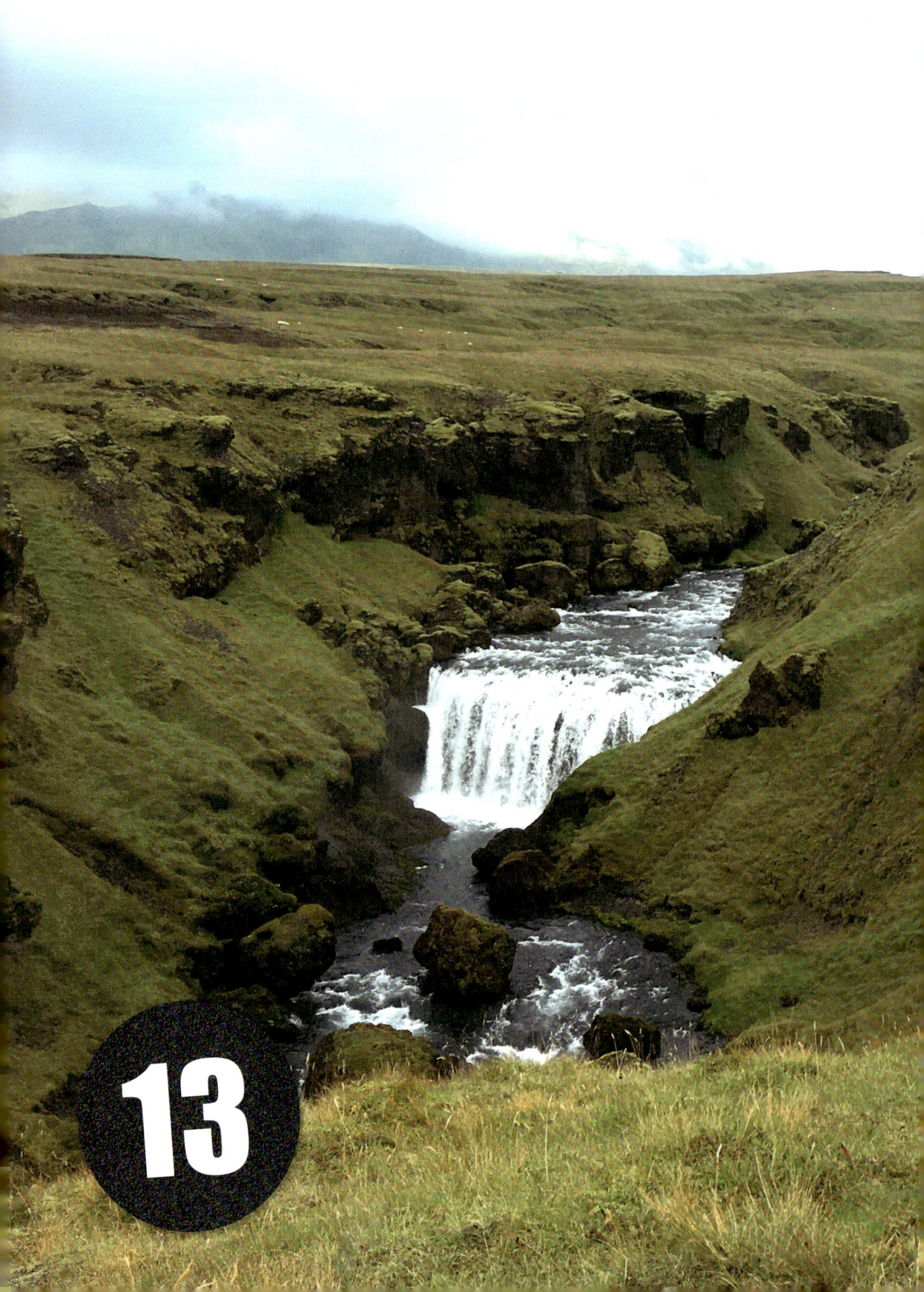

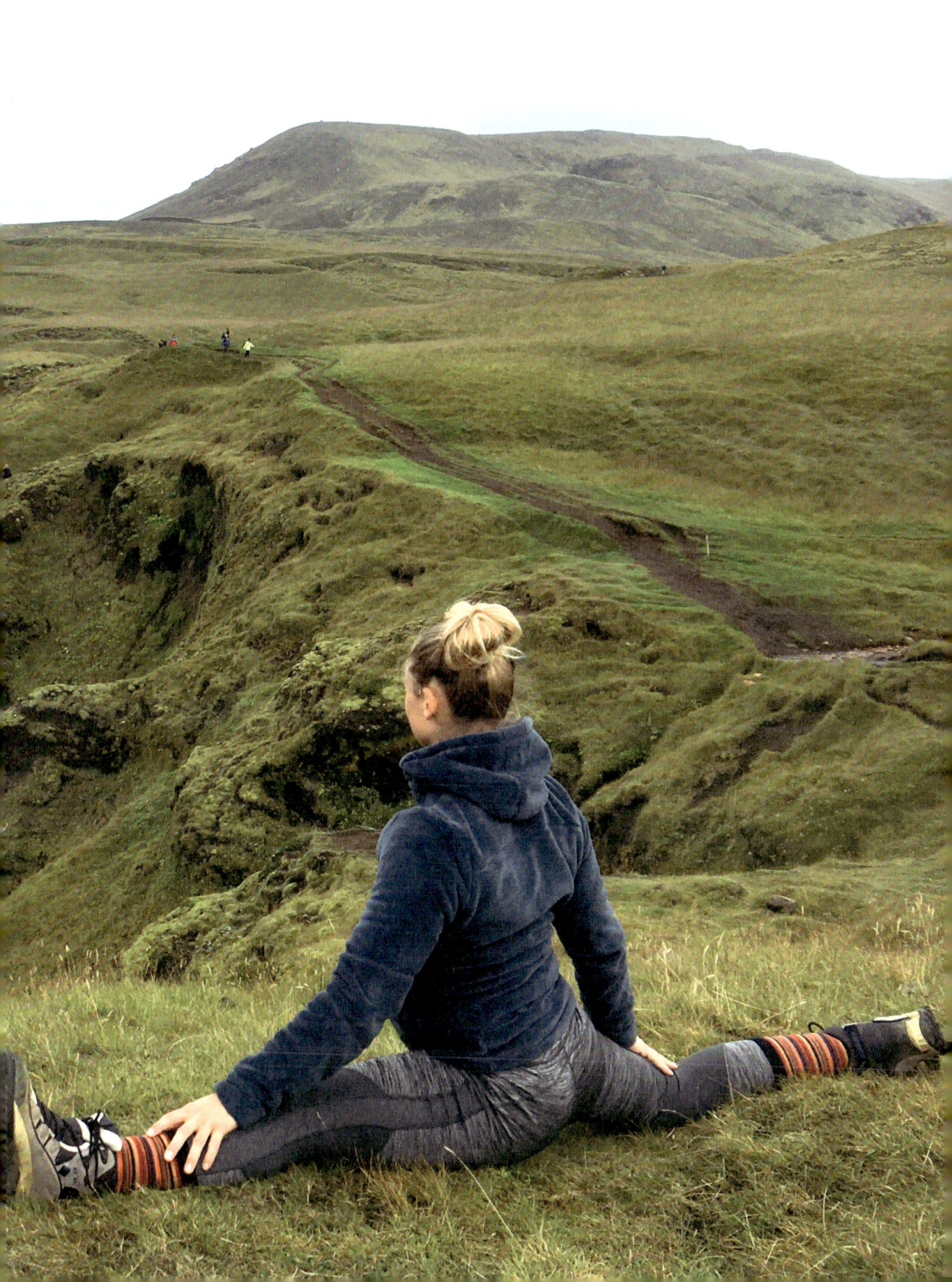

13 Goals, Time Investment, and Motivation

Before you dive headfirst into your training, I'd like to offer some thoughts for along the way.

Ask yourself the following four fundamental questions before embarking on the search for that one effective method.

1) WHAT do you want to achieve? What do you want your body, your physical awareness, or your performance to look like after a certain amount of time and with the use of willpower, self-discipline, strength, and patience, and *2) HOW* can you implement and achieve these goals?

If you simply want to lose weight and be thinner, even just changing some of your eating habits by cutting out fast-food, ready-made meals, and those little daily sins, like a cappuccino here and a soft drink there, can be helpful. But if you want to visibly strengthen your muscles, exercise is an essential companion on the way to your goal.

Here, the "it" depends on how much muscle mass you want to build and 3) **FOR WHAT?** Is it your goal to work on your aesthetics—to have a fit, muscular, and well-defined body? Or do you want to be able to do more with your body, get to know your body better, understand it, and make it functional? Your goals determine your training approach, your choice of the many training methods, and your diet.

And it's also a question of time. *4) HOW MUCH* time can you invest, and how easily can your training be integrated into your daily life and be reconciled with your job without adding more stress?

As Leon points out in section 2.8, "Why Stress Makes You Immobile," too much stress will make it harder not only to become more mobile but also to build more strength and muscle.

Goals, Time Investment, and Motivation

Always keep at it so you can reach the goal you set. It's a process that lowers the body's fitness level as soon as it's put on hold for a period of time. The body can't be made to achieve top performances in a matter of days, nor can it maintain a hard-earned fitness level without additional training.

A change in your approach to life can help you acquire a fit and healthy body. It takes time, energy, patience, self-control, and perseverance. Do you bring these qualities to the table, and are you prepared to bring positive change to your life? You'll gain a positive self-image, an overall healthier way of living, a lower risk of illness, and an optimistic lifestyle that will motivate you every day.

The choice is *yours*.

Now before you dive into the sport over-motivated by all this knowledge and without much of a plan, check your fitness level. Because you can determine the intensity of your next workout by your current performance level. If you've never exercised or have done so only rarely, at irregular intervals, start at zero and get into training slowly.

Even if you've been exposed to several other sports that have nothing to do with bodyweight strength training, there are a few things to remember to help you start off your training the right way. Only then will you stay pain-free long-term and enjoy training.

But the most-important thing is that you keep moving. It's like eating. What matters most is that you eat, but ultimately, the quality of your diet determines how healthy you are, remain, or become.

Quality beats quantity!

I don't want to give superfluous advice with motivational sayings like Just Keep Going, Never Give Up, or No Pain, No Gain. Instead, I want to motivate you intrinsically, by asking you to embrace awareness of your body and your health. Learn to take responsibility and act accordingly.

Adopt habits that are good for you, and live more responsibly. Exercise helps to move limits. Even in everyday life. You'll hardly exceed your maximum daily load simply because your sport requires discipline. What matters is finding solutions that will move you forward.

A sport will help you make decisions more consciously. Especially decisions about your body. You learn to set priorities, to structure your daily life, to optimize your health.

Sport, sleep, diet, and regeneration become more important and allow you to live healthier. I want to show you how important it is to take care of yourself and your body and inspire you to embrace an overall healthier lifestyle.

Always remember: You use your body every day and always and constantly carry it with you—everywhere. Only you have control over it. By combining the appropriate mobility and calisthenics exercises, a healthy diet, enough sleep, regeneration, strategies for stress management, and a healthy lifestyle, we make progress and rise to meet new challenges. That new approach to life is rewarded with impressive body control.

Have faith in yourself and your abilities, make exercise part of your value system, view nothing as unchangeable, and be aware that you alone are responsible for your improved performance.

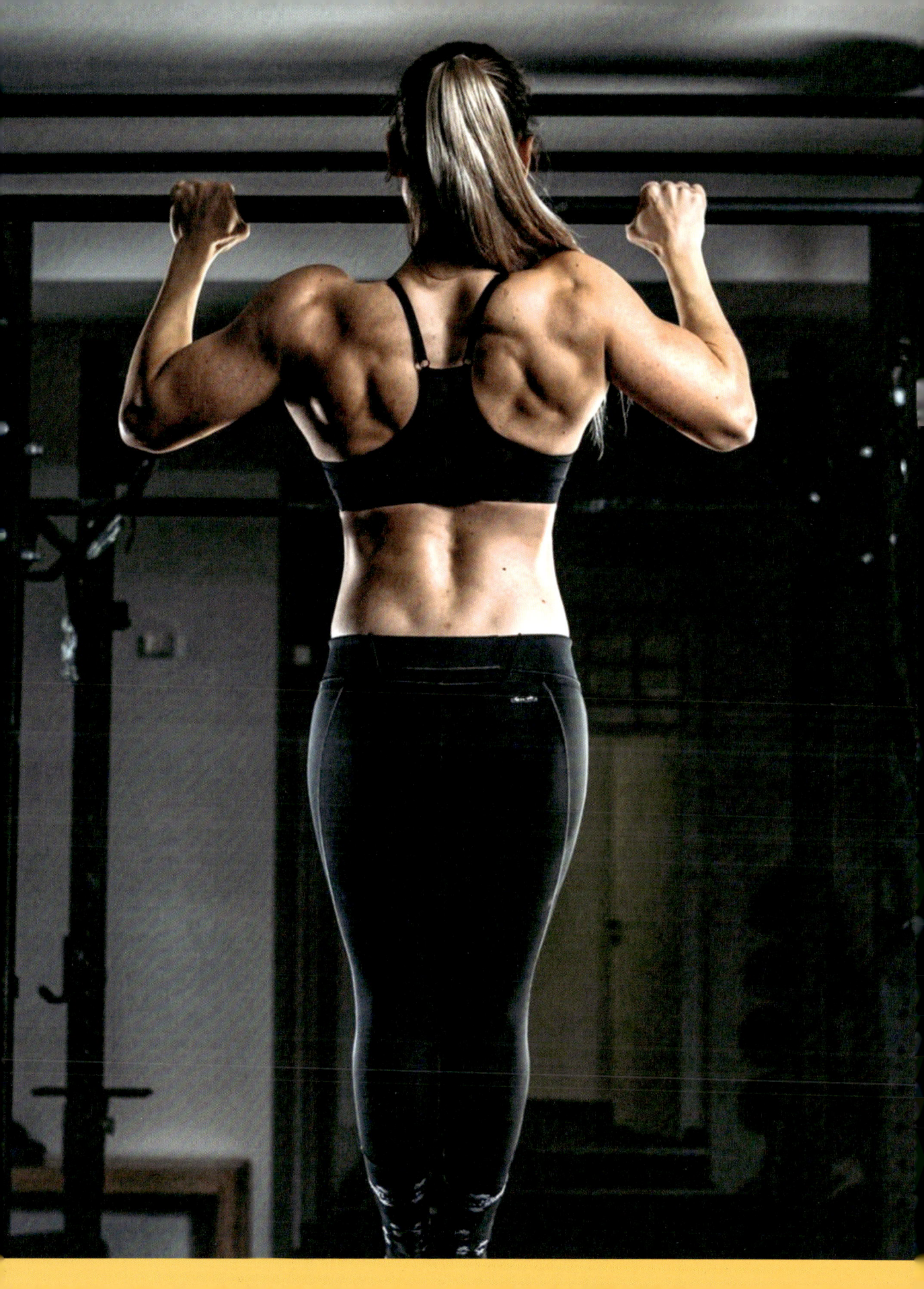

14 Acknowledgments

Books usually end with acknowledgments. But before we go far afield and thank all our supporters and those who accompanied us along the way, who helped us embark on this exercise journey, we want to thank you!

Thank you for the trust and curiosity that prompted you to buy this book and to hopefully put its content into practice.

Because those with all the knowledge aren't nearly as good as those with all the experience.

Even if we were very critical of some topics, it shouldn't stop you from trying things and finding out what works for you.

If you can think of someone you can help with the ideas, suggestions, and tips in this book, we'd like to encourage you to do so. The more people you can inspire, the healthier and happier you, too, will feel.

Last but not least, we'd like to dedicate these final lines to our supporters:

Thank you to David Dückers, who established contact between Monique and Meyer & Meyer Sport. At this point, I (Leon), would also like to thank Monique for bringing me on board to present with this book the symbiosis between calisthenics and mobility.

Of course, a big thank you goes to those at Meyer & Meyer Sport for lending their professional support. Robert Meyer's infinite patience and trust, in particular, helped us when we had to postpone the submission deadline for the book because we simply had too many ideas we wanted to include.

Acknowledgments

I (Monique) have to credit my former partner and cofounder of Calisthenics Parks with my passion for calisthenics. Thank you for showing me the beginnings of the sport and visiting European cities in search of undiscovered calisthenics spots and documenting them. Since then, every vacation has included visits to calisthenics spots and training at calisthenics facilities. I always bring some stickers to also represent the German calisthenics scene internationally and to bring attention to you.

Thank you to the Monkey Dad (@Ulrichstaege) for adorning and enhancing this book with your photos through your professional eye.

I (Leon) want to also thank the rest of my Monkey family: Mom, Anton, Heinz, and Omi—thank you for your support in all departments!

15 The Authors

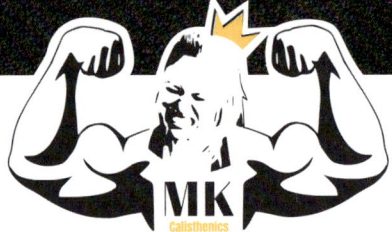

MONIQUE KÖNIG

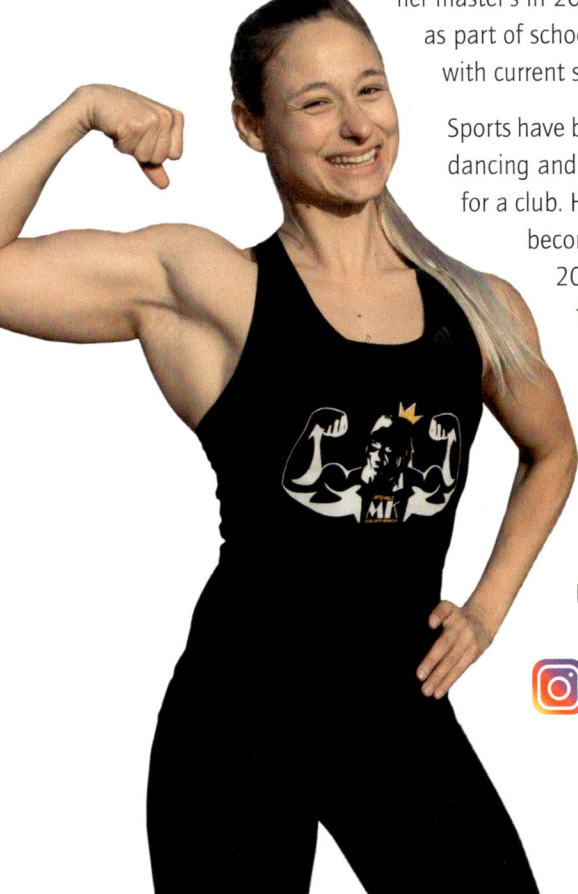

Monique König is thirty years old, and next to her work as a self-employed calisthenics trainer, she's currently an elementary school teacher in Germany. She majored in elementary education in Erfurt, with a minor in sports, which is why children are also part of her calisthenics target group, and she completed her master's in 2017. Her master's thesis focused on the possibility of calisthenics as part of school sports. It's scheduled to be published in a second book along with current studies.

Sports have been a part of Monique's life since early childhood. In addition to dancing and track and field, in her youth, she also competed as a triathlete for a club. Her passion for calisthenics began in October 2013 and has now become her vocation. She began teaching calisthenics workshops in 2016. She initially offered workshops for women only. Her goal was to make the male-dominated sport more accessible to women. She helps athletes get started with bodyweight training or achieve their calisthenics goals via online coaching and group-training units. Her mission: to get more people on the bar and thereby make the calisthenics sport popular in Germany so it eventually becomes part of school curricula.

She uses social-media networks (YouTube, Instagram, and Facebook) to impart her knowledge, to inspire, and to motivate.

@monique_koenig   @Monique König

@monique.calisthenics

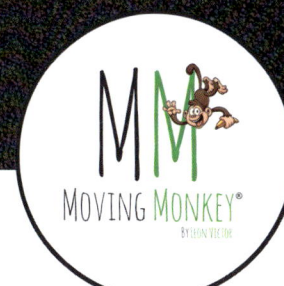

LEON VICTOR STAEGE: MOVING MONKEY

Leon began his athletic career at age three, with soccer, which he ended at age seventeen, when he graduated from high school. Since then, exercise and the human body have given him direction, whereupon he published his first book, titled *Pragmatisch Gesund in 2015*, after graduating from high school.

He began studying physical therapy in 2016 at Fresenius University of Applied Sciences in Cologne, Germany.

In 2016, Leon also established the online education platform Moving Monkey, which focuses on modern and science-based methods of mobility training and helps people to build more exercise into their largely sedentary daily lives. In addition, he trains many competitive and everyday athletes to make them strong, mobile, and pain-free long-term. Moving Monkey offers instructional and inspirational videos, which are enjoying a growing audience, on popular media and social-media platforms (YouTube, Instagram, Facebook, Spotify, and iTunes).

He teaches mobility and handstand workshops and also does speaking engagements.

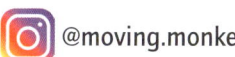 @moving.monkey   @Moving Monkey

 @movingmonkey   Moving Monkey Podcast

1 GLOSSARY

ACJ—acromioclavicular joint

Agonists—muscles that work in the same direction of movement

Animal moves—training concept that imitates animal movements and compiles them into workshops

Antagonists—muscles that work in opposing directions of movement

Arthrokinetic reflex—a reaction of the nervous system whereby joint movements trigger muscle inhibition or activation

Body map—model that describes the neuroplastic representation of one's joints and the contracting ability of the surrounding muscles in the brain

Bent-arm strength—the strength one needs from a bent arm or elbow in order to perform exercises like pull-ups, push-ups, or dips

Bilateral training—involving both arms or both legs in a movement or exercise

Cadence—speed of movement in an exercise (divided into different movement phases)

Calisthenics Parks—online platform where one can look at, rate, and find calisthenics parks around the world

CARs—controlled articular rotations; a controlled joint circle using the joint's full range of motion (FROM)

Cerebellum – area of the brain in charge of movement coordination and control

CS—cervical spine; area of the spine with segments C1–C7; C stands for the cervical area of the neck

Closing-angle joint pain—pain that can occur when the joint angle is narrowed

Concentric—phase overcoming gravity or load (muscles shorten)

Deep sensibility—stimuli that are transmitted to the brain by receptors inside the body (muscles, tendons, ligaments, joints, and organs)

Depression—lowering the shoulder blades

Eccentric—strength-receding phase (muscles get longer)

EFC Calisthenics—Calisthenics Club Erfurt, which Monique co-founded

Elevation—raising the shoulder blades

Exteroception—see surface sensibility

False joints—synarthrosis; classification of joints that don't possess the typical joint structure

Fast-twitch muscle fibers (FT 2)—have low fatigue tolerance and are thus primarily active during fast or explosive movements or loads

Frequency—how often exercises or training units are performed (per week)

FROM—full range of motion; describes the complete range of motion of a movement of a joint

GHJ—glenohumeral joint (upper-arm–scapula joint)

Hollow-body position—a basic body position in calisthenics used to improve body tension

Homeostasis—term for the state of equilibrium/balance of a system (here, the body)

Hypertrophy—describes the increase in the diameter of a muscle (muscle growth)

Impingement syndrome—condition where structures are pinched between two partner joints

Iron cross—gymnastics exercise

Isometric—holding phase (without change to muscle length)

Joint-by-joint approach—model that shows which area of the joint must be loaded or trained

LS—lumbar spine, area of the spine with segments L1–L5

Mechanoreceptors—sensory cells that transmit mechanical forces (e.g., pressure) as stimuli to the brain

Movement culture—established by Ido Portal, movement that cultivates expression, life, and the study of movement as a key element

Moving Monkey—established by Leon Victor Staege, a brand that spreads and teaches an exercise concept consisting of therapy and training that's heavily focused on mobility training via social media

Neuroathletics training—athletic training with emphasis on the brain and the central nervous system

Progression—expansion of an exercise or movement, with increased complexity

Proprioception—see deep sensibility

Protraction—moving the shoulder blades forward

Pointed toes—extending the toes so the feet and calves form a straight line

Posterior pelvic tilt—tilting the pelvis back, causing the pelvis to straighten and achieving reduction of lordosis (eliminating the physiological s-shape of the lumbar spine)

Reflexive stability—the body's basic tension resulting from the body reacting to an external stimulus

Regression—a simplification of an exercise or movement, with reduced complexity

Retraction—pulling the shoulder blades back

RTO—rings turned out; describes the movement that must be performed at the highest point of the support variation on the rings to achieve a full range of motion (FROM)

ROM—range of motion

SAID principle—specific adaptation on imposed demand; describes how the body adapts very specifically to the set stimulus, which means that to learn pull-ups you have to also practice pull-ups and not just body rows

Scapulothoracic groove—space between shoulder blade and ribcage

SCJ—sternoclavicular joint

Slow-twitch muscle fibers (FT 1)—have a high degree of fatigue tolerance and thus are primarily active during sustained and long holding movements or loads

SMART principle—specific, measurable, achievable, realistic, timed; concept for effective goal formulation

Sticking points or weak links—the part of a movement or exercise that's most difficult or where one has the greatest deficiencies
Straight-arm strength—the strength one needs from a straight arm in order to perform exercises like the handstand, a planche, and support positions on the rings

Stress bucket—model to describe stress factors and consequences of excessive stress; used for better stress management

Subacromial space—space between the acromion and the humeral head

Surface sensibility—stimuli perceived and transmitted to the brain by skin receptors

TS—thoracic spine with segments T1–T12

True joints—diarthroses; a classification of joints that possess the typical joint structure (two partner joints with a joint space and a surrounding multilayer joint capsule)

Unilateral training—using primarily one arm or one leg during a movement or exercise
Volume—the total workload completed during training (measured by weight moved or repetitions completed, totaled from all exercises and sets)

WSWCF—World Street Workout and Calisthenics Federation

2 FURTHER REFERENCES

Bowman, K. (2017). *Move your DNA. Restore your health through natural movement. Expanded edition.* Propriometrics Press.

Butler, D. S. & Moseley, G. L. (2003). *Explain pain.* NOI Group.

Hargrove, T. R. (2014). *A guide to better movement. The science and practice of moving with more skill and less pain.* Better Movement.

Lieberman, D. (2015). *Unser Körper. Geschichte, Gegenwart, Zukunft.* S. FISCHER.

Low, S. (2016). *Overcoming gravity. A systematic approach to gymnastics and bodyweight strength.* Battle Ground Creative.

Moseley, G. L. & Butler, D. S. (2013). *Explain Pain*. Noigroup Publications.

Myers, T. W. (2015). *Anatomy trains. Myofasziale Leitbahnen (für Manual- und Bewegungstherapeuten).* Elsevier.

Paulsen, F. & Waschke, J. (2017). *Sobotta, Atlas der Anatomie.* Elsevier.

Robbins, A. (2004). *Das Robbins Power Prinzip. Befreie die innere Kraft.* Ullstein.

Schmidt-Fetzer, U. & Lienhard, L. (2018). *Neuroathletiktraining. Grundlagen und Praxis des neurozentrierten Trainings.* Pflaum Verlag.

Starrett, K. & Starrett, J. (2016). *Deskbound. Standing up to a sitting world.* Victory Belt Publishing.

Starrett, K. & Cordoza, G. (2013). *Werde ein geschmeidiger Leopard. Die sportliche Leistung verbessern, Verletzungen vermeiden und Schmerzen lindern.* Riva.

Trepel, M. (2015). *Neuroanatomie. Struktur und Funktion.* Elsevier.

Tsatsouline, P. (2001). *Beyond stretching. Russain flexibility breakthroughs.* Dragon Door Publications.

Tsatsouline, P. (2001). *Realx into stretch*. Dragon Door Publications.

Waitzkin, J. (2008). *The art of learning. An inner journey to optimal performance.* Frees Press.

Voelpel, S. C. & Gerpott, F. H. (2016). *Der Positiv-Effekt. Mit einer Umstellung der Einstellung das Mangement revolutionieren.*

3 CREDITS

Cover and interior design: Annika Naas, Anja Elsen

Layout: Guido Maetzing, www.mmedia-agentur.de

Interior photos: Ulrich Staege

Photo p. 165: Leon Victor Staege

Interior illustrations: Leon Victor Staege

Illustrations p. 51, 191: © AdobeStock

Managing editor: Elizabeth Evans

Translation: www.AAATranslation.com

CALISTHENICS
4FCIRCLE®
This is how {movement} works

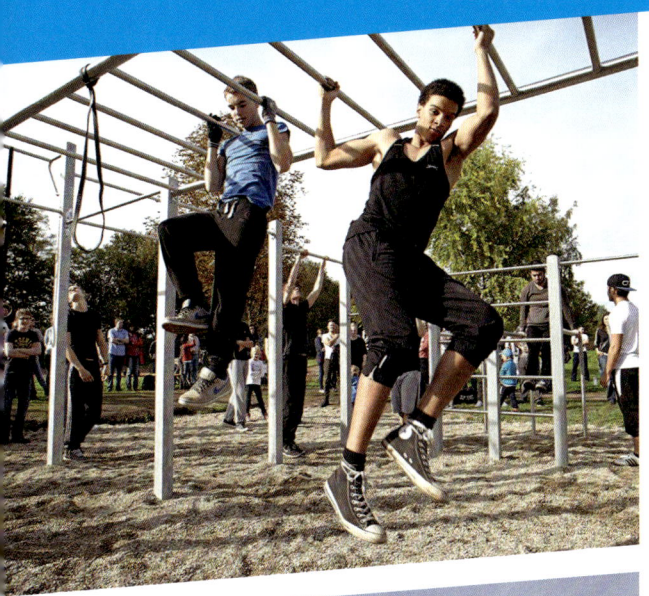
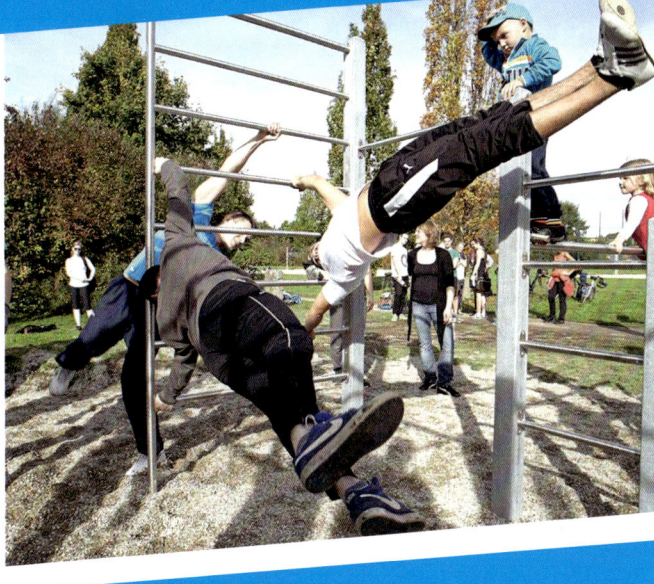
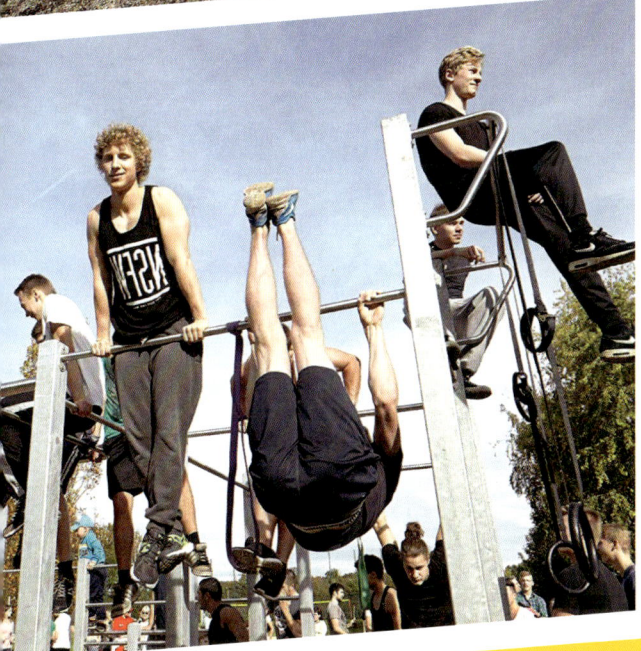

PARKS, EQUIPMENT, PLANNING, AND DESIGN
www.calisthenics-playparc.com

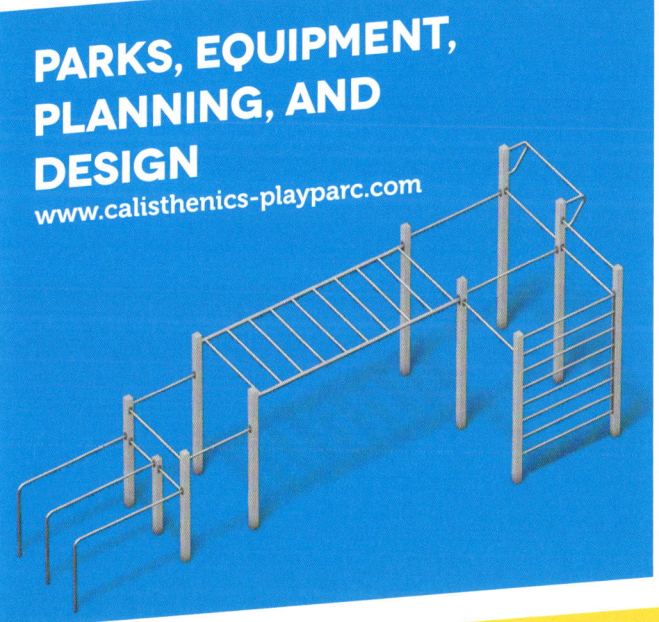

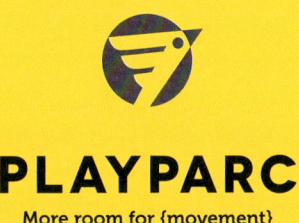

PLAYPARC
More room for {movement}

www.playparc.de

Subscribe to our free newsletter at www.m-m-sports.com

MORE GREAT FITNESS BOOKS FROM MEYER & MEYER!

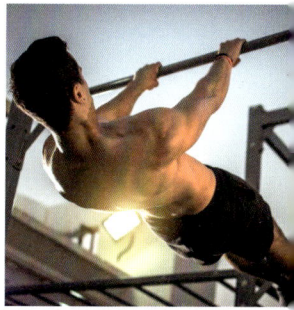

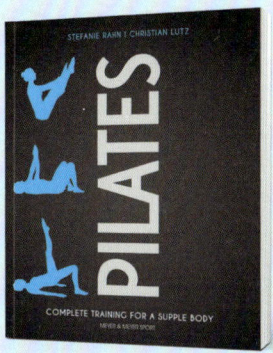

ISBN 978-1-78255-186-7
$29.95 US
384 p., in color
Paperback, 8 x 10"

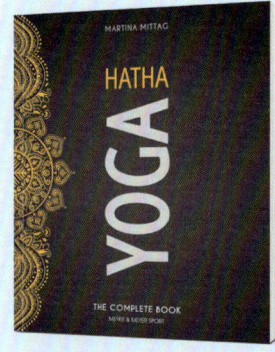

ISBN 978-1-78255-185-0
$34.95 US
424 p., in color
Paperback, 8 x 10"

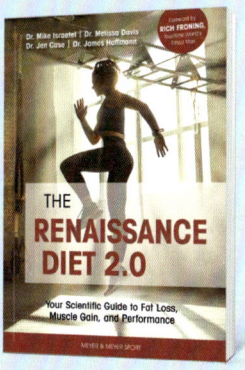

ISBN 978-1-78255-190-4
$26.95 US
344 p., b&w
Paperback, 6 x 9"

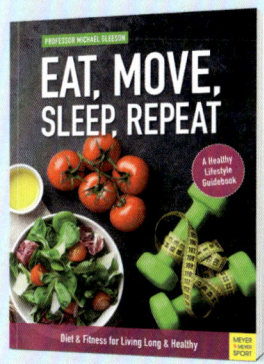

ISBN 978-1-78255-187-4
$29.95 US
400 p., b&w
Paperback, 7 x 10"

MEYER & MEYER
Fachverlag GmbH
Von-Coels-Str. 390
52080 Aachen

Telephone	02 41 - 9 58 10 - 13
Fax	02 41 - 9 58 10 - 10
E-Mail	sales@m-m-sports.com
Website	www.m-m-sports.com

You can buy our books online or at your local bookseller.

MEYER & MEYER SPORT